Common Toxicologic Issues in Small Animals

Guest Editors

SAFDAR A. KHAN, DVM, MS, PhD
STEPHEN B. HOOSER, DVM, PhD

VETERINARY CLINICS OF NORTH AMERICA: SMALL ANIMAL PRACTICE

www.vetsmall.theclinics.com

March 2012 • Volume 42 • Number 2

SAUNDERS an imprint of ELSEVIER, Inc.

W.B. SAUNDERS COMPANY
A Division of Elsevier Inc.

1600 John F. Kennedy Blvd. • Suite 1800 • Philadelphia, PA 19103-2899

http://www.vetsmall.theclinics.com

VETERINARY CLINICS OF NORTH AMERICA: SMALL ANIMAL PRACTICE Volume 42, Number 2
March 2012 ISSN 0195-5616, ISBN-13: 978-1-4557-3955-4

Editor: John Vassallo; j.vassallo@elsevier.com
Developmental Editor: Teia Stone

Veterinary Clinics of North America: Small Animal Practice (ISSN 0195-5616) is published bimonthly (For Post Office use only: volume 42 issue 1 of 6) by Elsevier Inc., 360 Park Avenue South, New York, NY 10010-1710. Months of issue are January, March, May, July, September, and November. Business and Editorial Offices: 1600 John F. Kennedy Blvd., Ste. 1800, Philadelphia, PA 19103-2899. Customer Service Office: 3251 Riverport Lane, Maryland Heights, MO 63043. Periodicals postage paid at New York, NY and additional mailing offices. Subscription prices are $283.00 per year (domestic individuals), $455.00 per year (domestic institutions), $138.00 per year (domestic students/residents), $375.00 per year (Canadian individuals), $559.00 per year (Canadian institutions), $416.00 per year (international individuals), $559.00 per year (international institutions), and $201.00 per year (international and Canadian students/residents). To receive student/resident rate, orders must be accompanied by name of affiliated institution, date of term, and the signature of program/residency coordinator on institution letterhead. Orders will be billed at individual rate until proof of status is received. Foreign air speed delivery is included in all *Clinics* subscription prices. All prices are subject to change without notice. **POSTMASTER:** Send address changes to *Veterinary Clinics of North America: Small Animal Practice,* Elsevier Health Sciences Division, Subscription Customer Service, 3251 Riverport Lane, Maryland Heights, MO 63043. Customer Service (orders, claims, online, change of address): Elsevier Periodicals Customer Service, Elsevier Health Sciences Division, Subscription Customer Service, 3251 Riverport Lane, Maryland Heights, MO 63043. Tel: 1-800-654-2452 (U.S. and Canada); 314-447-8871 (outside U.S. andCanada). Fax: 314-447-8029. E-mail: journalscustomerservice-usa@elsevier.com (for print support); journalsonlinesupport-usa@elsevier.com (for online support).

Reprints. For copies of 100 or more of articles in this publication, please contact the Commercial Reprints Department, Elsevier Inc., 360 Park Avenue South, New York, NY 10010-1710. Tel.: 212-633-3812; Fax: 212-462-1935; E-mail: reprints@elsevier.com.

Veterinary Clinics of North America: Small Animal Practice is also published in Japanese by Inter Zoo Publishing Co., Ltd., Aoyama Crystal-Bldg 5F, 3-5-12 Kitaaoyama, Minato-ku, Tokyo 107-0061, Japan.

Veterinary Clinics of North America: Small Animal Practice is covered in *Current Contents/Agriculture, Biology and Environmental Sciences, Science Citation Index, ASCA, MEDLINE/PubMed (Index Medicus), Excerpta Medica,* and *BIOSIS.*

Printed and bound by CPI Group (UK) Ltd, Croydon, CR0 4YY
Transferred to Digital Print 2012

Contributors

GUEST EDITORS

SAFDAR A. KHAN, DVM, MS, PhD
Diplomate, American Board of Veterinary Toxicology; Senior Director Toxicology Research, ASPCA Animal Poison Control Center, Urbana, Illinois

STEPHEN B. HOOSER, DVM, PhD
Diplomate, American Board of Veterinary Toxicology; Director, Animal Disease Diagnostic Laboratory; Professor of Toxicology, Department of Comparative Pathobiology, College of Veterinary Medicine, Purdue University, West Lafayette, Indiana

AUTHORS

KARYN BISCHOFF, DVM, MS
Diplomate, American Board of Veterinary Toxicology; Clinical Toxicologist, New York State Animal Health Diagnostic Center; Assistant Professor, Department of Population Medicine and Diagnostic Sciences, Cornell University, Ithaca, New York

ADRIENNE E. COLEMAN, DVM
Consulting Veterinarian in Clinical Toxicology, ASPCA Animal Poison Control Center, Urbana, Illinois

CAMILLE DECLEMENTI, VMD
Diplomate, American Board of Toxicology; Diplomate, American Board of Veterinary Toxicology; Senior Director, Medical Records and Senior Toxicologist, ASPCA Animal Poison Control Center; Adjunct Instructor, Department of Veterinary Biosciences, College of Veterinary Medicine, University of Illinois, Urbana, Illinois

PAUL A. EUBIG, DVM, MS
Diplomate, American Board of Toxicology; Research Assistant Professor, Department of Comparative Biosciences, College of Veterinary Medicine, University of Illinois at Urbana-Champaign, Urbana, Illinois

PATTI GAHAGAN, DVM
Novartis Animal Health US, Inc, Greensboro, North Carolina

SHARON GWALTNEY-BRANT, DVM, PhD
Diplomate, American Board of Toxicology; Diplomate, American Board of Veterinary Toxicology; Veterinary Information Network, Mahomet, Illinois

STEVEN R. HANSEN, DVM, MS, MBA
Diplomate, American Board of Toxicology; Diplomate, American Board of Veterinary Toxicology; ASPCA Animal Poison Control Center, Urbana, Illinois

CRISTINE L. HAYES, DVM
Consulting Veterinarian in Clinical Toxicology, ASPCA Animal Poison Control Center, Urbana, Illinois

STEPHEN B. HOOSER, DVM, PhD
Diplomate, American Board of Veterinary Toxicology; Director, Animal Disease Diagnostic Laboratory; Professor of Toxicology, Department of Comparative Pathobiology, College of Veterinary Medicine, Purdue University, West Lafayette, Indiana

SAFDAR A. KHAN, DVM, MS, PhD
Diplomate, American Board of Veterinary Toxicology; Senior Director Toxicology Research, ASPCA Animal Poison Control Center, Urbana, Illinois

MICHAEL KNIGHT, DVM
Senior Consulting Veterinary Toxicologist, ASPCA Animal Poison Control Center, Urbana, Illinois

MARY KAY MCLEAN, MS
ASPCA Animal Poison Control Center, Urbana, Illinois

IRINA MEADOWS, DVM
Diplomate, American Board of Toxicology; ASPCA Animal Poison Control Center, Urbana, Illinois

CHARLOTTE MEANS, DVM, MLIS
Diplomate, American Board of Toxicology; Diplomate, American Board of Veterinary Toxicology; Senior Toxicologist, ASPCA Animal Poison Control Center, Urbana, Illinois

VALENTINA M. MEROLA, DVM, MS
Diplomate, American Board of Toxicology; Diplomate, American Board of Veterinary Toxicology; Senior Toxicologist, ASPCA Animal Poison Control Center, Urbana, Illinois

LISA A. MURPHY, VMD
Diplomate, American Board of Toxicology; Department of Pathobiology, University of Pennsylvania School of Veterinary Medicine, Kennett Square, Pennsylvania

BIRGIT PUSCHNER, DVM, PhD
Diplomate, American Board of Veterinary Toxicology; Professor of Veterinary Toxicology, Department of Molecular Biosciences, School of Veterinary Medicine, University of California, Davis, California

WILSON K. RUMBEIHA, BVM, PhD
Diplomate, American Board of Toxicology; Diplomate, American Board of Veterinary Toxicology; Professor of Veterinary Toxicology, Veterinary Diagnostics and Production Animal Medicine, College of Veterinary Medicine, Iowa State University, Ames, Iowa

MARY SCHELL, DVM
Diplomate, American Board of Toxicology; Diplomate, American Board of Veterinary Toxicology; Senior Toxicologist, ASPCA National Animal Poison Control Center, Urbana, Illinois

BRANDY R. SOBCZAK, DVM
Consulting Veterinarian in Clinical Toxicology, ASPCA Animal Poison Control Center, Urbana, Illinois

LAURA A. STERN, DVM
Consulting Veterinarian in Clinical Toxicology, ASPCA Animal Poison Control Center, Urbana, Illinois

COLETTE WEGENAST, DVM
Consulting Veterinarian in Clinical Toxicology, ASPCA Animal Poison Control Center, Urbana, Illinois

CHRISTINA R. WILSON, PhD
Clinical Assistant Professor, Indiana Animal Disease Diagnostic Laboratory; Department of Comparative Pathobiology, Purdue University, School of Veterinary Medicine, West Lafayette, Indiana

TINA WISMER, DVM
Diplomate, American Board of Toxicology; Diplomate, American Board of Veterinary Toxicology; Medical Director, ASPCA Animal Poison Control Center, Urbana, Illinois

Contents

> Veterinary toxicology is a constantly evolving field. The authors use the ASPCA Animal Poison Control Center's medical record database to examine recent trends in veterinary toxicology/animal poisoning incidents received from 2002 to 2010. The demographics of animals exposed to potentially harmful substances, the types of substances ingested, changes/emerging trends in substance exposures, and trends in therapies used to treat exposures are discussed.

> Due to the potential implications of food-related illnesses in animals, recognition of pet food–related outbreaks is one of the many crucial roles of the veterinarian. This article describes the veterinarian's role in investigating and reporting food-related illnesses in cats and dogs. Recommendations regarding taking thorough case histories, appropriate sample collection, effective use of veterinary diagnostic laboratories, and recommendations for reporting such illnesses are described.

> Most pet foods are safe, but incidents of chemical contamination occur and lead to illness and recalls. There were 11 major pet food recalls in the United States between 1996 and 2010 that were due to chemical contaminants or misformulations: 3 aflatoxin, 3 excess vitamin D_3, 1 excess methionine, 3 inadequate thiamine, and 1 adulteration with melamine and related compounds and an additional 2 warnings concerning a Fanconi-like renal syndrome in dogs after ingesting large amounts of chicken jerky treat products. This article describes clinical findings and treatment of animals exposed to the most common pet food contaminants.

Intravenous lipid emulsion (ILE) infusions have become an emerging treatment modality in managing intoxications of veterinary patients. The advantages of ILE include an apparent wide margin of safety, relatively low cost, long shelf-life, and ease of administration. Based on limited case and anecdotal reports, ILEs have shown promise in the management of toxicoses from a variety of lipophilic agents, including drugs and pesticides. More studies are needed to determine optimum dosing regimens and identify potential adverse effects from the antidotal use of ILE in veterinary medicine.

The widespread use and availability of calcium channel blockers in human and veterinary medicine pose a risk for inadvertent pet exposure to these medications. Clinical signs can be delayed by many hours after exposure in some cases, with hypotension and cardiac rhythm changes (bradycardia, atrioventricular block, or tachycardia) as the predominant signs. Prompt decontamination and aggressive treatment using a variety of modalities may be necessary to treat patients exposed to calcium channel blockers. The prognosis of an exposed patient depends on the severity of signs and response to treatment.

Two types of drugs are generally used for treating attention-deficit/ hyperactivity disorder or attention-deficit disorder in humans: amphetamines or similar stimulants and the nonamphetamine atomoxetine. We describe the toxicity and treatment of both amphetamines and similar medications and atomoxetine in dogs and cats. Amphetamine intoxication can cause life-threatening stimulatory signs. Treatment is aimed at preventing absorption, controlling the stimulatory signs, and protecting the kidneys; prognosis is generally good. Atomoxetine also has a fast onset of action; stimulatory signs such as hyperactivity and tachycardia are often seen. There are little published data about treatment of atomoxetine toxicity in cats and dogs.

Nonsteroidal anti-inflammatory drugs (NSAIDs) are a group of heterogeneous compounds extensively used in both human and veterinary

medicine for their antipyretic, anti-inflammation, and analgesic properties. NSAIDs consist of a wide range of pharmacologically active agents
with different chemical structures, with similar therapeutic and adverse
effects. The ASPCA Animal Poison Control Center received 22,206
NSAID incidents in dogs and cats (3% of total cases; dogs [15,823] and
cats [1244]) during 2005 to 2010. This is roughly equivalent to 4%
NSAID incidents reported in humans. The most common NSAID
involved was ibuprofen, followed by aspirin, naproxen, deracoxib,
meloxicam, diclofenac, piroxicam, indomethacin, nabumetone, and
etodolac. This article provides a brief overview of classification, mechanism of action, pharmacologic and toxicologic properties, and treatment information involving frequently encountered human and veterinary NSAIDs in dogs and cats.

The sugar alcohol xylitol is a popular sweetener used in gums, candies,
and baked goods. While xylitol has a wide margin of safety in people
and most mammalian species, when ingested by dogs it is believed to
stimulate excessive insulin secretion leading to severe hypoglycemia,
potentially followed by acute hepatic failure and coagulopathies. Additional clinical findings may include thrombocytopenia, hypokalemia,
and hyperphosphatemia. The prognosis for recovery in dogs that
develop uncomplicated hypoglycemia is generally good with prompt
and aggressive veterinary care.

The macrocyclic lactones (MLs) are parasiticides able to kill a wide
variety of arthropods and nematodes. They have a high margin of safety
for labeled indications, and ivermectin has become the best-selling
antiparasitic in the world. Dogs of certain breeds and mixtures of those
breeds have a defect in the *ABCB1* gene (formerly *MDR1* gene) that
results in a lack of functional P-glycoprotein, which leads to accumulation
of the MLs in the central nervous system and a higher risk of adverse
effects when exposed. There is no specific antidote for ML toxicosis so the
most important part of treatment is good supportive care.

In the broadest definition, a pesticide (from fly swatters to chemicals) is
a substance used to eliminate a pest. Newer insecticides are much
safer to the environment, humans and non target species. These
insecticides are able to target physiologic differences between insects
and mammals, resulting in greater mammalian safety. This article briefly

reviews toxicity information of both older insecticides like organophosphates (OPs), carbamates, pyrethrins, and pyrethroids, as well as some newer insecticides.

This article focuses on the 3 most commonly used rodenticide types: anticoagulants, bromethalin, and cholecalciferol. It is important to verify the active ingredient in any rodenticide exposure. Many animal owners may use the term "D-con" to refer to any rodenticide regardless of the actual brand name or type of rodenticide. The EPA released their final ruling on rodenticide risk mitigation measures in 2008 and all the products on the market had to be compliant by June 2011, changing to consumer products containing either first-generation anticoagulants or nonanticoagulants including bromethalin and cholecalciferol. These regulations are likely to cause an increase in the number of bromethalin and cholecalciferol cases.

Intoxication with explosives or fireworks in dogs or cats is not common, but serious toxicosis can result from exposure to different types of explosives depending on the chemical class of explosive involved. This article will discuss the different types of materials/chemicals, clinical signs of toxicosis, and their treatment. Despite the complexities of explosives and plethora of different devices currently in use worldwide, the toxic potential is more easily explained by looking at the relatively short list of chemical classes used to produce these materials. This article combines structurally similar explosives into different groups and focuses on the toxicity of the most commonly available explosives.

Of the several thousand species of mushrooms found in North America, less than 100 are toxic. Species in the genus *Amanita* are responsible for the vast majority of reported mushroom poisonings. In general, the number of reported mushroom poisonings in animals is low, most likely because toxicology testing is available for a limited number of mushroom toxins and thus many cases are not confirmed or reported. Also, only a limited number of mushrooms are submitted for identification purposes. Mushroom intoxications require tremendous efforts from clinicians and toxicologists in terms of making a diagnosis and treatment, and management is challenging.

This table outlines common toxicologic versus nontoxicologic rule outs based on clinical abnormalities seen in an acutely ill animal. The purpose is to provide an initial guideline for considering toxicologic versus nontoxicologic rule outs when a patient is presented to a practicing veterinarian. Major clinical abnormalities followed by common toxicologic rule outs and non-toxicologic rule outs have been listed so that practicing veterinarians can narrow down an etiology quickly. Based on history, physical examination findings, and blood work changes, once a reasonable etiology has been narrowed down or established, the reader is encouraged to review a more detailed discussion on management of the particular poisoning or disease listed in this or other references.

Different antidotes counteract the effect of a toxicant in several different ways. Antidotes can reverse, decrease, or prevent action of a toxicant. They can also help in achieving stabilization of vital signs, directly or indirectly, and promote excretion of a toxicant. However, overreliance on an antidote can be unrealistic and dangerous. While expectations of rapid recovery from antidotes are usually high, in a real life situation, there are many impediments in achieving this goal. The timing of its use, availability, cost, and sometimes adverse effects from the antidote itself can influence the results and outcome of a case. The majority of toxicants do not have a specific antidote therapy indicated and patients in these cases equally benefit from supportive care. In this chapter, commonly used antidotes and reversal agents in small animals are listed in a table form. The table lists generic name along with brand name of an antidote/reversal agent whenever available, main indications for their use, and provides comments or cautions in their use as needed. After stabilizing the patient and establishing the etiology, the clinicians must review more detailed management of that particular toxicant discussed here or in other references.

THE CLINICS ARE NOW AVAILABLE ONLINE!

Access your subscription at:
www.theclinics.com

Preface

Common Toxicologic Issues in Small Animals

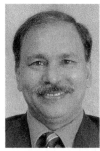 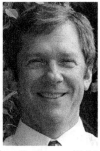

Safdar A. Khan, DVM, MS, PhD   Stephen B. Hooser, DVM, PhD
Guest Editors

Acknowledgment and dedication from Dr Safdar Khan:

"Dedicated to my father who, through education and participation in sports, strived to enrich the lives of his children and grandchildren."

Compiling information for this issue, editing, and working with peers and friends, has been a great honor and humbling experience. Thanks to my most wonderful colleagues and friends at the ASPCA and administration who contributed directly or indirectly for providing me time and facilities and for their untiring support and encouragement in completing this task. And most importantly, thanks to my family for their patience, support, and understanding, without which this project could not be completed.

Acknowledgment from Dr Stephen Hooser:

"As always, I would like to acknowledge the unwavering support of my wife, daughter, and son, without whom I would never have done this much or gone this far."

Animals, small and large, are continually exposed to chemicals in their environment. Each individual animal is exposed to chemicals from the earliest point in its existence, ie, the moment when the egg that will someday develop into that individual is formed in the ovary of its mother while she is still in the uterus of its grandmother. Therefore, it is important that we periodically review trends in toxicology to see what is out there and keep the veterinary community informed. This current volume of *Veterinary Clinics of North America: Small Animal Practice* continues this vital task.

Vet Clin Small Anim 42 (2012) xi–xii
doi:10.1016/j.cvsm.2012.01.005
0195-5616/12/$ – see front matter © 2012 Elsevier Inc. All rights reserved.

vetsmall.theclinics.com

Although our grandmothers were exposed to heavy metals and organochlorine insecticides such as DDT, these have largely been eliminated or replaced by newer and safer compounds over the years. Although still important, heavy metals such as lead have been replaced with other compounds or eliminated from use when possible. Organophosphate insecticides are being phased out in favor of pyrethroids and other pesticides that have lower mammalian toxicity. The chemicals have changed, and in relation, the acute poisonings affecting small animals have changed as well.

As veterinary toxicologists have observed over the years, and as are described in the articles of this current volume, trends in small animal toxicoses have changed. They reflect the changes not only in the chemicals being used but also in the relationship of domestic animals with their owners. While exposure and possible toxicoses related to insecticides, rodenticides, household chemicals, and plants still occur, there are now many more reports of exposures and toxicoses related to ingestion of human medications. Pets play important roles in our lives; they bring pleasure, calmness, and joy to us and to our children. They are often now considered important members of our families. This integration into our homes has increased opportunities for pets to get exposed accidently to many agents easily available in their environment. Instead of being exposed to highly toxic pesticides, pets are now more likely to be exposed to human medications and suffer serious consequences. Many types of medications such as attention deficit and hyperactivity disorder, non-steroidal anti-inflammatory drugs, and heart medications are commonly available in many households. As needed, analytical techniques for diagnosis of newly introduced compounds are developed. Reports of adverse pet food-related events have led to increased surveillance activities to identify possible contaminants. The assistance of highly trained canines to detect explosives has led to increased ingestion of explosives by dogs. New therapies, including intralipid therapy for the treatment of toxicoses due to exposure to fat-soluble chemicals, are being used. Discussions of these types of intoxications, plus articles on differential diagnoses and antidotal therapy, are presented here. To strengthen evidence, characterize sensitivities and trends, and identify clinical syndromes, information retrieved from the ASPCA Animal Poison Control Center toxicology database has been included whenever needed. As the world changes, veterinary toxicologists will continue to help monitor, follow, and understand those changes so that evolving toxicological problems can be controlled, treated, or eliminated.

Safdar A. Khan, DVM, MS, PhD
ASPCA Animal Poison Control Center
1717 South Philo Road, Suite 36
Urbana, IL 61802, USA

Stephen B. Hooser, DVM, PhD
Animal Disease Diagnostic Laboratory
406 South University Street, ADDL
Purdue University
West Lafayette, IN 47907, USA

E-mail addresses:
safdar.khan@aspca.org (S.A. Khan)
shooser1@purdue.edu (S.B. Hooser)

An Overview of Trends in Animal Poisoning Cases in the United States: 2002–2010

Mary Kay McLean, MS*, Steven R. Hansen, DVM, MS, MBA

KEYWORDS
- Veterinary • Toxicology • Toxicants
- Animal poisoning incidents/trends

Each year the ASPCA Animal Poison Control Center (APCC) receives thousands of reports of suspected animal poisonings. By utilizing AnTox, an electronic medical record database maintained by the APCC, data on current trends in animal poisoning cases can be mined and analyzed. This article explores recent trends in the field of veterinary toxicology including the types of animals and breeds that are most commonly exposed to different toxicants, seasonal and geographic distribution of poisoning incidents, the therapies that are most commonly administered, and trends in agents that are most frequently involved in poisonings.

MATERIALS AND METHODS

The APCC is a 24-hour service that receives calls from the United States and Canada regarding animal exposures to a variety of man-made and natural substances. When a call is received, the APCC veterinary staff collects information about the animal's signalment, medical history, exposure history, onset time, types, and duration of clinical signs, treatment information, and laboratory findings. If needed, follow-up calls are made to track the progression of clinical signs, the animal's response to and the effectiveness of treatments implemented, laboratory changes, and the final outcome. The electronic medical records from over 900,000 animal poisoning cases reported to the APCC were reviewed. Data collected from January 1, 2002, to December 31, 2010 were retrieved and analyzed.

WHERE AND WHEN EXPOSURES/POISONINGS OCCUR

Suspected animal exposures/poisonings occur year round across the country. The data collected from 2002 to 2010 show that calls regarding animal exposures to various agents are distributed throughout the year relatively evenly. The highest

The authors have nothing to disclose.
ASPCA Animal Poison Control Center, 1717 South Philo Road, Suite 36, Urbana, IL 61802, USA
* Corresponding author.
E-mail address: marykaymclean@aspca.org

Seasonal Trends 2002-2010

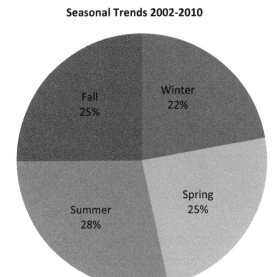

Fig. 1. Seasonal distribution of exposure reports from 2002 to 2010.

number of calls (28%) was reported in summer months followed by Fall and Spring, with 25% of the calls each. Twenty-two percent of calls were received during winter months (**Fig. 1**). The largest volume of calls occurs in July (9.7% of calls) and the least number of calls occurs in February (6.6%).

Exposures/poisonings occur at all hours of the day. A review of 2010 case data shows that the highest numbers of calls occurs from 7 to 8 pm CST with 7.97% of exposures being reported during that hour (**Fig. 2**). The slowest call volume occurs overnight from 4 to 5 am CST with only 0.61% of the cases being reported at that time. The increase of poisoning reports in the early evening hours is most likely related to the fact that many pet owners return home from work and discover that their pet had been exposed to a substance during the day when they were home alone.

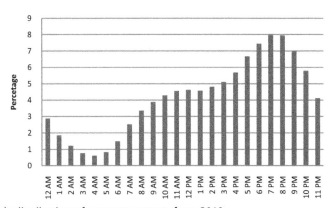

Fig. 2. Hourly distribution of exposure reports from 2010.

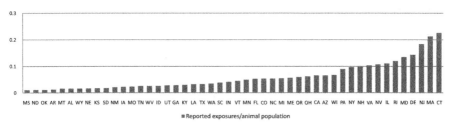

Fig. 3. Percentage of reported exposures by animal population in each state in 2006.

Although poisoning cases also occur overnight, the owner's may not know about it until the morning when they wake up and then call the APCC about it.

Information on the state (geographic information) from which a poisoning report originated was collected from 2006 cases. The data were then compared to the total population of dogs and cats in each state as reported by the American Veterinary Medical Association.[1] The highest frequency of calls per dog and cat population was from Connecticut where an estimated 0.23% of pets had a suspected poisoning reported to the APCC (**Fig. 3**). The lowest frequency was reported from Mississippi, where 0.01% of pets had a suspected poisoning reported. Regionally, the New England states had the highest reported incidents of suspected poisoning per pet, and the East South Central states had the lowest reported incidents. This information could be dependent on a variety of factors including the public's awareness of the APCC, and because the APCC is a fee-based, cost-recovery service, many poisoning incidents may go unreported.

TYPES OF ANIMALS INVOLVED IN POISONING CASES

The species of animals involved in poisonings reported to the APCC has remained consistent over the past 8 years. Canines account for 76% of the incidents reported, followed by felines at 13%, equines at 0.46%, and birds at 0.42% (**Table 1**).

Since 2006, Labradors and Labrador mixes, Golden Retrievers, Chihuahuas, Yorkshire Terriers, Shih Tzus, German Shepherds, Beagles, Miniature Dachshunds, and Boxers have consistently topped the list of dogs breeds involved in poisonings, while reports on Pit Bulls and Pit Bull mixes have slowly increased. Labradors have accounted for an average of 14% of dog cases followed by Golden Retrievers and Chihuahuas, which each accounted for about 4.5% of reports (**Table 2**).

When compared to American Kennel Club (AKC) registration statistics, in 2010 Labrador Retrievers topped the list of the most registered dogs followed by German Shepherds, Yorkshire Terriers, Beagles, Golden Retrievers, Bulldogs, Boxers, Dachshunds, Poodles, and Shih Tzus. While most breeds remained steady on the AKC registration list, Bulldogs increased from 21st most common breed in 2000 to 6th most common in 2010. Although bulldogs are not very commonly reported as being involved in poisonings cases to the APCC, as their popularity has increased they went from being involved in 0.13% of canine poisonings in 2002 to 0.38% of canine poisonings in 2010. The largest discrepancy between the number of AKC registrations and the number of reported exposures to the APCC is for Parson Russell Terriers. Although they only accounted for 0.14% of AKC registrations in 2006, they accounted for 2.3% of the canine cases reported to the APCC.[2]

Animal signalment data were retrieved from cases reported from 2009 through 2010. Most exposures reported to the APCC involved dogs and cats under 1 year of

Species	%
Table 1	
Percentage of species reported by total number of reports from 2002 to 2010	
Canine	76.5
Feline	13.1
Equine	0.5
Bird	0.4
Lagomorph	0.2
Ferret	0.2
Bovine	0.1
Rodent	0.1
Fish	0.07
Caprine	0.06
Porcine	0.05
Lizard	0.02
Ovine	0.02
Poultry	0.02
Turtle	0.02
Snake	0.02
Nonhuman primate	0.01
Marsupial	0.01
Canine wild	0.01
Camelid	0.008
Feline wild	0.003
Frog	0.003
Cervid	0.002
Salamander	0.001
Sea mammal	0.001
Bear	0.001

age (34% and 36%, respectively). For dogs, most weighed between 0 and 5 kg (24%) and most cats weighed 5 kg (26%). Distribution of males and females for both dogs and cats are fairly equally represented. A majority of male dogs are neutered (78%) and a majority of female dogs are spayed (80%). A majority of male cats are neutered (89%) and a majority of female cats are spayed (85%).

TRENDS IN THE TYPES OF TOXICANTS INVOLVED

As a result of curiosity and indiscriminant eating habits, animals are exposed to a variety of agents in their environment. While many exposures occur accidentally, some exposures occur maliciously, or when owners administer agents with good intentions not knowing they can actually cause harm. Consistently over the past 8 years, human medications have topped the list accounting for almost 25% of exposures. Other top categories included insecticides like flea control spot-ons, rodenticides, human food, veterinary medications, chocolate, household toxicants like bleach and cleaning supplies, plants, herbicides, and outdoor products like antifreeze and ice melts.

Table 2
Yearly distribution (percentage) of the top 10 dog breeds reported in 2006, 2008, and 2010

2006		2008		2010	
Breed	**%**	**Breed**	**%**	**Breed**	**%**
Labrador retriever	14.8	Labrador retriever	14.1	Labrador retriever	13.7
Golden retriever	4.9	Golden retriever	4.7	Golden retriever	4.6
Chihuahua	3.6	Chihuahua	4.2	Chihuahua	4.6
German shepherd	3.6	Yorkshire terrier	3.6	Yorkshire terrier	3.9
Beagle	3.1	German shepherd	3.4	Shih tzu	3.4
Yorkshire terrier	3.1	Shih tzu	3.2	German shepherd	3.3
Boxer	2.9	Beagle	3.2	Beagle	3.2
Miniature dachshund	2.8	Boxer	2.8	American pit bull terrier	3.0
Shih tzu	2.8	Miniature dachshund	2.8	Boxer	2.8
Cocker spaniel	2.7	Cocker spaniel	2.7	Miniature dachshund	2.7

The most common human medication exposures reported to the APCC involved acetaminophen accounting for 5.1% of all exposures in 2009 followed by ibuprofen (2.1%) and loratadine (1.3%) (**Table 3**). Acetaminophen and ibuprofen are available over the counter and are commonly used for pain management. In humans, acetaminophen is primarily metabolized by conjugation to a nontoxic glucruonide. Because cats are deficient in glucuronyl tranferase, they have a lower capacity to glucuronidate acetaminophen so it is instead metabolized via sulfation and to N-acetyl-*para*-benzoquinoneimine (NAPQUI) when sulfate is depleted. NAPQUI is a toxic metabolite that causes methemoglobinemia and hypatotoxicity. Ibuprofen is a nonsteroidal anti-inflammatory drug (NSAID) inhibiting both cyclooxygenase (COX)-1 and COX-2 isoenzymes. Among other functions, COX-1 promotes the production of the natural mucus lining of the stomach so even at therapeutic doses; the inhibition of COX-1 can cause GI ulcerations. At higher doses, ibuprofen can cause renal damage and/or failure. Loratadine is a second-generation H1 histamine antagonist used to treat allergies that have been available for over-the-counter use since 2002.

Table 3
Information regarding the most common human medication exposures reported in 2009 (percentage of reported exposures)

Human Medication	%
Acetaminophen	5.10
Ibuprofen	2.08
Vitamin D	1.31
Loratidine	1.28
Lisinopril	1.26
Aspirin	1.21
Iron	1.05
Levothyroxine	1.02
Hydrocodone bitartrate	1.00

Table 4	
Top 10 most common pesticide exposures reported in 2009 and the percentage of reported exposures by the total number of cases	
Pesticide	**%**
Permethrin	6.73
S-Methoprene	3.65
Abamectin	3.21
Fipronil	2.68
Pyrethrins	2.46
Ivermectin	2.12
Indoxacarb	1.85
Dinotefuran	1.25
Hydramethylnon	0.78
Cyphenothrin	0.78

In dogs and cats, exposure to loratadine can cause mild lethargy or hyperactivity, and tachycardia.

The most common pesticide exposures reported to the APCC involved permethrin, accounting for 6.73% of exposures in 2009, followed by S-methoprene (3.7%) and abamectin (3.2%) (**Table 4**). Permethrin is a common ingredient in many spot-on flea and tick preventatives for canines and is also available as a premise spray or granules for household use. Although permethrin has low mammalian toxicity, cats are considered to be very sensitive to it. It is believed that cats may be more sensitive because of their limited ability to glucoronide the permethrin metabolites prolonging the detoxification process. Methoprene is an insect growth regulator that acts on the larval stage of insects, preventing them from reaching the adult stage and reproducing. Methoprene is found in shampoos, spot-ons, ant baits, collars, and sprays and has a wide margin of safety in mammals. Abamectin is a general use pesticide found in low concentrations in many ant and roach baits available for use in residential homes. Abamectin is relatively low in toxicity to mammals as it affects a specific type of neurologic synapse in the insect's brain.

The most common plant exposures reported to the APCC involve *Lilium* and *Hemerocallis* spp, accounting for 0.42% of all exposures in 2010, followed by *Spathiphyllum* spp (0.18%) and *Cycas revolute* (0.13%) (**Table 5**). Cats are unusually sensitive to an unidentified toxic principle(s) in *Lilium* and *Hemerocallis* spp, and even minor exposures to plant material including pollen appears to result in renal failure in some cats.[3] *Spathiphyllum* spp, also known as Peace Lilies, will not cause renal failure in cats but contain insoluble calcium oxalate crystals.[3] When chewed, cells release sharp needle-shaped crystals that cause oral pain and irritation in all species. All parts of the *Cycas revolute* or Sago palms are considered toxic, but especially the seeds.[4] If eaten, Sago palms can cause hepatic damage and coagulopathy in dogs and cats.[4]

Over the past few years there have been some notable trends in animal exposures most likely due to regulatory changes, new product availability, and the increase or decrease of popularity of certain agents. One notable increase in both the number of exposures and the severity of the toxicity resulting from the exposure involves vitamin D and cholecalciferol cases. In 2002, these cases accounted for only 0.56% of exposures reported to the APCC (**Table 6**). In 2010, the frequency of exposures

Table 5
Top 10 most common plant exposures reported in 2010 and the percentage of reported exposures by the total number of cases

Plant Species	%
Lilium and Hemerocallis sp	0.42
Spathiphyllum sp	0.18
Cycas revoluta	0.13
Hydrangea sp	0.12
Dracaena	0.10
Philodendron sp	0.09
Tulipa sp	0.09
Zantedeschia sp	0.08
Hibiscus sp	0.08
Epipremnum aureum	0.07

increased to 2.97% of all reported exposures. This increase in exposures is most likely due to the increase in the publicity of health benefits of vitamin D. In humans, vitamin D at appropriate dosages promotes bone health, increases immunity, treats tuberculosis, and prevents cancer.[5] In dogs and cats, however, high doses of vitamin D can cause hypercalcemia and renal failure.[6] Prescription-strength vitamin D supplements are available in tablets as high as 50,000 IU (1250 μg; 40 IU of vitamin D = 1 μg). The availability of higher strength vitamin D supplements may contribute to the severity of clinical signs (hypercalcemia, renal failure) seen in some animals after exposures to these increasing doses. Some of the affected animals with hypercalcemia may require days and weeks of treatment.

In addition to the increased popularity of vitamin D supplements, new Environmental Protection Agency (EPA) guidelines may increase the availability of cholecalciferol-based rodenticides, further contributing to the increase in reports of exposures in animals. On May 28, 2008, the EPA released their final ruling on rodenticide risk mitigation measures. These measures required all products on the market satisfy the new guidelines by June 2011.[7] The purpose of the regulatory changes are to reduce ecological effects and exposure risk to children, wildlife, and pets to

Table 6
Yearly percentage of cholecalciferol exposures per total case volume from 2002 to 2010

Year	Cholecalciferol Exposures (%)
2002	0.57
2003	0.82
2004	1.17
2005	1.45
2006	1.38
2007	1.79
2008	2.02
2009	2.49
2010	2.97

Table 7
Yearly percentage of bromethalin exposures per total case volume from 2002 to 2010

Year	Bromethalin Exposures (%)
2002	0.07
2003	0.07
2004	0.07
2005	0.11
2006	0.10
2007	0.12
2008	0.13
2009	0.14
2010	0.16

second-generation anticoagulants rodenticides like brodifacoum, bromadiolone, dife-thiolone, and difenacoum by eliminating them from consumer products and requiring the use of bait stations for agricultural products. Although it is too soon to see a decreasing trend in second-generation anticoagulant exposures, the APCC has seen a slight increase in bromethalin-based rodenticide exposures. In 2002, bromethalin accounted for only 0.07% of cases, and that number increased to 0.16% in 2010 (**Table 7**).

Other noticeable trends in exposures come from the increased popularity of dark chocolates containing high percentages of cocoa and therefore methylxanthine content, and the increased availability of synthetic cannabinoids or K2. In 2002 dark chocolate exposures accounted for 0.09% of exposures reported to the APCC, which increased to 0.62% in 2007. Since then, the number has decreased slightly to 0.58% of exposures in 2010. Although K2 is rumored to have first been sold in the early 2000s, the APCC did not receive a reported exposure until 2010 when 5 exposures occurred. As of September 2011, a total of 31 exposures were reported. Clinical signs reported from K2 exposures are similar to those reported from marijuana exposures and can include ataxia, bradycardia, lethargy, depression, somnolence, hypothermia, urinary incontinence, and vomiting.[8]

The top classes of agents reported between 2002 and 2010 that cause death in animals include pyrethrin insecticides, accounting for death in 0.038% of all reported exposures, carbamate insecticides (0.022%), and organophosphate insecticides (0.012%). The off-label application of concentrated permethrin-containing products can result in death in cats.[9] Since 2009, there has been a decrease in the number of deaths caused by molluscicides. Molluscicides generally contain either methaldehyde or ferric phosphate. Methaldehyde is rapidly absorbed and causes ataxia, convulsions, hypersalivation, muscular rigidity, and death.[10] Ferric phosphate, although still potentially toxic, has a wider margin of safety. The decrease in reported deaths from metaldehyde may be possibly due to the increased use of ferric phosphate–containing products or due to increased awareness about the risks of methaldehyde, particularly in dogs.

TRENDS IN THERAPIES

Although there have been some recent additions to the therapies used to treat different toxicities, common mainstay medications and treatment recommendations included methocarbamol, use of fluids (both intravenous and subcutaneous),

Table 8		
Number of times lipid fat emulsion therapy was reported as being administered annually and the frequency compared to the total number of reported exposures		
	Lipid Fat Emulsion Therapy	
Year	Count	%
2007	3	0.002
2008	60	0.047
2009	285	0.219
2010	475	0.358

famotadine (Pepcid), sucralfate, acepromazine, monitoring of blood work profiles (blood chemistries and CBCs), and cyproheptadine. Decontamination with activated charcoal and induction of emesis also remains effective, especially in the dog. The use of activated charcoal in dogs and cats has decreased over the years. For example, in 2006, activated charcoal was administered in 3.6% of canine exposures but in only 2.5% of exposures in 2010. The decrease in the use of activated charcoal may be also because of potentials of hypernatremia developing after the administration of activated charcoal in some dogs. Clearly, the use of activated charcoal in appropriate exposures is beneficial but, as with all therapies, clinicians must weigh risk versus benefit before using it.

There have been some changes in the agents used to induce emesis in animals. Although it was a more popular emetic in the past, the risk associated with the use of syrup of ipecac in animals has caused a decline in its popularity. In 2006 syrup of ipecac was used in 0.04% of cases but decreased to 0.01% in 2010. Risks and poor efficacy in animals associated with the use of syrup of ipecac include a delay in the onset of vomiting, protracted vomiting, and risk of cardiotoxicity.[11]

The use of intravenous lipid fat emulsion in veterinary toxicology has become popular in recent years. The benefits of and mechanism of action are still being studied, but there have been many anecdotal reports and some published data on efficacy when treating patients acutely exposed to a lypophilic substances. It has been proposed that lipid emulsion therapy may be effective because small lipid particles have a high binding capacity, allowing them to trap highly lipid soluble substances; the lipids may activate calcium channels reversing intoxications from calcium channel blocking agents; or lipids can help overcome a decrease in fatty acid transport.[12] In 2002, intravenous fat emulsion therapy was administered in 0.002% of reported exposures but increased to 0.358% in 2010 (**Table 8**).

SUMMARY

Like every science, the field of veterinary toxicology is constantly evolving. While the demographics of animals exposed to different toxicants remains relatively steady, changes in society norms have an effect on the potential substances to which animals are exposed. Dogs are the species most commonly exposed to potentially toxic substances, and exposures are more often reported during summer months in the early evening. Current trends show that human medications continue to be a common risk for pets and that there has been an increase in the number of vitamin D exposures reported. As veterinary medicine advances, new and more effective therapies will continue to affect how suspected exposures to toxic substances are treated.

Decontamination remains an important therapy to lessen the risk for signs after an exposure, and although its effectiveness remains debatable, the experimental use of intravenous lipid fat emulsion has risen. The continued monitoring of medical record databases will ensure clinicians are up to date and well informed of emerging trends in toxicology.

REFERENCES

1. American Veterinary Medical Association. All pets. In: U.S. Pet Ownership and Demographics Sourcebook. Schaumburg: American Veterinary Medical Association; 2007. p. 7–12.
2. American Kennel Club. AKC Dog registration statistics. Available at: http://www. akc.org/reg/dogreg_stats_2006.cfm. Accessed September 23, 2011.
3. Volmer PA. Easter lily toxicosis in cats. Vet Med 1999;94:331.
4. Youssef H. Cycad toxicosis in dogs. Vet Med 2008;103:242–4.
5. Grant W, Holick M. Benefits and requirements of vitamin D for optimal health: a review. Altern Med Rev 2005;10:94–111.
6. Morrow C. Cholecalciferol poisoning. Vet Med 2001;96:905–11.
7. US Environmental Protection Agency. Risk mitigation decision for ten rodenticides. Washington, DC: United States Environmental Protection Agency; 2008.
8. AnTox Database. Urbana (IL): ASPCA Animals Poison Control Center; 2001–2011.
9. Richardson J. Permethrin spot-on toxicosis in cats. J Vet Emerg Crit Care 2000;10: 103–9.
10. Dolder L. Metaldehyde toxicosis. Vet Med 2003;98:213–5.
11. Manoguerra A, Cobaugh D; Members of the Guidelines for the Management of Poisonings Consensus Panel. Guideline on the use of ipecac syrup in the out-of-hospital management of ingested poisons. Clin Toxicol 2005;1:1–10.
12. O'Brien T, Clark-Price S, Evans E, et al. Infusion of a lipid emulsion to treat lidocaine intoxication in a cat. J Am Vet Med Assoc 2010;237:1455–8.

Investigative Diagnostic Toxicology and the Role of the Veterinarian in Pet Food–Related Outbreaks

Christina R. Wilson, PhD[a,b,]*, Stephen B. Hooser, DVM, PhD[a,b]

KEYWORDS
- Food-related illness • Pet food • Outbreak • Pet food recall
- Diagnostic testing

More than 90% of cats and dogs are being fed commercial pet food by their owners.[1] Even though some of these animals receive varying amounts of other food stuffs (eg, table scraps), more than 50% of their dietary intake is through consumption of commercial pet food products. However, more recently, some pet owners are electing to feed more noncommercial foods, such as home-prepared foods, to their companion animals.[1] This may be due in part to the occurrences of adulterated commercial pet food that have been widely reported in the media over the past several years. While the great majority of manufactured pet foods are safe, there have been a few instances in which chemical or bacterial contamination has caused outbreaks of illness in companion animals.

PET FOOD–RELATED OUTBREAKS AND RECALLS

Contaminants in pet food resulting in animal illness can be due to several factors, such as incorrect formulation of the nutritional components in the food, insufficiencies in analytical testing of food for toxins or toxicants, mixing errors during the production process, or incorporation of contaminated raw materials (eg, grains, meats, or other feed components) into the product. While industry quality control measures and voluntary recalls by pet food manufacturers usually preclude incidents of adverse health events in animals, there have been a few instances in which pet food contamination have occurred causing morbidity or mortality in dogs and cats. For

The authors have nothing to disclose.
[a] Indiana Animal Disease Diagnostic Laboratory, Purdue University, 406 South University, West Lafayette, IN 47907, USA
[b] Department of Comparative Pathobiology, Purdue University, School of Veterinary Medicine, 725 Harrison Street, West Lafayette, IN 47907, USA
* Corresponding author. Indiana Animal Disease Diagnostic Laboratory, Purdue University, 406 South University Street, West Lafayette, IN 47907-1175.
E-mail address: wilsonc@purdue.edu

example, in 2006 and 2010, mixing errors resulted in incorrect formulations of vitamin D in a pet food product. In the 2010 incident, the ingredient supplier for the pet food manufacturer produced a vitamin D supplement immediately prior to preparing ingredients for the pet food. Residual vitamin D in the manufacturing process carried over into the pet food ingredients causing cross-contamination of product. According to the US Food and Drug Administration (FDA), the 2010 recall resulted in 36 reported cases of nephrotoxicity nationwide.[2,3]

Adulteration of pet food products has also occurred due to contamination during general food processing. In 2006, *Salmonella enterica* serotype Schwarzengrund was responsible for widespread recalls of dry dog and cat food.[4] The number of affected animals in this outbreak, which was reported in 19 states, totaled 79. Contamination was thought to be due to the presence of the *Salmonella* strain in a flavoring room where the manufacturer sprayed the product to enhance palatability. Voluntary recalls due to suspect *Salmonella* contamination in pig ear products, pet treats, and canned or dry dog and cat food happen occasionally and are usually initiated before food-borne illness is reported.

Another example of pet food-related illness occurred in 2005 when approximately 19 varieties of dog food were recalled due to contamination with aflatoxin.[5] Animals in 23 states and 29 other countries to which the product was exported were affected. It was later discovered that corn and corn products contaminated with aflatoxin were inadvertently incorporated into commercial dog food. This error was likely due to the company not adhering to its own quality control guidelines for aflatoxin testing in shipments of corn to be used in the product.

Possibly the most notable pet food–related outbreak was the occurrence of renal failure in dogs and cats exposed to food adulterated with melamine and cyanuric acid. In 2007, there was a massive recall of melamine-contaminated pet food in the United States. In this incident, it was discovered that wheat and rice gluten incorporated into pet food was artificially contaminated with melamine and cyanuric acid in order to increase the apparent protein concentration of the product. Exposure to toxic amounts of these chemicals resulted in the formation of yellow-brown melamine-cyanuric acid crystals in renal tubules, resulting in proximal tubular epithelial necrosis and related nephrotoxicity in exposed cats and dogs.[6] More than 1000 commercial pet foods were recalled due to this adulteration.[7] Approximately 450 cases of renal failure were reported in cats and dogs, of which approximately 100 animals died.[7,8]

THE ROLE OF THE VETERINARIAN AND THE HUMAN ELEMENT

It is evident that the veterinarian plays a crucial role in recognizing these adverse events and the severity of animal health risk. While these occurrences have a tremendous impact on animal health, the veterinarian must also be cognizant of the potential human health risk. For example, human exposure to *Salmonella* Schwarzengrund–contaminated pet food (through handling) resulted in the first case of human salmonellosis linked to use of dry cat and dog food.[9] In this outbreak, 79 people were infected. Of these 79 people, 48% were children under the age of 2 years. This case emphasizes the importance of the veterinarian in educating households on the proper handling and storage of pet foods. It also underscores the need for veterinarians to have an awareness of potential human exposure in client households, in addition to being attentive to animal health.

Also highlighting the importance of the role of the veterinarian is the fact that animals can serve as sentinels for human exposure to toxins or toxicants. An example of this was underscored when nephrotoxicity had occurred in dogs and cats due to melamine-cyanuric acid–contaminated pet foods in 2007. Recognition of this pet food contamination event probably expedited making the correlation that nephrolithiasis and acute kidney injury in children was linked to melamine-cyanuric acid–contaminated infant formula in 2008. Due to this unfortunate event, an estimated 53,000 children were affected and 6 deaths were reported.[10,11] Therefore, the potential for human health risk and the global implications of these incidents highlight the significance of the veterinarian with respect to both animal and human health.

ESTABLISHING A CAUSAL RELATIONSHIP BETWEEN CLINICAL SIGNS AND SUSPECT FOODSTUFF
Obtaining a Thorough Case History

Recent changes in food or treats that coincide chronologically with changes in the animal's eating behavior or with onset of health-related problems can be suggestive of a food contamination issue. Documenting a thorough case history is the most crucial, initial step in successfully establishing a causal relationship between the animal's clinical signs and the suspect food source. This will also help ascertain whether other toxicology differentials should be considered during the diagnostic work-up for the case. Working in collaboration with the pet owner, the veterinarian should begin the case history at a point in time preceding the owner's first discovery that there was a problem and then progress chronologically from that point. A thorough case history should include detailed information about the animal(s) exposed as well as the pet food product in question. A list of items that should be included in the case history are as follows:

Regarding the Animal Exposed

1. Signalment (sex, breed, age, weight of animal)
2. Animal's complete medical history (including vaccinations, medications, and treatments given)
3. Results of any diagnostic testing or clinical pathology performed (complete blood count, chemistries, urinalysis, serology, etc)
4. Description of the progression of clinical signs (onset time, duration, and types of clinical signs exhibited by the pet)
5. Number of animals affected in the household
6. Number of animals and humans potentially exposed
7. How the owner stored/handled the pet food
8. Duration of exposure
9. Timeframe between feeding product and onset of clinical signs/change in behavior
10. Approximate amount of the food product the animal consumed
11. Description of possibilities for exposure to other toxins/toxicants/drugs.

Regarding the Pet Food Product in Question

12. Brand name of product and product description from the label
13. Purchase date and purchase location and total amount purchased
14. Type of product container (can, pouch, bag, etc)
15. Name of the manufacturer of the product
16. Lot number and expiration date (best by or best before date)
17. UPC code (barcode)
18. Product date and product code
19. Amount of food product used and the amount unused owner still has
20. Where and how the product was stored.

The preceding case information obtained by the attending veterinarians must be documented in case records with time and date. Once the case history has been completed, the veterinarian can use the pet food product information to query the FDA Center for Veterinary Medicine (CVM)'s pet food recall products list. This will help to establish whether the pet food product in question has already been recalled due to contamination or other adulteration. The pet food recall products list can be accessed at their website (http://www.accessdata.fda.gov/scripts/newpetfoodrecalls/). Other useful resources regarding pet food recalls, case consultation, or information include contacting the state veterinarian, the Veterinary Information Network, the ASPCA Animal Poison Control Center, the Pet Poison Helpline, or veterinary diagnostic laboratories.

EFFECTIVE USE OF VETERINARY DIAGNOSTIC LABORATORIES
Collecting Appropriate Samples for Diagnostic Testing

After the case history is thoroughly documented, narrowing down the differential diagnoses will likely begin with performing diagnostic tests. Therefore, collecting the appropriate samples from the affected animal(s) and saving as much of the suspect pet food product as possible will be the key to arriving at an accurate diagnosis. After doing some fact finding, particularly if a recall has been initiated, the veterinarian may already have knowledge of the contaminant/adulterant of concern. In this case, the veterinarian can query the American Association of Veterinary Laboratory Diagnosticians' website (http://www.aavld.org/) to investigate which veterinary diagnostic laboratory would be appropriate for consulting. This will direct the veterinarian to which veterinary diagnostic laboratory can perform analytical testing for that specific analyte and obtain guidance regarding which sample(s) are recommended for submission. Additionally, the FDA or the manufacturer of the pet food product can be contacted regarding guidance for analytical testing. It is likely that the FDA or the manufacturer of the product will want to perform follow-up testing on the foodstuff in question.

As part of the diagnostic investigative toxicology work-up, it is imperative that the client or veterinarian retains as much of the food product as possible. This includes storing the product in its original packaging (no sub-sampling from the bag, can, pouch, etc). There are some adulterants or contaminants for which diagnostic testing of biological samples is limited. For example, aflatoxin M_1 was detected in 7 out of 8 submitted livers from one of the feed-related aflatoxin outbreaks in dogs.[5] Although aflatoxin M_1 was detected in this case, diagnostic methods for testing aflatoxins in tissues have not been developed or validated to the extent that veterinary diagnostic laboratories could offer it as a routine diagnostic test. However, there are sensitive, accurate methods for quantitating aflatoxins in foodstuffs. Therefore, it is imperative to save as much of the pet food product as this may be the only sample that can be analyzed for the case in question. Approximately 1 kilogram of dry food or 4 cans of food should be saved for analysis and some should be saved for future reference. Food should be properly identified and labeled (date and time of collection) and stored frozen or at room temperature in an airtight bag/jar. Other source material can be collected, such as water (eg, from their water bowl) and other foodstuffs the animal has eaten within the timeframe of onset of clinical signs.

In addition to saving the suspect food source, collecting biological samples from affected animals is also essential. Antemortem samples should be collected as soon as possible after exposure and stored at the appropriate conditions. A list of recommended, antemortem samples to collect is described in **Table 1**. Whole blood collected should be stored refrigerated until analysis. Although the remaining antemortem samples listed

Table 1	
Recommended antemortem and postmortem samples to collect for diagnostic testing	
Antemortem	**Postmortem**
Suspect pet food product[a]	Suspect pet food product[a]
Whole blood (EDTA)	Brain (half in 10% formalin and the other half frozen)
Serum or plasma	Eyeball or ocular fluid[b]
Vomitus or ingesta[b]	Ingesta[b]
Urine[b]	Liver (one set in 10% formalin and one set frozen)
Samples for infectious disease testing	Kidney (one set in 10% formalin and one set frozen)
Other source material[c]	Intestinal contents Urine[b] Samples for infectious disease testing Other source material[c] Fix representative tissue samples in 10% formalin

[a] Save entire suspect pet food product in the original package (bag, can, pouch, etc).
[b] Store chilled or frozen.
[c] Collect other source material such as other food sources or water.

can be stored refrigerated for several days; it is recommended that they be stored frozen until analysis.

In circumstances in which animal mortality has occurred, performing a complete necropsy on the animal is highly recommended. While the practitioner can perform a necropsy and collect the appropriate tissue samples for testing, submitting the animal for a complete necropsy to a veterinary diagnostic laboratory would be optimal. At the diagnostic laboratory, a thorough gross and histopathologic examination can be performed by a veterinary pathologist. Pathology results can help refine the differential diagnoses or direct further testing. If the practitioner performs the necropsy, the postmortem samples recommended for collecting are listed in **Table 1**. It is important to document any remarkable, gross anatomical observations noted during the necropsy. After fixing representative tissue samples in 10% formalin for histopathology, the remaining samples procured by the practitioner can be refrigerated; however, for long-term storage, samples should be kept frozen. Ideally, 2 sets of tissue samples should be prepared. One set should be composed of thinly sliced tissues stored in 10% formalin for histologic examination. The other set should include large, frozen tissues (50–100 g each if possible) for toxicologic analysis.

Investigative toxicology testing is often limited by inadequate sample size or submission of an inappropriate sample; therefore, it is important to collect as much of each sample as possible to maximize diagnostic testing efforts, particularly if testing in multiple laboratories is warranted. Being cognizant of the fact that the causative agent or contaminant may not be toxicologically relevant (ie, an infectious agent) is another reason to be thorough and complete in collecting samples from affected animals for diagnostic testing.

REPORTING A PET FOOD COMPLAINT
Agencies Regulating Commercial Pet Foods

The Association of American Feed Control Officials (AAFCO) works in collaboration with the US FDA to ensure the safety of commercial pet foods. The AAFCO regulations on pet food products are intended to address the nutrient content of pet foods and label claims on the product in an effort to guarantee uniform consistency and enforcement of these claims.[12] The US FDA's role involves regulating health claims on pet food products, particularly regarding the safety of new ingredients or food additives. In 2007, The Food and Drug Administration Amendments Act was passed, giving the FDA more jurisdiction over taking action against pet food contamination or safety issues.[12] The FDA CVM is the primary authority for regulating health claims on pet food labels.

How to Report a Pet Food Complaint

Veterinarians should not wait for all diagnostic testing to be completed before reporting a pet food-borne illness. If the practitioner has reasonable suspicion that the adverse health event was due to pet food contamination, he or she should initially contact the manufacturer of the food product. The manufacturer may be able to provide insight into the potential issue and will also need that information to trace increased occurrences associated with a particular product or ascertain if there is an outbreak associated with a specific geographic location. If there is heightened suspicion that a contaminant in pet food is the source of illness (eg, diagnostic tests are completed or most differentials are eliminated), then the veterinarian should report a pet food complaint to the FDA CVM. A complaint can be reported electronically through the FDA's "Safety Reporting Portal" or it can be reported by calling the FDA Consumer Complaint Coordinator in that state. By accessing the FDA CVM website (https://www.safetyreporting.hhs.gov/), the "Safety Reporting Portal" can be accessed electronically and information regarding the clinical case history and pet food product can be entered. If reporting by telephone, the FDA CVM website (http://www.fda.gov/Safety/ReportaProblem/ConsumerComplaintCoordinators/default.htm) has a "FDA Consumer Complaint Coordinators" directory that lists the telephone number for the coordinators in each state. The practitioner can also contact their state veterinarian, the Office of the State Chemist, or its equivalent in that state or notify veterinary diagnostic laboratories to make them aware of the issue. If human exposure is suspected, then the state department of human health should be notified.

SUMMARY

Although pet food products are generally safe and incidences of contamination rare given the enormous quantities of pet foods manufactured and sold, there are still some instances in which pet food–borne illness occurs in dogs and cats. The veterinarian plays a crucial role in recognizing these adverse events, including assessing the severity of animal and human health risk. Due to the potential global implications of these outbreaks, proper reporting and consultation with government and state agencies are crucial. Accurate diagnoses and identifying the source of illness in these outbreaks are promising when thorough case histories are documented, appropriate samples are collected, and state and federal agencies such as veterinary diagnostic laboratories and the FDA are used effectively.

REFERENCES

1. Michel KE, Willoughby KN, Abood SK, et al. Attitudes of pet owners toward pet foods and feeding management of cats and dogs. JAVMA 2008;233:1699–703.
2. Press release. Blue Buffalo Company, Ltd. recalls limited production code dates of dry dog food because of possible excess vitamin D. Available at: http://www.fda.gov/AnimalVeterinary/default.htm. Accessed December 6, 2011.
3. Refsal K, Schenck P. Pet food illness in dogs results in a national recall. Q Newsl DCPA Health News 2010;4:2.

4. Centers for Disease Control and Prevention. Update: recall of dry dog and cat food products associated with human Salmonella Schwarzengrund infections: United States. Morb Mortal Wkly Rep 2008; 57:1200–2.

5. Stenske KA, Smith JR, Newman SJ, et al. Aflatoxicosis in dogs dealing with suspected contaminated commercial foods. JAVMA 2006;228:1686–91.

6. Brown CA, Jeong K, Poppenga RH, et al. Outbreaks of renal failure associated with melamine and cyanuric acid in dogs and cats in 2004 and 2007. J Vet Diagn Invest 2007;19:525–31.

7. Rumbeiha WK, Agnew D, Maxie G, et al. Analysis of a survey database of pet food-induced poisoning in North America. J Med Toxicol 2010;6:172–84.

8. Puschner B, Reimschuessel R. Toxicosis caused by melamine and cyanuric acid in dogs and cats: uncovering the mystery and subsequent global implications. Clin Lab Med 2011;31:181–99.

9. Behravesh CB, Ferraro A, Deasy, M, et al. Human Salmonella infections linked to contaminated dry dog and cat food, 2006-2008. Pediatrics 2010;126:477–83.

10. Bhalla V, Grimm PC, Chertow GM, et al. Melamine nephrotoxicity: an emerging epidemic in an era of globalization. Kidney Int 2009;75:774–9.

11. Xin H, Stone R. Chinese probe unmasks high-tech adulteration with melamine. Science 2008;322:1310–1.

12. Chase LP, Daristotle L, Hayek MG, et al. History and regulation of pet foods. In: Canine and feline nutrition: a resource for companion animal professionals. 3rd edition. Maryland Heights (MO): Mosby; 2011. p. 121–9.

Pet Food Recalls and Pet Food Contaminants in Small Animals

Karyn Bischoff, DVM, MS[a,b],*, Wilson K. Rumbeiha, BVM, PhD[c]

KEYWORDS

- Aflatoxin • Cholecalciferol • Cyanuric acid • Melamine
- Thiamine • Vitamin B_1 • Vitamin D

Most pet foods are safe. Only 1.7% of reported poisonings in dogs and cats have been attributed to pet foods.[1] Incidents of contamination occur through microbial action, mixing error, or intentional adulteration. Although rare, the effects of pet food contamination can be physically devastating for companion animals and emotionally devastating and financially burdensome for their owners. Whereas most people consume a diet from various sources, for companion animals a single bag of food or cans from a single brand/lot will likely be the major or sole source of nutrition until that food has been completely consumed. Thus, the effects of food contaminants in people is diluted by the varied diet, but the uniform diet of most dogs and cats, although preferred for nutritional reasons, increases the risk of adverse effects if a contaminant is present in their food. As the companion animal veterinarian is aware, many animal owners consider their dog or cat to be a vulnerable family member that needs to be protected.[2] Based on the authors' experiences, pet owners often experience seemingly disproportionate guilt when pets become sickened or die after being unknowingly fed contaminated pet foods. Some owners have described feeling responsible for poisoning their pet during pet food contamination incidents.

When pet food is contaminated or adulterated there is usually a food recall. There are 3 types of recalls involving chemical contaminants: Class I—reasonable probability that the contaminated food will cause adverse health consequences or death; Class II—the contaminated food can cause temporary or medically reversible adverse

The authors have nothing to disclose.
[a] New York State Animal Health Diagnostic Center, PO Box 5786, Room A2, 232, Ithaca, NY 13081, USA
[b] Department of Population Medicine and Diagnostic Sciences, Cornell University, PO Box 5786, Room A2 232, Ithaca, NY 14853-5786, USA
[c] Veterinary Diagnostics and Production Animal Medicine, College of Veterinary Medicine, Iowa State University, 2659 Vet Med, Ames, IA 50011, USA
* Corresponding author. Department of Population Medicine and Diagnostic Sciences, Cornell University, PO Box 5786, Room A2 232, Ithaca, NY 14853-5786.
E-mail address: KLB72@cornell.edu

Vet Clin Small Anim 42 (2012) 237–250
doi:10.1016/j.cvsm.2011.12.007
0195-5616/12/$ – see front matter © 2012 Elsevier Inc. All rights reserved.

health consequences but is unlikely to cause serious adverse health effects; and Class III—the contaminated food is unlikely to cause adverse health consequences. There were 22 Class I and II pet food recalls in the United States over a 12-year period (1996 to 2008), and 6 were due to chemical contaminants.[3] Of these 6, 2 were due to aflatoxin (a mycotoxin), 3 were due to feed mixing or formulation errors (2 excess vitamin D_3 and 1 excess methionine), and 1 was due to adulteration of food ingredients with melamine and related compounds.[3]

Since 2008, there have been 3 cat foods and 1 dog food recalled due to mixing or formulation errors (inadequate thiamine in the cat foods, excessive vitamin D_3 in the dog food) and 1 dog and cat food recall due to contamination with aflatoxin. There have also been 2 US Food and Drug Administration (FDA) warnings and one from the Canadian Veterinary Medical Association since 2007 concerning a Fanconi-like renal syndrome in dogs after ingestion of large amounts of chicken jerky treat products, manufactured in China, over time.[4,5] Similar warnings have occurred in Australia.[6] Despite extensive testing, the cause of the adverse health effects (Fanconi-like syndrome) associated with consumption of chicken jerky has not been determined.

Pet food contamination incidents due to adulteration are rare but occurred with melamine and cyanuric acid. The melamine contamination investigation in 2007 led to the discovery that other cases of melamine poisoning had happened in companion and agricultural animals in the Republic of Korea, Japan, Thailand, Malaysia, Singapore, Taiwan, the Philippines, South Africa, Spain, China, and Italy.[7-11]

There have been several other international pet food contamination incidents. Aflatoxin contamination of dog food has been mentioned in news stories from South Africa and Israel since 2006. The use of sulfur dioxide, which destroys thiamine, in processing pet foods has been associated with repeated outbreaks of polioencepha-lomalacia in dogs and cats in Australia.[12-14] Also in Australia, there was a unique recall of irradiated cat food in 2008–2009, after it was found to cause severe central nervous system damage to cats. The proximate cause of the neurological disorder that afflicted cats fed irradiated pet food in Australia has not been determined to date.

The FDA is charged with ensuring the wholesomeness of pet foods. The US Congress passed the FDA Amendments Act of 2007 (FDAAA) to improve responsive-ness to contamination of pet foods and other products after the adulteration of pet food with melamine and related compounds was identified that year. The FDAAA requires manufacturers to report incidents of possible contamination to the FDA within 24 hours, investigate the cause, and report findings of the investigation. When contamination is confirmed, the pet food is recalled. Recall initiation is usually voluntary by the manufacturer at the request of the FDA. The FDA can secure a court order to issue a recall if the manufacturer is reluctant, but this is rare because of the bad publicity and increased potential for litigation should a manufacturer refuse to initiate a recall.[1]

Veterinarians must be involved for the FDAAA to work properly. This involves examining and treating animals that are suspected to have had adverse effects from pet foods, documenting pertinent findings, collecting appropriate samples, advising pet owners, and contacting the FDA and pet food manufacturers. Samples for laboratory analysis include the suspected food and its packaging (or, if unavailable, lot numbers, manufacturing codes, and other identifying information), and samples from the pet such as blood, serum, urine, vomitus or gastric lavage fluids, and feces. A full necropsy with postmortem sample collection for histopathology and analytical chemistry includes fresh urine, adipose tissue, and heart blood, fresh and fixed brain, liver, and kidney, and fixed lung, spleen, and bone marrow. These samples are often required to rule in or out toxins when the affected animal dies or is euthanized. Often the pet food manufacturer will help with associated costs of treatment and testing; thus, it is in the interests of the pet owner and veterinarian to contact them as soon as contamination is suspected. Manufacturer contact information is usually found on product packaging. Consumer complaints can be reported to local FDA consumer complaint coordinators or online (http://www.fda.gov/cvm/petfoods.htm). Local government agriculture or food safety agencies should also be alerted when contamination of a commercial product is suspected.

The rest of this text gives some details concerning major pet food contamination or formulation errors that have been associated with morbidity and mortality in pets in the United States, with mention of some minor contaminants and a formulation error that occurred in Asia. The most common natural contaminant of pet food is aflatoxin, a fungal metabolite. The common conditions that have been associated with misformulation include hypervitaminosis D and polioencephalomalacia. Last, included in the category of adulterants are melamine and related cyanuric acid.

NATURAL CONTAMINANTS

The most common natural contaminants in pet foods are mycotoxins (fungal metabolites). Aflatoxins are the most common mycotoxins to cause pet food recalls in the United States, but other mycotoxin contaminants have been reported. There was a recall of dog food due to contamination with the mycotoxin deoxynivalenol (DON) in 1995. DON is produced on grain by *Fusarium* spp under temperate conditions. Pet food DON concentrations of greater than 4.5 ppm and 7.7 ppm were associated with feed refusal in dogs and cats, respectively, and concentrations of 8 ppm or greater cause vomiting in both species.[15,16] Animals recover quickly once the food is replaced, although supportive care is needed if gastroenteritis is severe.[16]

Aflatoxin

Aflatoxicosis in dogs was first described in 1952 as "hepatitis X" and reproduced in experimental dogs using contaminated feed in 1955, then by dosing with purified aflatoxin B_1 in 1966. Moldy corn poisoning in swine in the 1940s and turkey X disease in turkeys fed peanut meal were also linked to aflatoxin.

Aflatoxins are a group of related compounds *sometimes* produced as metabolites of various fungi, *Aspergillus parasiticus, A flavus, A nomius*, some *Penicillium* spp, and others. Names of common aflatoxins are derived from the colors that fluoresce: aflatoxins B_1, the most common and potent form, and B_2 fluoresce blue and G_1 and G_2 both fluoresce green. High energy foods, such as corn, peanuts, and cottonseed, are most often affected. Rice, wheat, oats, sweet potatoes, potatoes, barley, millet, sesame, sorghum, cacao beans, almonds, soy, coconut, safflower, sunflower, palm kernel, cassava, cowpeas, peas, and various spices can also be affected.[17,18] Aflatoxin production can occur on field crops or in storage. Temperature, humidity, drought stress, insect damage, and handling techniques influence mycotoxin production.[17] Use of aflatoxin-contaminated food commodities in the manufacture of pet foods have caused intoxication in pets. Improper storage of dog food and ingestion of moldy garbage have been implicated in aflatoxicosis.[19]

Both dogs and cats are very sensitive to aflatoxin.[18] The oral median lethal dose (LD_{50}) for aflatoxin in dogs is between 0.5 and 1.5 mg/kg.[20] The experimental oral LD_{50} for cats is 0.55 mg/kg, although no field cases of aflatoxicosis have been identified in cats to the authors' knowledge.[18] It is difficult to determine the total dose of aflatoxin received in field cases, where the period of exposure and amount fed are not always available. Aflatoxin concentrations of 60 ppb in dog food have been implicated in aflatoxicosis.[20] Factors associated with increased susceptibility to aflatoxicosis include genetic predisposition, concurrent disease, age, and sex, with young males and pregnant females considered particularly susceptible.[20,21]

Aflatoxin is highly lipophilic and absorbed rapidly and almost completely, particularly in young animals, mostly in the duodenum. Aflatoxin enters the portal circulation and is highly protein bound in the blood. The unbound fraction is distributed to the tissues, with highest concentrations accumulating in the liver.[17] The liver is the primary site of metabolism, although some metabolism takes place in other tissues, including the kidneys and small intestine. Phase I metabolism of aflatoxin B_1 by cytochrome P450 enzymes produces the reactive intermediate aflatoxin B_1 8,9-epoxide. Some aflatoxin B_1 is eventually metabolized to aflatoxin M_1.[21] During phase II metabolism, aflatoxin B_1 8,9-epoxide is conjugated to glutathione in a reaction catalyzed by glutathione S-transferase.[22] Metabolites of aflatoxin are excreted in the urine and bile, primarily as M_1 in dogs. More than 90% of metabolized aflatoxin detected in canine urine is excreted within the first 12 hours, and urine aflatoxin is below detectable concentrations within 48 hours.[23] Conjugated aflatoxin is excreted mostly in bile.[17]

Aflatoxin B_1 8,9-epoxide, produced by metabolism of aflatoxin B_1, is a potent electrophile and binds readily to cellular macromolecules such as nucleic acids, proteins, and constituents of subcellular organelles.[24] Formation of DNA adducts modifies the DNA template and the ability of DNA polymerase to bind, affecting cellular replication, and binding to ribosomal translocase effects protein production.[20,25] These changes can lead to necrosis in hepatocytes and, less frequently, other metabolically active cells such as renal tubular epithelium.[21] Coagulopathy results from synthetic hepatic failure and decreased prothrombin and fibrinogen.[26] No carcinogenic effects have been reported in cats and dogs, although aflatoxins are known to be carcinogenic in some species, including rats, ferrets, ducks, trout, swine, sheep, and rats, and are classified by the International Agency for Research on Cancer (IARC) as Class I human carcinogens.[18,25]

The presentation of aflatoxicosis in small animals may be acute or chronic. Exposure to contaminated foods can occur for weeks or months before dogs become clinically affected; indeed, in one author's experience, contaminated food was removed from the diet of a dog approximately 3 weeks before clinical aflatoxicosis was evident. Many dogs die within a few days of initial clinical signs, but illness can be protracted for up to 2 weeks.[21] Early clinical signs of aflatoxicosis in dogs include feed refusal or anorexia, weakness and obtundation, vomiting, and diarrhea. Later, dogs become icteric, often with melena or frank blood in the feces, hematemesis, petechia, and epistaxis.[18,27] Experimentally poisoned cats died within 3 days of onset of signs.[18]

Complete blood cell count, serum chemistry, including bile acids, and urinalysis are helpful to support the diagnosis of aflatoxin poisoning and rule out other causes of liver failure. Total bilirubin is increased in aflatoxicosis and hepatic enzyme concentrations, including alanine aminotransferase (ALT), aspartate aminotransferase (AST), alkaline phosphatase (ALP), and gamma-glutamyl transpeptidase (GGT), are variably elevated.[20,21] Liver function tests are often more helpful in supporting the diagnosis. Prothrombin time is increased due to decreased synthesis of clotting factors, and serum albumin, protein C, antithrombin III, and cholesterol concentrations are decreased.[27]

Diagnosis of aflatoxicosis is usually based on history, clinical signs, clinical pathology findings, and postmortem changes. The primary differential diagnosis for dogs in recent food-contamination related cases of aflatoxicosis was often

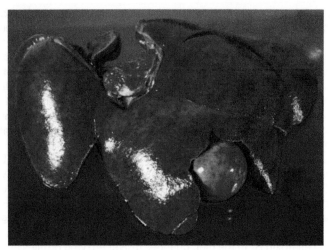

Fig. 1. Liver from a dog with aflatoxicosis. (*Courtesy of* S.P. McDonough.)

leptospirosis, but other differential diagnoses include parvovirus and anticoagulant rodenticide toxicosis based on the severe gastrointestinal hemorrhage, and a variety of hepatotoxic agents including acetaminophen, xylitol, microcystin from cyanobacteria (blue-green algae), amanitin and phalloidin from mushrooms, toxins associated with cycad palms, phosphine, and iron.[20,27,28] Necropsy is helpful in confirming the diagnosis and ruling out other conditions. Common gross findings include icterus, hepatomegaly with evidence of lipidosis (**Fig. 1**), ascites, gastrointestinal hemorrhage, and multifocal petechia and ecchymosis.[20,26,27] The primary histologic changes of canine aflatoxicosis are associated with the liver, although pigmentary nephrosis and necrosis of the proximal convoluted renal tubules have been reported.[21,26] Liver lesions in acute toxicosis include fatty degeneration of hepatocytes with one to numerous lipid vacuoles. Centrilobular necrosis and canalicular cholestasis with mild inflammation are commonly reported.[19,26,27] Dogs with subacute toxicosis still have fatty degeneration, canalicular cholestasis, and multifocal to locally extensive necrosis, often with neutrophilic inflammation and evidence of regeneration. Fibrosis is more prominent, with bridging of portal triads, bile ductule proliferation, and obfuscation of the central vein by dilated sinusoids. Chronic aflatoxicosis is characterized by less fatty degeneration, marked fibrosis, and regenerative nodules, causing disruption of the normal hepatic architecture.[26] Experimental cats with aflatoxicosis had hepatomegaly with petechiation, minimal hepatocystic glycogen storage, and, in cats surviving more than 72 hours, bile duct hyperplasia was also present.[18]

Laboratory testing of dog food or other implicated material helps to confirm the diagnosis, but due to the extended time between exposure and onset of aflatoxicosis, the food is most often unavailable. Before the 2005 dog food recall, a veterinarian submitted dog food from each of 3 households, 2 of which had dogs with clinical aflatoxicosis, to a laboratory. The single sample that contained aflatoxin in toxicologically significant concentrations was from the household of a dog that had no clinical signs of toxicosis until weeks later.

Commercial grain is routinely screened for aflatoxin, but sampling error is possible due to the uneven distribution of mold within the grain and other commodities. Current analytical techniques use enzyme-linked immunosorbent assays, high-performance liquid chromatography, and liquid chromatography/mass spectrometry to detect aflatoxin. Some laboratories can test for aflatoxin M_1 in the urine, but urinary excretion is very rapid in dogs.[23] Urine may be useful for a period of up to 48 hours post exposure. Serum or liver can be tested, but due to the rapid metabolism and excretion of aflatoxin, this testing is often of limited usefulness.[20]

The prognosis for dogs with clinical aflatoxicosis is guarded. Early intervention improves the prognosis, but many cases fail to respond to treatment.[19,20,27] Patient assessment and stabilization are the first steps in management. Remove access to contaminated food and replace it with a high-quality protein containing diet if the dog continues to eat. Supportive care includes hydration and correcting electrolyte imbalances with intravenous fluids, which can be supplemented with B vitamins, vitamin K, and dextrose.[21] Plasma transfusions improve coagulation ability.[20] Sucralfate, famotidine, and sometimes parenteral nutrition have been used for anorexic dogs and those with severe gastroenteritis.[20,25]

Liver protectants, such as silymarin (a mix of silybin and other flavolignans from milk thistle), have been used clinically and experimentally. When silymarin was given to chickens fed aflatoxin B_1 in the diet, changes in liver enzyme profiles and histologic lesions were decreased compared to controls on clean diets.[24] Proposed mechanisms of action for silybin include inhibition of phase I metabolism of aflatoxin B_1, thus decreasing epoxide production.[24,29] S-Adenosylmethionine (SAMe), which can act as a sulfhydryl donor, has been used as a hepatoprotectant in aflatoxicosis cases.[20,27] N-Acetylcysteine, a commonly used sulfhydryl donor, is given parenterally rather than orally for severely affected dogs. Experimentally, N-acetylcysteine (Mucomyst) has been shown to enhance elimination of aflatoxin B_1 and prevent liver damage in poultry.[22]

MISFORMULATION

As noted earlier, misformulation is a common cause of adverse reactions to pet foods in cats and dogs. Hypervitaminosis D and thiamine deficiency are discussed in detail later. Other misformulations have involved methionine, which caused a US recall, and excessive vitamin A in Thailand. Excessive methionine was associated with anorexia and vomiting.[3] Misformulation of a feline research diet in Thailand in 2009 resulted in evident hypervitaminosis A (Dr Rosama Pusoonthornthum, personal communication, 2009). Hypervitaminosis A in cats and dogs causes osteopathy, commonly affecting the axial skeleton, and often presents as lameness, paresis, or paralysis due to entrapment of spinal nerves.[30,31] Some animals with hypervitaminosis A, even those severely affected, recover in the long term after they are placed on a new diet.

Hypervitaminosis D

Of the essential vitamins, vitamin D is the one that has been most frequently involved in pet food recalls. Vitamin D serves many physiologic roles, and regulation of calcium and phosphorous metabolism is one of the major roles. Other physiologic roles include immunomodulation and improved reproduction in animals. There are 2 major active forms of vitamin D in mammals. These are ergocalciferol (vitamin D_2) and cholecalciferol (vitamin D_3). There is also increasing use of 25-hydroxy vitamin D_3 in animal feeds, particularly poultry and swine feeds. Oversupplementation and unintentional cross contamination have all caused vitamin D_3 excess in pet food.

There have been 3 pet food recalls triggered by excessive vitamin D_3 in the past 15 years. In 1999, DVM Nutri-Balance and Golden Sun Feeds Hi-Pro Hunter dog food was recalled due to excessive amounts of cholecalciferol. In 2006, 4 products of ROYAL CANIN Veterinary Diet were recalled also due to excessive amount of cholecalciferol. More recently, in 2010, Blue Buffalo dog food was recalled due to contamination with 25-hydroxy vitamin D. Apparently this vitamin ingredient was intended for livestock feed, as it is not supposed to be used in the manufacture of dog food. HyD is a 25-hydroxy vitamin D product made for use in poultry feed, but there is inadequate information to determine the source of the 2010 pet food contamination with 25-hydroxy vitamin D. This incident, however, led to the discovery of a new phenomenon, the apparent physiologic interaction between 25-hydroxy vitamin D and cholecalciferol. The latter was present at recommended concentrations in the recalled dog food and yet clinically affected dogs had elevated serum ionized calcium and 25-hydroxy vitamin D and suppressed intact parathyroid hormone (PTH), all hallmarks of vitamin D toxicosis. In all these cases involving pet food, vitamin D poisoning occurred following prolonged ingestion of the contaminated food, usually weeks of exposure.

Following ingestion, cholecalciferol is rapidly absorbed and transported to the liver where it is rapidly broken down to 25-hydroxy vitamin D_3. This is further metabolized primarily to 1,25-dihydroxy vitamin D_3 (calcitriol) and 24,25-dihydroxy vitamin D_3 in renal proximal convoluted tubular epithelium. Calcitriol is the vitamin D metabolite that is most important in calcium-phosphorus metabolism; thus, imbalances in these macrominerals are important to the pathophysiology of vitamin D toxicosis.

Commonly reported clinical signs of vitamin D poisoning in pets include depression, weakness, anorexia polyuria, and polydipsia. Often these are the only clinical signs noticed but are significant enough to prompt pet owners to seek veterinary care for their pets. Diagnosis of vitamin D poisoning consists of clinical signs consistent with vitamin D poisoning and serum vitamin D toxicity profile: serum intact PTH, total and ionized serum calcium, and serum 25-hydroxy vitamin D_3. In animals with vitamin D toxicosis, a significant increase in serum calcium and phosphorus levels occurs and intact PTH is suppressed. In pets that have died, finding elevated 25-hydroxy vitamin D_3 in the kidney, on top of histopathology characterized by metastatic soft tissue mineralization, is usually sufficient to confirm vitamin D poisoning. However, in cases of 25-hydroxy vitamin D poisoning, as in the case of Blue Buffalo recall, analysis for 25-hydroxy vitamin D_3 could have been helpful, although reference values have yet to be established in dogs and cats.

In episodes of vitamin D toxicosis triggered by pet food contamination, switching diets is often sufficient to correct the problem. Patience is required, though, as it may take weeks before indices of vitamin D poisoning return to normal. Aggressive therapy includes use of salmon calcitonin, pamidronate disodium, corticosteroids, and furosemide diuretic among others. Treatment of vitamin D poisoning has been discussed more extensively elsewhere.

Thiamine Deficiency

As noted in the introduction, there have been 3 recent cat food recalls due to inadequate thiamine. Thiamine is a required B vitamin (B_1). Monogastric animals like cats and dogs cannot synthesize thiamine, and because it is a water-soluble vitamin, there is no long-term storage in the body. Factors such as age and diet affect the thiamine requirements for dogs and cats.[12] Thiamine is absorbed predominantly in the small intestine via a carrier molecule.[32] The vitamin is required as a coenzyme for pyruvate dehydrogenase, alpha-ketoglutarase, translocase, and other enzymes required for carbohydrate metabolism and energy production.[12] Pet foods should contain at least 5 mg/kg and 1 mg/kg thiamine on a dry matter basis, for cats and dogs, respectively.[13,33] Thiamine deficiency in cats has been associated with a food containing 0.56 mg thiamine/kg dry matter.[34]

Thiamine is found in meat, liver, and some cereal grains. Causes of thiamine deficiency in small animals include feeding of meat preserved with sulfur compounds that cleave thiamine, cooking and processing, which destroys 40 to 50% of thiamine, and natural thiaminases found in raw fish.[12,14,34] Absence of thiamine impairs cerebral energy metabolism, producing focal lactic acidosis and neuronal ischemia.[32,33]

Polioencephalomalacia describes the lesion associated with thiamine deficiency. Clinical signs described in experimental cats studied by Everett (1944)[35] began after 2 to 4 weeks on the deficient diet and included anorexia, which is responsive to thiamine injection, and weight loss. Progressive neurologic signs seen soon after included ataxia with a wide-based stance, circling, dilated pupils, positional ventro-flexion of the head, and seizures, which may be spontaneous or secondary to stimulus. These signs remain responsive to thiamine supplementation. Eventually (after a month or more) cats become unable to walk and exhibit extensor tone in all limbs, which fails to respond to thiamine supplementation, followed by coma and death.[35] Positional ventroflexion of the head, sometimes termed "the praying sign," is active and caused by vestibular dysfunction rather than muscle weakness. This sign can be observed when the cat is held by the hindquarters and the front end is moved toward the tabletop. The chin will drop to near the sternum.[36] Cats presented during the 2009 recall had similar clinical signs, including anorexia, head tilt, dilated pupils, apparent blindness, circling, ataxia, extensor rigidity of the front legs and positional ventral flexion of the head, and seizures. All cats in the 2009 case were responsive to thiamine treatment except one with marked extensor rigidity. A study of puppies found that the first signs occurred after nearly 2 months on a thiamine-deficient diet and included inappetence, poor growth or weight loss, coprophagia, and neurologic signs similar to those seen in cats, although some puppies died before the abrupt onset of neurologic signs.[37]

Bilaterally symmetric changes have been observed in affected dogs and cats using magnetic resonance imaging, with lesions documented in the cerebellar nodulus, caudal colliculi, and periaqueductal grey matter, and in dogs the red nuclei and vestibular nuclei, and in cats the facial nuclei and medial vestibular nuclei.[14,33] Diagnostic testing is infrequently used. Functional tests are considered sensitive indicators of thiamine deficiency.[32] The most common is erythrocyte transketolase activity, which has been used in humans and dogs, but no reference values are available for cats.[12,32-34] The reported thiamine pyrophosphate concentration is 32 μg/dL in feline blood and 8.4 to 10.4 μg/dL in blood from healthy canines.[37,38] Cats in the 2009 outbreak had blood thiamine pyrophosphate concentrations ranging from 2.1 to 3.9 μg/dL, but no samples from unaffected cats were analyzed.

Postmortem lesions associated with thiamine deficiency–induced polioencepha-lomalacia in cats and dogs include bilaterally symmetric areas of petechia in the brainstem and elsewhere, corresponding to the areas seen on magnetic resonance imaging. Histologically, lesions include spongiform degeneration with reactive changes, including vascular hypertrophy, macrophage infiltrate, and gliosis.[12,37]

As noted previously, most animals respond to therapy with thiamine hydrochloride, given parenterally at a dose of 100 to 250 mg for cats and 5 to 250 mg/day for dogs.[39] After 5 days of parenteral dosing in a cat, oral thiamine at 25 mg/d was continued for 1 month.[33] Improvement is usually rapid, with significant improvement observed within a few days and often complete within 1 to 12 weeks.[14,32,34,40] However persistent, ataxia, hearing loss, and positional nystagmus are reported.[32,40]

ADULTERATION

Adulteration of pet foods is rare but was responsible for the largest pet food recall in US history. Melamine was intentionally added to pet food ingredients to enhance the apparent protein content. Protein in pet foods is estimated based on the nitrogen content, which is usually measured using the Kjeldahl method. Because melamine is 67% nitrogen based on the molecular weight, its addition to foodstuff increases the nitrogen content and thus the estimated protein content.

Melamine and Cyanuric Acid

Melamine, or 1,3,5-triazine-2,4,6-triamine, has found numerous uses in manufacturing. It can be used in yellow pigments, dies, and inks or can be polymerized with formaldehyde to produce a variety of durable resins, adhesives, cleansers, and flame retardants. Cyanuric acid is an intermediate produced during melamine manufacture or degradation and is used to stabilize chlorine in swimming pools.

Early in 2007, there were several reports of renal failure in cats and dogs consuming commercial pet foods in the United States. Clinical signs included inappetence, vomiting, polyuria, polydipsia, and lethargy. A large number of affected cats were on feeding trials at a laboratory.[41] A recall was initiated on March 15 and melamine was detected in the cat food 2 weeks later, but at the time melamine was believed to have low oral toxicity based on early studies in rodents and dogs. Later, cyanuric acid, ammelide, and ammeline were detected. These are intermediates in the production of melamine from urea. The FDA investigation determined that wheat gluten and rice protein concentrates used in pet food production were intentionally mislabeled by Chinese exporters and actually contained wheat flour and poor quality rice protein mixed with melamine.[10] Eventually, more than 150 pet food products were identified, containing up to 3200 ppm melamine and 600 ppm cyanuric acid, and recalled.[41,42] Samples of imported wheat gluten contained 8.4% melamine, 5.3% cyanuric acid, and 2.3% and 1.7% ammelide and ammeline, respectively.[3] Estimates of the numbers of pets affected range from hundreds to thousands.

Many consider the 2007 pet food recall a sentinel event.[10,43] A year later, contamination of Chinese baby formula and other milk-based products was detected. Melamine concentrations ranged from 2.5 to 2563 ppm in 13 commercial brands of milk powder.[7] More than 52,000 Chinese children were hospitalized and 6 died. There is evidence that children in Taiwan, Hong Kong, and Macau were also affected.[42,44,45] Due to global marketing of food products and ingredients, melamine-contaminated foods were found in almost 70 countries, including the United States.

The oral LD_{50} of melamine is 3200 mg/kg in male rats, 3800 mg/kg in female rats, 3300 mg/kg in male mice, and 7000 mg/kg in female mice. Long-term dietary administration of melamine to laboratory rats at concentrations ranging from 0.225% to 0.9% produced urolithiasis and urinary bladder lesions, including transitional cell carcinoma and, in females, lymphoplasmcytic nephritis and fibrosis.[46] Sheep were given single (217 mg/kg) or multiple (200 to 1,351 mg/kg/d for up to 39 days) doses of melamine. Clinical signs, including anorexia, anuria, and uremia, developed after 5 to 31 days after the first exposure in a dose-dependent manner.[47] A study involving dogs fed 125 mg/kg melamine reported crystalluria but no other adverse effects were identified.[48] Cyanuric acid by itself has similarly low toxicity but is known to produce degenerative changes in the kidneys in guinea pigs at doses of 30 mg/kg body weight for 6 months, rats fed 8% monosodium cyanurate in the diet for 20 weeks, and in dogs fed 8% monosodium cyanurate in the diet. Lesions included ectasia of the distal collecting tubules and multifocal epithelial proliferation.[49] The combination of melamine and cyanuric acid is markedly more toxic to most animals than either compound alone. Cats fed up to 1% melamine or cyanuric acid in the diet had no evidence of clinical abnormalities, but when fed diets containing 0.2% each of melamine and cyanuric acid, the cats had evidence of acute renal failure within 48 hours. Lesions were typical of those associated with the recalled pet food.[50] A pig fed 400 mg/kg melamine and 400 mg/kg cyanuric acid daily had transient bloody diarrhea within 24 hours. Necropsy revealed perirenal edema and round golden-brown crystals with radiating striations in the kidneys. Similar lesions were present in tilapia, rainbow trout, and catfish dosed with 400 mg/kg each of melamine and cyanuric acid daily for 3 days, although most survived the renal damage.[51]

Melamine and cyanuric acid form crystals in distal convoluted tubules of the kidney when given together by binding to form a lattice structure at pH 5.8.[7,10] Renal pathology most likely results from intratubular obstruction and increased intrarenal pressure. Interestingly, cyanuric acid did not contribute to the formation of melamine-containing urinary calculi in children.[52] Calculi in children were produced by a similar interaction between melamine and uric acid. Infants and many primates lack uricase, an enzyme that converts uric acid to allantoin and thus excrete uric acid via the kidneys.[51] Urinary pH less than 5.5 is associated with the formation of urate crystals, and children with melamine/urate renolith formation were determined to have low urine pH.[52]

Melamine is minimally metabolized and does not accumulate in the animal body. It is about 90% eliminated within 1 day by the kidneys with a half-life for urinary elimination of 6 hours in dogs.[23,48] Therefore, melamine should be almost completely excreted within 2 days; however, crystals were seen microscopically in feline kidneys 8 weeks after dietary exposure to melamine and cyanuric acid.[41]

Cats and dogs had evidence of renal failure after ingesting recalled foods. Clinical signs included inappetence, vomiting, polyuria, polydipsia, and lethargy. Urine specific gravities less than 1.035 and elevated serum urea nitrogen and creatinine concentrations were seen in these cats. Circular green-brown crystals were observed in urine sediment (**Fig. 2**). Postmortem examinations of animals that died or were

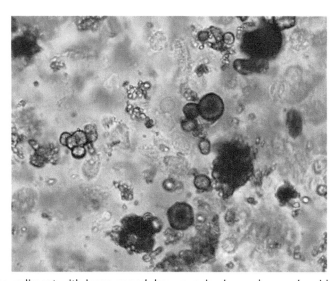

Fig. 2. Urine sediment with large, round, brown melamine and cyanuric acid crystals with adial striations. (*Courtesy of* R.E. Goldstein.)

euthanized typically noted bilateral renomegaly and evidence of uremia. Microscopic lesions were primarily localized primarily to the kidneys: renal tubular necrosis, tubular rupture, and epithelial regeneration. In the distal convoluted tubules, there were large golden-brown birefringent crystals (15 to 80 μm in diameter) with centrally radiating striations, sometimes in concentric rings, and smaller amorphous crystals.[41,53] Crystals from kidneys and urine contained 70% cyanuric acid and 30% melamine based on infrared spectra.[10,53] The outbreak of melamine-induced nephropathy in children differed from that in domestic animals by the absence of cyanuric acid. Uroliths associated with nephrotoxicosis in infants contained melamine and uric acid at a molar ratio of 1:1–2, respectively.[42,54]

Treatment regimens for crystalluria and urolithiasis related to melamine ingestion in veterinary and pediatric patients included fluid therapy and supportive care.[54,55] Oral and parenteral fluid therapy increased urine output. Because low urinary pH is associated with crystal formation in infants, urine pH was maintained between 6.0 and 7.8 in affected children by adding sodium bicarbonate or potassium citrate to intravenous fluids. Most children recovered with conservative management.[52,54]

Analysis of 451 cases matching the definition of melamine toxicosis found that 65.5% were cats and 34.4% were dogs. The case mortality rates were 73.3% and 61.5% for affected dogs and cats, respectively. Older animals and those with preexisting conditions were less likely to survive.[3] However, more than 80% of exposed cats during the original feeding trials survived with supportive care.[41]

SUMMARY

With myriad possible contaminants, ranging from fungal metabolites like aflatoxin and vomitoxin, to misformulations producing hypervitaminoses and other nutritional excesses and deficiencies, to adulteration with industrial chemical such as melamine and related compounds, it is impossible to predict the cause of the next pet food recall. Indeed, the definitive cause of Fanconi syndrome in dogs associated with consumption of jerky treats for dogs has also not been found. Vigilance is our major line of defense.

ACKNOWLEDGMENTS

The authors would like to thank Drs Sanderson and Gluckman for their work with the aflatoxin dogs, Dr McDonough for his pathology work and for contributing **Fig. 1**, Drs Woosley and Hubbard for their work with the polioencephalomalacia cats, Dr Kang for his thiamine analysis, Dr Rosama Pusoonthornthum for information about hypervitaminosis A, and Dr Goldstein for his work with melamine-poisoned cats and for contributing **Fig. 2**.

REFERENCES

1. Dzanis D. Anatomy of a recall. Top Comp Anim Med 2008;23:133–6.
2. Feng T, Keller LR, Wang L, et al. Product quality risk perception and decisions: contaminated pet food and lead-painted toys. Risk Anal 2010;30:1572–89.
3. Rumbeiha W, Morrison J. A review or class I and class II pet food recalls involving chemical contaminants from 1996 to 2008. J Med Toxicol 2011;7:60–6.
4. Anonymous. Jerky treats from China could be causing illness in pets. J Am Vet Med Assoc 2007;231:1183.
5. May K. Remain vigilant for illness possibly linked to chicken jerky treat consumption. Available at: http://atwork.avma.org/2011/06/17/remain-vigilant-for-illness-possibly-linked-to-chicken-jerky-treat-consumption/. Accessed December 6, 2011.

6. Thompson MF, Fleeman LM, Arteaga A, et al. Proximal renal tubulopathy in dogs exposed to a common dried chicken treat: a retrospective study of 99 cases (2007–2009) [abstract 1]. Small Animal Medicine chapter meeting at ACVSc Science Week. Surfers Paradise, Australia, July 2009. p. 1.

7. Bhalla V, Grimm PC, Chertow GM, et al. Melamine nephrotoxicity: an emerging epidemic in an era of globalization. Kidney Int 2009;75:774–9.

8. Cocchi M, Vascellari M, Galina A, et al. Canine nephrotoxicosis induced by melamine-contaminated pet food in Italy. J Vet Med Sci 2010;72:103–7.

9. Gonzalez J, Puschner B, Perez V, et al. Nephrotoxicosis in Iberian piglets subsequent to exposure to melamine and derivatives in Spain between 2003 and 2006. J Vet Diagn Invest 2009;21:558–63.

10. Osborne CA, Lulich JP, Ulrich JL. Melamine and cyanuric acid-induced crystalluria, uroliths, and nephrotoxicity in dogs and cats. Vet Clin N Am Sm Anim 2008;39:1–14.

11. Yhee JY, Brown C, Yu CH, et al. Retrospective study of melamine/cyanuric acid-induced renal failure in dogs in Korea between 2003 and 2004. Vet Pathol 2009;46: 348–54.

12. Singh M, Thompson M, Sullivan N. Thiamin deficiency in dogs due to the feeding of sulphite-preserved meat. Aust Vet J 2005;85:412–7.

13. Steel R. Thiamin deficiency in a cat associated with the preservation of 'pet meat' with sulfur dioxide. Aust Vet J 1997;75:719–21.

14. Studdert VP, Lubac RH. Thiamin deficiency in cats and dogs associated with feeding meat preserved with sulfur dioxide. Aust Vet J 1991;68:54–7.

15. Hughs DM, Gahl MJ, Graham CH, et al. Overt signs of toxicity to dogs and cats of dietary deoxynivalenol. J An Sci 1999;3:693–711.

16. Puschner B. Mycotoxins. Vet Clin N Am Small Anim 2002;32:409–19.

17. Meerdink GL. Mycotoxins. In: Plumlee KH, editor. Clinical veterinary toxicology. St Louis (MO): Mosby; 2004. p. 231.

18. Newbern PM, Butler WH. Acute and chronic effects of aflatoxin on the liver of domestic and laboratory animals: a review. Cancer Res 1969;29:236.

19. Liggett AD, Colvin BM, Beaver BW, et al. Canine aflatoxicosis: a continuing problem. Vet Hum Toxicol 1986;28:428–30.

20. Stenske KA, Smith JR, Shelly JN, et al. Aflatoxicosis in dogs and dealing with suspected contaminated commercial foods. J Am Vet Med Assoc 2006;228:1686.

21. Hooser SB, Talcott PA. Mycotoxins. In: Peterson ME, Talcott PA, editors. Small animal toxicology. 2nd edition. St Louis (MO): Elsevier Saunders; 2006. p. 888–97.

22. Valdivia AG, Martinez A, Damian FJ, et al. Efficacy of N-acetylcysteine to reduce the effects of aflatoxin B_1 intoxication in broiler chickens. Poultry Sci 2001;80:727.

23. Bingham AK, Huebner HJ, Phillips TD, et al. Identification and reduction of urinary aflatoxin metabolites in dogs. Food Chem Toxicol 2004;42:1851.

24. Tedesco D, Steidler S, Gallette S, et al. Effects of silymarin-phosphide complex in reducing the toxicity of aflatoxin B_1 in broiler chickens. Poultry Sci 2004;83:1839–43.

25. Miller DM, Wilson DE. Veterinary diseases related to aflatoxins. In: Eaton DL, Groopman JD, editors. The toxicology of aflatoxins. San Diego (CA): Academic Press; 1994. p. 347–64.

26. Bastianello SS, Nesbit JW, Willliams MC, et al. Pathological findings in a natural outbreak of aflatoxicosis in dogs. Onderspoort J Vet Res 1987;64:635.

27. Dereszynski DM, Center S, Randolph JF, et al. Clinical and clinicopathologic features of dogs that consumed foodborne hepatotoxic aflatoxins: 72 cases (2005-2006). J Am Vet Med Assoc 2008;232:1329–37.

28. Bischoff K, Ramiah SK. Liver toxicity. In Gupta RC, editor. Veterinary toxicology basic and clinical principles. New York: Elsevier; 2007. p. 145–60.

29. Rastogi R, Srivastava AK, Rastogi AK. Long term effects of aflatoxin B(1) on lipid peroxidation in rat liver and kidney: effect of picroliv and silymarin. Phytother Res 2001;15:307–10.
30. Cho DY, Frey RA, Guffy MM, et al. Hypervitaminosis A in the dog. Am J Vet Res 1975;36:1597–603.
31. Polizopoulou ZS, Patsikas MN, Roubies N. Hypervitaminosis A in the cat: a case report and review of the literature. J Feline Med Surg 2005;7:363–8.
32. Garosi LS, Dennis R, Platt SR, et al. Thiamine deficiency in a dog: clinical, clinicopath-ologic, and magnetic resonance imaging findings. J Vet Intern Med 2003;17:719–23.
33. Penderis J, McConnell JF, Calvin J. Magnetic resonance imaging features of thiamine deficiency in a cat. Vet Rec 2007;160:270–2.
34. Davidson M. Thiamin deficiency in a colony of cats. Vet Rec 1992;130:94–7.
35. Everett G. Observations on the behavior and neurophysiology of acute thiamin deficient cats. Am J Physiol 1944;141:439–48.
36. Malik R, Sibraa D. Thiamin deficiency due to sulfur dioxide preservative in 'pet meat': a case of deja vu. Aust Vet J 2005;83:408–11.
37. Read DH, Harrington DD. Experimentally induced thiamine deficiency in beagle dogs: clinical observations. Am J Vet Res 1981;42:984–91.
38. Rubin L. Atlas of veterinary ophthalmoscopy. Philadelphia (PA): Lea & Febiger; 1974. p. 258.
39. Plumb D. Veterinary drug handbook. 4th edition. White Bear Lake (MN): PharmaVet Publishing; 2002. p. 788–9.
40. Leow FM, Martin CL, Dunlop RH, et al. Naturally-occurring and experimental thiamin deficiency in cats receiving commercial cat food. Can Vet J 1970;11:109–13.
41. Cianciolo RE, Bischoff K, Ebel JG, et al. Clinicopathologic, histologic, and toxicologic findings in 70 cats inadvertently exposed to pet food contaminated with melamine and cyanuric acid. J Am Vet Med Assoc 2008;233:729–37.
42. Skinner CH, Thompson JD, Osterloh JD. Melamine toxicity. J Med Toxicol 2010;6: 50–5.
43. Lewin-Smith MR, Kalasinsky JF, Mullick FG, et al. Melamine containing crystals in the urinary tract of domestic animals: sentinel event? Arch Pathol Lab Med 2009;133: 341–2.
44. Hau AK, Kwan TH, Lee PK. Melamine toxicity in the kidney. J Am Soc Nephrol 2009;20:245–50.
45. Reimschussel R, E Evans E, Andersen WC, et al. Residue depletion of melamine and cysnuric acid in catfish and rainbow trout following oral administration. Vet Pharmacol Ther 2009;33:172–82.
46. Melnick RL, Boorman GA, Haseman JK, et al. Urolithiasis and bladder carcinogenicity of melamine in rodents. Toxicol Appl Pharmacol 1984;72:292–303.
47. Clark R. Melamine crystalluria in sheep. J S Afr Vet Med Assoc 1966;37:349–51.
48. Lipschitz WL, Stokey E. The mode of action of three new diuretics: melamine, adenine, and formoguanamine. J Pharmacol Exp Ther 1945;82:235–49.
49. Canelli E. Chemical, bacteriological, and toxicological properties of cyanuric acid and chlorinated isocyanurates as applied to swimming pool disinfection, a review. Am J Public Health 1974;64:155–62.
50. Puschner B, Poppenga RH, Lowenstine LJ, et al. Assessment of melamine and cyanuric acid toxicity in cats. J Vet Diagn Invest 2007;19:616–24.
51. Reimschuessel R, Gieseker CM, Miller RA, et al. Evaluation of the renal effects of experimental feeding of melamine and cyanuric acid to fish and pigs. Am J Vet Res 2008;69:1217–28.

52. Gao J, Shen Y, Sun N, et al. Therapeutic effects of potassium sodium, hydrogen citrate on melamine-induced urinary calculi in China. Chinese Med J 2010;123: 1112–6.
53. Thompson ME, Lewin-Smith MR, Kalasinsky VF, et al. Characterization of melamine-containing and calcium oxalate crystals in three dogs with suspected pet food-induced nephrotoxicosis. Vet Path 2008;55:417–26.
54. Anonymous. Specialists confer about the pet food recall. J Am Vet Med Assoc 2007;233:1603.
55. Wen JG, Li ZZ, Zhang H, et al. Melamine related bilateral renal calculi in 50 children: single center experience in clinical diagnosis and treatment. J Urol 2010;183:1533–8.

Use of Intravenous Lipid Emulsions for Treating Certain Poisoning Cases in Small Animals

Sharon Gwaltney-Brant, DVM, PhD[a],*, Irina Meadows, DVM[b]

KEYWORDS

- Poisoning • Antidote • Lipid emulsion • Intralipids
- Fat emulsion • Intoxication

The use of intravenous (IV) lipid emulsion (ILE; Intralipids, Liposyn, Medialipid) in the resuscitation of human patients poisoned by accidental local anesthetic overdoses has become a common practice in the human medicine arena over the past decade.[1] More recently, ILE therapy has been used in the veterinary world for the management of a variety of toxicoses.[2] Although further clinical studies are needed to determine the safety and effectiveness and risk:benefit ratio of this modality, a growing number of experimental studies and case reports suggest that ILE may become valuable addition to the veterinary clinician's emergency drug arsenal.

ILE is composed of neutral, medium to long-chain triglycerides derived from combinations of plant oils (eg, soybean, safflower), egg phosphatides, and glycerin. Formulated primarily a source of essential fatty acids for patients requiring parenteral nutrition, ILE is available in formulations ranging from 10% to 30% lipid; the latter is for compounding use and not for direct infusion.[3] ILE is stored at room temperature, and an unopened container will have a shelf life of up to 2 years.[2,3] Once opened and/or mixed with other fluids, ILE should be refrigerated between uses and used within 24 hours.[3] ILE can be administered via peripheral or central venous catheter.[3] ILE have a high margin of safety, with an estimated IV LD_{50} in rats of 67 mL/kg.[5]

BACKGROUND

The use of ILE as an antidotal procedure evolved from the discovery that administration of lipid solutions could attenuate the cardiotoxicosis of bupivacaine in rats.[6] A study in dogs demonstrated that IV overdoses of bupivacaine (10 mg/kg) resulted in

The authors have nothing to disclose.
[a] Veterinary Information Network, 501 North Dorchester Court, Mahomet, IL 61853, USA
[b] ASPCA Animal Poison Control Center, 1717 South Philo Road, Suite 36, Urbana, IL 61802, USA
* Corresponding author.
E-mail address: Sharon@vin.com

deaths in all dogs receiving open-chest cardiac massage but no deaths in dogs receiving open-chest cardiac massage along with infusion of 20% ILE.[7] Although one porcine model failed to show similar positive benefits of ILE in bupivacaine,[8] there were concerns expressed regarding the cardiac effects of anesthetic drugs used on the pigs prior to administration of cardiotoxic levels of bupivacaine.[9] Another study performed on pigs showed that ILE reversed bupivacaine-induced cardiac electrophysiologic abnormalities.[10] Based on these results, it was proposed that ILE may be a potentially useful treatment for local anesthetic systemic toxicosis (LAST) in humans, a condition that tends to be resistant to conventional modes of resuscitation.[1]

Subsequently, numerous human case reports emerged showing positive results of the use of ILE in resuscitation of patients experiencing the cardiac effects of LAST. In one case, an elderly woman received 3 bupivacaine injections for peripheral and spinal nerve blocks.[11] Three minutes after third injection, she became nonverbal and had a seizure. The patient received 1.5 mL/kg of ILE within 2 minutes and seizure activity ceased; she regained consciousness within 3-4 minutes. In another case, a 17 year-old adolescent male experienced seizures and became pulseless after receiving 20 mL of 0.5% bupivacaine for postoperative analgesia.[12] He was treated with midazolam and 8 mL/kg of 20% ILE. The patient's cardiac status normalized following ILE infusion. In a final case, a 58 year-old man developed a tonic-clonic seizure 30 seconds following injection of bupivacaine for a brachial plexus nerve block.[13] Asystole occurred 90 seconds later; following 20 minutes of unsuccessful chemical, mechanical, and electrical attempts at resuscitation, the patient was being prepared for cardiopulmonary bypass when ILE was suggested. Within a few seconds of initiation of administration of 20% ILE, a single sinus beat appeared and progressed to normal sinus rhythm within 15 seconds. The patient fully recovered with no adverse effects.

Despite these and several similar cases, the use of ILE for LAST remained controversial due to the inability to demonstrate conclusively that ILE, and not adjunctive resuscitation measures (cardiac compression, electroconversion, other drugs, etc), were responsible for the recoveries.[14,15] Critics have also pointed out that the case reports reflected only those cases in which the ILE treatment was successful, noting that unsuccessful treatments did not merit reporting, so the actual efficacy of ILE therapy was not known. Criticisms aside, sufficient evidence of the potential of ILE to result in a positive outcome in LAST patients existed such that this treatment modality has been recommended for management of LAST by a number of human medical organizations, including the Association of Anaesthetists of Great Britain and Ireland, the American Society of Critical Care Anesthesiologists, the American Society of Anesthesiologists Committee on Critical Care Medicine, the Resuscitation Council of the UK, and the American Society of Regional Anesthesia.[1]

Recognizing that randomized controlled trials may not be possible given the catastrophic nature of situations where ILE are used in human intoxications, an international collaboration of clinical investigators has developed an online registry (http://www.lipidregistry.org) for reporting cases where ILE has been used antidotally.[1] This LIPAEMIC (Lipid Injection for the Purpose of Antidotal Effect in Lipophilic Medicine Intoxication) Study Group is attempting to collate clinical experiences of efficacy and adverse events associated with the antidotal use of ILE. Additionally, physicians and veterinarians can post their experiences with ILE as an antidote on the "Lipid Rescue" website (http://www.lipidrescue.org).

PROPOSED MECHANISMS OF ACTION

The mechanism(s) by which ILE improves cardiac function in patients with LAST has not yet been entirely elucidated. Several theories have been proposed, of which 2 are currently considered to be the most feasible: a metabolic effect from the lipid and a sequestration effect ("lipid sink") effect of the lipid.[16]

The metabolic theory proposes that increasing the serum concentration of free fatty acids via ILE infusion results in increased fatty acid uptake by myocardial cells, providing fodder for beta-oxidation and ATP production.[16] The myocardium derives 80% to 90% of its ATP from the oxidative phosphorylation of fatty acids. Bupivacaine decreases fatty acid transport through the inhibition of carnitine-acylcarnitine translocase, resulting in decreases in fatty acid transport into the myocardium. Suppression of mitochondrial function and decreased ATP formation within the myocardium result in depletion of myocardial ATP and myocardial failure. By providing fatty acids for beta-oxidation, ILE helps the heart to overcome the bupivacaine-induced metabolic inhibition and may improve the potential for successful cardiac resuscitation. Additionally, improved myocardiocyte contractility may be due to ILE-induced increase in intracellular calcium levels.[1]

The sequestration effect theory proposes that the expanded lipid phase in the plasma provided by ILE serves as a discrete compartment that sequesters lipophilic compounds and prevents them from reaching their sites of action.[16] This "lipid sink" action may be so strong as to draw local anesthetics from heart and brain. Evidence of this "sink" action has been shown using studies that demonstrated that drugs such as bupivacaine, amiodarone, and clomipramine preferentially isolate to the lipid phase of the plasma from animals treated with ILE infusions.[17–19] ILE has also been shown to accelerate the removal of radiolabeled bupivacaine from myocardial tissues.[17] The "sink" theory is also supported by the clinical impressions that toxicoses from lipophilic drugs appear to respond better to ILE than more hydrophilic drugs. In studies on animals administered beta-blockers, ILE infusions resulted in superior improvement of hemodynamic parameters administered toxic doses of propranolol when compared to animals receiving similar toxic levels of the more hydrophilic beta-blockers metoprolol and atenolol.[20–22]

One question that can arise as one considers the "lipid sink" theory is whether the drugs sequestered in the lipid layer might be suddenly "released" at a future time, resulting in recrudescence of the toxidrome. A single case report exists of a 33-year-old man who developed cardiotoxicity following bupivacaine injection and whose cardiac asystole was successfully managed via administration of 500 mL of 20% ILE.[23] Although the patient had an initial positive response to ILE therapy, within 40 minutes following cessation of the ILE infusion, the patient's cardiovascular status deteriorated, necessitating antiarrhythmic therapy, as additional ILE was not available. The authors indicate that the amount of ILE administered (500 mL) was less than the 1000 mL recommended by the Association of Anesthetists of Great Britain and Ireland in their "Guidelines for the Management of Severe Local Anaesthetic Toxicity" and speculate that recurrence may have been due to a combination of factors related to insufficient ILE, including redistribution of bupivacaine, decrease in serum ILE levels due to redistribution and metabolism, and prolongation of bupivacaine half-life. The authors note that this episode reinforces that importance of appropriate dosing and close monitoring of patients treated with antidotal ILE. Another question that arises with the "lipid sink" theory of ILE action is "Where do the drugs go once they have been taken up into the lipid?" As a component of parenteral nutrition, triglycerides in ILE are thought to be cleared in a manner similar to chylomicrons, that is, cleared through lymphatics and ultimately taken up by cells (especially skeletal muscle) for use as energy.[3,4] Lipophilic drugs internalized along with the lipid would be broken down in the cytosol or sequestered in lysosomes, effectively removing the drugs from the circulation.

BEYOND LOCAL ANESTHETIC TOXICOSES

Although metabolic effects from ILE may play some role in the improved cardiac function seen in LAST patients, the fact that ILE infusions have been used to successfully manage toxicoses from lipophilic, noncardiac drugs appears to make the "lipid sink" theory the key component in the antidotal uses of ILE. Controlled studies are lacking in human medicine, but there is a growing volume of case reports on the use of ILE in humans to successfully manage toxicoses due to a variety of drugs including lamotrigine, dosulepin, lamotrigine and bupropion, quetiapine and sertraline, verapamil, and beta-blockers.[24–28]

Studies in animals have found that ILE is effective in the management of toxicosis associated with a variety of drugs (**Table 1**). In the veterinary literature, a few case reports have been published on the successful use of ILE in the management of toxicoses in a clinical setting. In one case, a 3.2-kg puppy that ingested an overdose of moxidectin became comatose and bradycardic and required mechanical ventilatory support.[32] Within 2 hours of an initial infusion of 20% ILE (6.5 mL bolus followed by 12 mL/h for 4 hours), the puppy was able to be removed from the ventilator, although it remained unconscious. The puppy was able to be extubated at 11 hours after ILE therapy, although it remained laterally recumbent and developed tonic-clonic muscle activity. A constant-rate infusion (CRI) of IV diazepam was administered for the seizure activity along with a second ILE infusion (48 mL over 30 minutes). Within 30 minutes following the cessation of the lipid infusion, the puppy was ambulatory and its behavior normalized over the subsequent 6 hours. The rapid recovery of this puppy is in contrast to the usual clinical course of moxidectin toxicosis in dogs, which typically requires several days or longer (depending on the dose) for recovery in moderate to severe intoxications.[32] Another case report of 3 dogs with suspected (2 dogs had access to ivermectin-based horse dewormers and showed typical clinical signs) and witnessed (1 dog administered 0.165 mg/kg) ivermectin toxicosis showed no improvement following the use of ILE.[51] All 3 dogs were homozygous for the ABCB-1-1Δ gene mutation that codes for a defective P-glycoprotein, resulting in a defective blood-brain barrier that allows normally excluded xenobiotics (eg, ivermectin) into the central nervous system (CNS). All 3 dogs' signs progressed to significant CNS depression, including coma in 1 dog. Administration of 20% ILE at 1.5–mL/kg boluses followed by slow IV infusion of 7.5 to 15 mL/kg over 30 minutes failed to result in improvement of the neurologic status of any of the dogs. The authors hypothesize that the P-glycoprotein defect shared by these dogs may have resulted in brain concentrations of ivermectin that were unable to be overcome by ILE and that the P-glycoprotein defect may have impaired biliary clearance mechanisms necessary for optimum ILE function. An additional factor to consider when comparing the results of the moxidectin and ivermectin cases is that moxidectin is reported to be 100 times more lipophilic than ivermectin and therefore may be more readily removed from the CNS into the "lipid sink."[52]

A recent presentation at a veterinary emergency and critical care conference indicated that successful outcomes had been anecdotally reported by veterinarians with the use of ILE for intoxications by the following compounds: local anesthetics, calcium channel blockers, avermectin parasiticides, baclofen, bupropion, loperamide, permethrin (cats), and sertraline.[2] Additionally, the ASPCA Animal Poison Control

Table 1
Use of ILEs to manage drug-related toxicoses in animals

Species	Description	Outcome	References
Cat	ILE effect on accidental lidocaine toxicosis (case report)	Accidental SC administration of 20 mg/kg lidocaine hydrochloride; developed profound lethargy, respiratory distress, poor-quality pulses with severe hypotension, pulmonary edema; oxygen and lactated Ringer's solution administered followed by 20% ILE over 30 min; caused "dramatic improvement in cardiovascular and behavioral variables" and appeared to speed recovery	[29]
Dog	ILE vs standard resuscitation (NS, calcium atropine) in severe verapamil toxicosis	ILE increased ST (>120 min vs 75 min with NS); increased survival rate (100% vs 14% with NS); increased MAP; no difference in HR	[30]
	ILE vs insulin in treatment of verapamil toxicosis	No difference in survival time (191 min with ILE vs 187 min with insulin); no difference in MAP or HR	[31]
	ILE vs NS in bupivacaine toxicosis	ILE increased survival (6 of 6 vs 0 of 6 with NS); ILE increased MAP (93 mm Hg vs 10 mm Hg with NS); ILE increased HR (126 bpm vs 0 pbm with NS)	[7]
	ILE effect on accidental moxidectin toxicosis (case report)	Appeared to rapidly reverse signs of toxicosis and speed recovery	[32]
	ILE effect on accidental ivermectin toxicosis in 3 dogs (case report)	All 3 dogs homozygous for MDR-1 defect; 1 dog administered 0.165 mg/kg ivermectin, other 2 suspected exposure; infusion of ILE did not result in improvement of any dog; MDR-1 status may alter efficacy of IFE	[33]
Pig	ILE vs VE in bupivacaine-induced cardiac arrest	Survival: VE = 5 of 5, ILE 0 of 5 VE superior for coronary perfusion	[34]
	ILE effect on amiodarone-induced hypotension and sequestration of amiodarone	Amiodarone was largely sequestered within the lipid-rich plasma and prevented changes in MAP during amiodarone infusion	[18]
	Long-chain triglyceride vs mixture of long-chain and short-chain triglyceride emulsions in bupivacaine toxicosis	Both lipid emulsions reversed bupivacaine-induced cardiac electrophysiologic abnormalities	[10]
	ILE vs NS following resuscitation attempts with chest compression, epinephrine and vasopressin	No improvement of rates of return to spontaneous circulation (3 of 10 for ILE, 4 of 9 for NS)	[8]

(continued on next page)

Table 1
(continued)

Species	Description	Outcome	References
Rabbit	ILE vs NS effect on metoprolol toxicosis	No difference between ILE and NS	[21]
	ILE vs NS effect on atenolol toxicosis	No difference in MAP or HR between ILE and NS	[22]
	ILE vs NaHCO₃ in clomipramine toxicosis	ILE more rapidly and completely reversed drug-induced hypotension; Survival: ILE 4 of 4, NaHCO₃ 0 of 4	[35]
	ILE vs NS on propranolol-induced hypotension in rabbits	ILE treatment resulted in increased MAP (69 mm Hg vs 53 mm Hg with NS)	[20]
	Determine distribution of clomipramine in plasma and peritoneal diasylate following resuscitation from clomipramine-induced hypotension with ILE	ILE reduced initial clomipramine Vd and increased clomipramine plasma levels compared to NS-treated rabbits; peritoneal dialysis with ILE enhanced clomipramine extraction; results consistent with intravascular drug-lipid sequestration	[19]
	ILE effect on thiopental anesthesia	ILE increased initial CNS depression; no difference in duration of anesthesia	[36]
	ILE vs insulin in severe propranolol toxicosis	High-dose insulin resulted in greater improvement of hematologic parameters. No difference in survival.	[61]
	ILE vs 5% XY vs NI 15 min prior to IV chlorpromazine overdose (25 and 30 mg/kg);	Survival at 25 mg/kg (# of rabbits): NI 0 of 6 vs XY 6 of 7 vs ILE 7 of 7 Survival at 30 mg/kg (No. of rabbits): NI, XY = 0 of 6 vs ILE 7 of 7	[37]
Rat	ILE vs NS effect in amitriptyline toxicosis	No difference in mortality	[38]
	Pretreatment (15 min prior) with ILE vs NS on propranolol-induced hypotension	ILE resulted in higher MAP at 15 and 30 min after intoxication but no difference at 60 min	[39]
	ILE vs NS on propranolol toxicosis	ILE increased ST (47 min vs 18.75 min with NS); ILE had less HR reduction and QRS width change than NS	[40]
	ILE vs NS effect on nifedipine overdose	Median ST increased from 34 min with NS to 81 min with ILE	[41]
	ILE vs epinephrine vs NS pretreatment effect on bupivacaine toxicosis	ILE superior to other treatments in model of cardiac resuscitation; epinephrine treatment not significantly better than NS	[42]
	Pretreatment with ILE vs NS 2 h prior to verapamil infusion in severe verapamil toxicosis	Increased ST with ILE (53 min vs 39 with NS), no difference in MAP at any time; HR lower by 53 bpm at 30 min but no difference at other times	[43]

(continued on next page)

Table 1 (continued)			
Species	Description	Outcome	References
	Determine optimal dose ILE for treatment of severe verapamil toxicosis	Survival greatest at ILE dosage of 18.6 mL/kg; greatest benefit to HR, MAP at 24.8 mL/kg; optimal dosage in rat determined to be 18.6 mL/kg	[44]
	Effect of infusion rate of ILE on survival in severe verapamil toxicosis	Increase in survival with faster infusions: infusion in ≤30 min had mean survival rate of 182 min vs 108 min for infusions ≥45 min	[45]
	Corn oil and cotton seed oil emulsions vs nonlipid infusion effects on thiopental anesthesia	Oil emulsions shortened anesthesia duration	[46]
	ILE vs NS on verapamil toxicosis	Increased ST with ILE (44 ± 21 min vs 24 ± 9 min); increased LD_{50} in ILE (25.7 mg/kg vs 13.6 mg/kg); less marked reduction in HR with ILE	[47]
	ILE vs vasopressin vs epinephrine treatment of bupivacaine-induced asystole	ILE > epinephrine >> vasopressin in resuscitation	[48]
	ILE vs in bupivacaine toxicosis	ILE pretreatment shifts dose response, lowers toxicity (LD_{50} raised from 12.5 mg/kg in control to 18.5 mg/kg in ILE-treated rats)	[6]
	ILE vs NS effect in clomipramine toxicosis	Survival: ILE 80%, NS 0%	[49]
	ILE vs epinephrine vs NS in bupivacaine overdose	Return of spontaneous circulation occurred in 2 of 5 NS-, 4 of 5 epinephrine-, and 5 of 5 ILE-treated rats; ILE caused improved hemodynamic parameters compared to epinephrine and NS; epinephrine no better than NS	[50]

Abbreviations: bpm, beats per minute; HR, heart rate; MAP, mean arterial pressure; NI, no infusion; NS, normal saline solution; ST, survival time; Vd, volume of distribution; VE, vasopressin-epinephrine; XY, xylitol.

Center (APCC) has recommended the judicious use of ILE in cases of severe intoxication with certain lipophilic drugs for more than 3 years and has reported favorable results with the use of ILE to manage intoxications with the following drugs: amlodipine, baclofen, benzocaine, bromethalin, bupropion, CCNU, chlorpyrifos, diltiazem, doramectin, endosulfan, ivermectin, moxidectin, minoxidil, marijuana, permethrin, and phenobarbital (ASPCA Animal Poison Control Center (APCC). AnTox, unpublished data, 2010). Preliminary observations made by the APCC toxicologists indicate lack of adequate response of cholecalciferol overdoses to ILE administration although this is not conclusive. For a list of other potential medications where IV fat emulsion treatment can be considered, see Fernandez and colleagues.[53]

Anecdotal reports of successful use of ILE in the management of veterinary patients are becoming more commonplace, but until controlled clinical studies are published caution should be taken to avoid viewing ILE as a "silver bullet" with guaranteed results.[54] Anecdotal reports on the antidotal use of ILE have the drawbacks of lack of controls for comparison, potential for subjective bias in determining clinical improvement, frequent uncertainty of identity or amount of toxicant, lack of analytical confirmation of toxicant exposure, coadministration of drugs for symptomatic care (eg, anticonvulsants for seizures), and inconsistency of treatment protocols. Also, data regarding the potential for adverse effects of the antidotal use of ILE are lacking. Until further information is available, ILE should be considered an "experimental" treatment, and in most cases it should be reserved for severe intoxications.

CLINICAL APPLICATION OF ILE IN VETERINARY MEDICINE

Not all toxicants will respond to ILE and even those that might respond may not require ILE therapy to make a full recovery. For example, a dog or cat with mild ivermectin toxicosis (mydriasis, ataxia) will likely recover within a few days with no special care other than confinement to prevent trauma; in this case, the use of ILE cannot be justified due to its experimental status. Conversely, an ivermectin toxicosis resulting in seizures and/or coma may take days or even weeks to recover, necessitating special care (frequent turning, enteral/parenteral nutrition sources, IV fluids, etc) that is costly and time consuming; in these cases it is not uncommon for financial concerns to result in a decision for euthanasia to be made. In the latter case, the potential for ILE to assist in shortening the duration and severity of signs, thereby decreasing costs of treatment, outweighs its experimental status and the use of ILE should be considered.

In all cases ILE should be used in addition to, not instead of, standard symptomatic and supportive care. Optimal treatment protocols will likely vary between toxicants and, possibly, species; however, currently this information is not available. Several different ILE infusion protocols have been published and some of the more commonly used ones are listed in **Table 2**. All protocols use 20% lipid solutions. ILE infusions are generally given as a slow bolus over several minutes followed by a CRI for 30 to 60 minutes via peripheral or central venous catheter. The serum should be monitored every 2 hours and additional infusions considered if the patient is still symptomatic and the serum is clear of lipemia. Do not repeat ILE if the serum is very orange or yellow.[54] If no improvement is noted after 3 doses (bolus and CRI), discontinue ILE therapy.[54] Patients should be kept under veterinary care and monitored until clinical signs have resolved and the serum is no longer lipemic in case signs return once the lipid has been metabolized.

Potential adverse effects from ILE infusions include the following:

- *Interference with drugs administered for symptomatic or supportive care.*[1] To date this has not been reported, but the potential for ILE to trap desirable drugs (eg, anticonvulsants) must be considered when lipid solutions are being used.
- *Pancreatitis due to persistent lipemia.* A 33-year-old man resuscitated using ILE developed elevations in serum amylase suggesting pancreatic injury, although symptoms of pancreatitis did not develop.[23] ILE should be used with caution in patients with a history of prior pancreatic disease, and ILE should not be administered in patients with lipemic serum. The common adverse effects reported to the APCC include hyperlipidemia and pancreatitis associated with IV emulsion therapy.
- *Hypersensitivity due to ILE constituents.* Many ILE formulations contain traces of soybean proteins, which may trigger hypersensitivity reactions in allergic patients.[59]

Table 2
Various dosing protocols of ILEs in veterinary and human patients

Bolus	Infusion	Notes; Reference
Veterinary Applications		
1.5 mL/kg over 2–3 min	CRI of 0.25 mL/kg/min for 30–60 min	Check serum q2h until it becomes clear; repeat as needed; if no improvement after 3 doses, discontinue; APCC[53]
1.5 mL/kg over 5–15 min	CRI of 0.25 mL/kg/min for 1–2 h	Can repeat in several hours if signs return; do not administer if serum is lipemic; Johnson[2]
None	1.5 mL/kg over 30 min	Used in feline lidocaine toxicosis; O'Brien et al[29]
2.0 mL/kg	CRI of 0.06 mL/kg/min for 4 h; then 0.5 mL/kg/min for 30 min	Used in canine moxidectin toxicosis; second infusion given 11 hours after first; Crandell and Weinberg[32]
Human Applications		
1.0 mL/kg × 3 doses	CRI of 0.25 mL/kg/min for 30–60 min	Bolus could be repeated 1–2 times; Weinberg[55]
1.2 mL/kg	CRI of 0.5 mL/kg/min	Used in resuscitation of LAST patient; Rosenblatt et al[56]
1.5 mL/kg over 1 min	CRI of 0.25 mL/kg/min for 30–60 min	For severe intoxications and cardiac asystole: repeat bolus twice at 5-min intervals if adequate circulation has not been restored; after another 5 minutes, increase infusion rate to 0.5 mL/kg/min; POISINDEX[57]
2.0 mL/kg	CRI of 0.2 mL/kg/min	Used in resuscitation of LAST patient; Litz et al[58]

Abbreviations: APCC, ASPCA Animal Poison Control Center; CRI, constant rate infusion; LAST, local anesthetic systemic toxicosis.

- *Lipid emboli in neonatal animals.* Pulmonary lipid emboli have been reported in pediatric humans in association with ILE used for parenteral nutrition. Studies of the antidotal use of ILE in numerous species have failed to produce similar pulmonary lesions.[1] Pulmonary and hepatic abnormalities were noted in rats administered 60 and 80 mL/kg of 20% ILE over 30 minutes.[5]
- *Interference with laboratory tests due to lipemia.* ILE causes false elevations in blood glucose concentrations with certain glucose analyzers.[60]
- *Adverse reactions due to product contamination* (inappropriate handling, non-sterile techniques, microbial or particulate contamination).[53]
- *Delayed or subacute reactions due to excessive administration volumes or high administration rates* known as "fat overload syndrome (FOS)" in humans. FOS can lead to hyperlipidemia, hepatomegaly, embolism, icterus, and hemolysis.[53] The APCC received one report of hemolysis associated with IV fat emulsion treatment in a dog. The dog recovered after blood transfusion and other supportive care.

SUMMARY

IV fat emulsion holds promise as an antidote for toxicosis from certain highly lipophilic drugs. Investigational and clinical evidence supports this concept, but experimental controlled studies in laboratory and target animal species demonstrating its safety and efficacy and more clinical evidence are necessary before IV fat emulsion becomes a routine part of the management of toxicoses. Clinicians must be aware of potential adverse effects of using IV lipid emulsion. The overall safety profile of lipids is promising. In addition, lipids are inexpensive, require no special storage, and have shelf lives of up to 2 years. It is important to remember that IV fat emulsion is not a substitute for standard supportive and symptomatic care when managing poisoned patients.

REFERENCES

1. Rothschild L, Bern S, Oswald S, et al. Intravenous lipid emulsion in clinical toxicology. Scand J Trauma Resusc Emerg Med 2010;18:51.
2. Johnson T. Intravenous lipid emulsion (IVLE) therapy for selected toxicoses. In: Proceedings of the International Veterinary Emergency and Critical Care Symposium. San Antonio (TX), September 11, 2011.
3. Intralipid® 30% [package insert]. Deerfield (IL): Baxter Healthcare Corporation; 2000.
4. LiposynII® 20% [package insert]. Lake Forest (IL): Hospira; 2005.
5. Hiller DB, Di Gregorio G, Kelly K, et al. Safety of high volume lipid emulsion infusion: a first approximation of LD_{50} in rats. Reg Anesth Pain Med 2010;35:140–4.
6. Weinberg GL, VadeBoncouer T, Ramaraju GA, et al. Pretreatment or resuscitation with a lipid infusion shifts the dose-response to bupivacaine-induced asystole in rats. Anesthesiology 1998;88:1071–5.
7. Weinberg G, Ripper R, Feinstein DL, et al. Lipid emulsion infusion rescues dogs from bupivacaine-induced cardiac toxicity. Reg Anesth Pain Med 2003;28:198–202.
8. Hicks SD, Salcido DD, Logue ES, et al. Lipid emulsion combined with epinephrine and vasopressin does not improve survival in a swine model of bupivacaine induced cardiac arrest. Anesthesiology 2009;111:138–46.
9. Woehlck HJ, El-Orbany M. Anesthetic effects and lipid resuscitation protocols. Anesthesiology 2010;112:499–500.
10. Candela D, Louart G, Bousquet PJ, et al. Reversal of bupivacaine-induced cardiac electrophysiological changes by two lipid emulsions in anesthetized and mechanically ventilated piglets. Anesth Analg 2010;110:1473–9.
11. Whiteside J. Reversal of local anaesthetic induced CNS toxicity with lipid emulsion. Anaesthesia 2008;63:203–4.
12. Markowitz S, Neal JM. Immediate lipid emulsion therapy in the successful treatment of bupivacaine systemic toxicity. Reg Anesth Pain Med 2009;34:276.
13. Corman SL, Skeldar SJ. Use of lipid emulsion to reverse local anesthetic-induced toxicity. Ann Pharmacother 2007;41:1873–7.
14. Aya AG, Ripart J, Sebbane MA, et al. Lipid emulsions for the treatment of systemic local anesthetic toxicity: efficacy and limits. Ann Fr Anesth Reanim 2010;29:464–9.
15. Rosenberg P. Lipid emulsion for the treatment of severe local anesthetic toxicity in adults – probably useful, but evidence is lacking. Rev Esp Anestesiol Reanim 2008;55:67–8.
16. Bern S, Akpa BS, Kuo I, et al. Lipid resuscitation: a life-saving antidote for local anesthetic toxicity. Curr Pharm Biotechnol 2011;12:313–9.
17. Weinberg GL, Ripper R, Murphy P, et al. Lipid infusion accelerates removal of bupivacaine and recovery from bupivacaine toxicity in the isolated rat heart. Reg Anesth Pain Med 2006;31:296–303.
18. Niiya T, Litonius E, Petaja L, et al. Intravenous lipid emulsion sequesters amiodarone in plasma and eliminates its hypotensive action in pigs. Ann Emerg Med 2010;56:402–8.
19. Harvey G, Cave G, Hoggett K. Correlation of plasma and peritoneal dialysate clomipramine concentration with hemodynamic recovery after intralipid infusion in rabbits. Acad Emerg Med 2009;16:151–6.

20. Harvey G, Cave G. Intralipid infusion ameliorates propranolol-induced hypotension in rabbits. J Med Toxicol 2008;4:71–6.
21. Browne A, Harvey M, Cave G. Intravenous lipid emulsion does not augment blood pressure recovery in a rabbit model of metoprolol toxicity. J Med Toxicol 2010;6:373–8.
22. Cave G, Harvey M. Lipid emulsion may augment early blood pressure recovery in a rabbit model of atenolol toxicity. J Med Toxicol 2009;5:50–1.
23. Marwick PC, Levin AI, Coetzee AR. Recurrence of cardiotoxicity after lipid rescue from bupivacaine-induced cardiac arrest. Anesth Analg 2009;108:1344–6.
24. Castanares-Zapatero D, Wittebole X, Huberlant V, et al. Lipid emulsion as rescue therapy in lamotrigine overdose. J Emerg Med 2011. [Epub ahead of print].
25. Boegevig S, Rothe A, Tfelt-Hansen J, et al. Successful reversal of life threatening cardiac effect following dosulepin overdose using intravenous lipid emulsion. Clin Toxicol (Phila) 2011;49:337–9.
26. Sirianni AJ, Osterhoudt KC, Calello DP, et al. Use of lipid emulsion in the resuscitation of a patient with prolonged cardiovascular collapse after overdose of bupropion and lamotrigine. Ann Emerg Med 2008;51:412–5.
27. Finn SD, Uncles DR, Willers J, et al. Early treatment of a quetiapine and sertraline overdose with Intralipid. Anaesthesia 2009;64:191–4.
28. Dolcourt B, Aaron C. Intravenous fat emulsion for refractory verapamil and atenolol induced-shock: a human case report. NACCT. Clin Toxicol 2008;46:620.
29. O'Brien TQ, Clark-Price SC, Evans EE, et al. Infusion of a lipid emulsion to treat lidocaine intoxication in a cat. J Am Vet Med Assoc 2010;237:1455–8.
30. Bania TC, Chu J, Perez E, et al. Hemodynamic effects of intravenous fat emulsion in an animal model of severe verapamil toxicity resuscitated with atropine, calcium, and saline. Acad Emerg Med 2007;14:105–11.
31. Bania T, Chu J, Perez E, et al. Hemodynamic effects of intravenous fat emulsion versus high dose insulin euglycemia in a model of severe verapamil toxicity. Acad Emerg Med 2008;15(Suppl 1):S93.
32. Crandell DE, Weinberg GL. Moxidectin toxicosis in a puppy successfully treated with intravenous lipids. J Vet Emerg Crit Care 2009;19:181–6.
33. Wright HM, Chen AV, Talcott PA, et al. Intravenous fat emulsion (IFE) for treatment of ivermectin toxicosis in 3 dogs. In: American College of Veterinary Internal Medicine forum. Denver (CO): American College of Veterinary Internal Medicine; 2011.
34. Mayr VD, Mitterschiffthaler L, Neurauter A, et al. A comparison of the combination of epinephrine and vasopressin with lipid emulsion in a porcine model of asphyxial cardiac arrest after intravenous injection of bupivacaine. Anesth Analg 2008;106:1566–71.
35. Harvey M, Cave G. Intralipid outperforms sodium bicarbonate in a rabbit model of clomipramine toxicity. Ann Emerg Med 2007;49:178–85.
36. Kazemi A, Harvey M, Cave G, et al. The effect of lipid emulsion on depth of anaesthesia following thiopental administration to rabbits. Anaesthesia 2011;66:373–8.
37. Krieglstein J, Meffert A, Niemeyer D. Influence of emulsified fat on chlorpromazine availability in rabbit blood. Experimentia 1974;30:924–6.
38. Bania T, Chu J. Hemodynamic effect of intralipid in amitriptyline toxicity. Acad Emerg Med 2006;13:S177.
39. Bania T, Chu J, Wesolowski M. The hemodynamic effect of intralipid on propranolol toxicity. Acad Emerg Med 2006;13:S109.
40. Cave G, Harvey M, Castle C. The role of fat emulsion therapy in a rodent model of propranolol toxicity: a preliminary study. J Med Toxicol 2006;2:4–7.
41. Chu J, Medlej K, Bania T, et al. The effect of intravenous fat emulsions in nifedipine toxicity. Acad Emerg Med 2009;16:S226.

42. DiGregorio G, Schwartz D, Ripper R, et al. Lipid emulsion is superior to vasopressin in a rodent model of resuscitation from toxin-induced cardiac arrest. Crit Care Med 2009;37:993–9.

43. Medlej K, Bania T, Chu J, et al. Delayed effects of intravenous fat emulsion on verapamil toxicity. Acad Emerg Med 2008;15(Suppl. 1):S93.

44. Perez E, Bania T, Medlej K, et al. Determining the optimal dose of intravenous fat emulsion for the treatment of severe verapamil toxicity in a rodent model. Acad Emerg Med 2008;15(Suppl 1):s92–3.

45. Perez E, Medlej K, Bania T, et al. Does the infusion rate of intravenous fat emulsion in severe verapamil toxicity affect survival and hemodynamic parameters? Acad Emerg Med 2009;16:S154.

46. Russell R, Westfall B. Alleviation of barbiturate depression by fat emulsion. Anesth Analg 1962;41:582–5.

47. Tebbutt S, Harvey M, Nicholson T, et al. Intralipid prolongs survival in a rat model of verapamil toxicity. Acad Emerg Med 2006;13:134–9.

48. Weinberg G, Ripper R, Kelly K, et al. A rodent model comparing lipid and pressor treatment of bupivacaine-induced asystole. Anesthesiology 2007;107:A23.

49. Yoav G, Odelia G, Shaltiel C. A lipid emulsion reduces mortality from clomipramine overdose in rats. Vet Hum Toxicol 2002;44:30.

50. Weinberg G, Gregorio GD, Ripper R, et al. Resuscitation with lipid versus epinephrine in a rat model of bupivacaine overdose. Anesthesiology 2008;108:907–13.

51. Wright HM, Chen AV, Talcott PA, et al. Intravenous fat emulsion (IFE) for treatment of ivermectin toxicosis in 3 dogs. In: American College of Veterinary Internal Medicine forum. Denver (CO): American College of Veterinary Internal Medicine; 2011. Abstract: 21754775.

52. Gokbulut C, Nolan AM, McKellar QA. Plasma pharmacokinetics and faecal excretion of ivermectin, doramectin and moxidectin following oral administration in horses. Equine Vet J 2001;33:494–8.

53. Fernandez AL, Lee JA, Rahilly L, et al. The use of intravenous liquid emulsion as an antidote in veterinary toxicology. J Vet Emerg Crit Care 2011;21:309–20.

54. Felice K, Schumann H. Intravenous lipid emulsion for local anesthetic toxicity: a review of the literature. J Med Toxicol 2008;4:184–91.

55. Weinberg G. Reply to Drs. Goor, Groban, and Butterworth—lipid rescue: caveats and recommendations for the 'silver bullet'. Reg Anaesth Pain Med 2004;29:74.

56. Rosenblatt MA, Abel M, Fischer GW, et al. Successful use of a 20% lipid emulsion to resuscitate a patient after a presumed bupivacaine-related cardiac arrest. Anesthesiology 2006;105:217–8.

57. POISINDEX® System. Intravenous lipid emulsion therapy for overdose [database on CD-ROM]. Version 5.1. Greenwood Village (CO): Thomson Reuters (Healthcare); 2011.

58. Litz RJ, Popp M, Stehr SN, et al. Successful resuscitation of a patient with ropivacaine-induced asystole after axillary plexus block using lipid infusion. Anaesthesia 2006;61:800–1.

59. Weidmann B, Lepique C, Heider A, et al. Hypersensitivity reactions to parenteral lipid solutions. Support Care Cancer 1997;5:504–5.

60. Heijboer AC, Bouman AA, Blankenstein MA, et al. Intralipid causes falsely increased glucose concentrations with the Hemocue glucose analyzer. Clin Chem Lab Med 2010;48:737–8.

61. Harvey M, Cave G, Lahner D, et al. Insulin versus lipid emulsion in a rabbit model of severe propranolol toxicity: a pilot study. Crit Car Res Pract 2011;2011:361737.

Calcium Channel Blocker Toxicity in Dogs and Cats

Cristine L. Hayes, DVM*, Michael Knight, DVM

KEYWORDS
- Calcium channel blocker • Verapamil • Diltiazem
- Dihydropyridine

Calcium channel blockers (CCBs) are a commonly used group of drugs in both human medicine since the 1960s and in veterinary medicine since the 1980s.[1,2] They are defined by their ability to block the slow, or long-lasting (L-type), calcium channel, which is found primarily in cardiac and arterial smooth muscle tissue and to a much lesser extent in other tissues as well.[3] They have been commonly used for the treatment of hypertension, cardiac disease including hypertrophic cardiomyopathy (and in human medicine, angina and congestive heart failure), and cardiac arrhythmias, and they have also been suggested for other uses such as premature labor in humans and acute renal failure in companion animals.[1,3,4]

Several classes of CCB currently exist; of these, the most widely used are the phenylalkylamine verapamil (Calan; Verelan; Verelan PM; Isoptin; Isoptin SR; Covera-HS), the benzothiazepine diltiazem (Cardizem; Dilacor; Tiazac), and the dihydropyridines amlodipine (Norvasc), felodipine (Plendil), isradipine (Dynacirc), nicardipine (Cardine; Cardine SR), nifedipine (Adalat; Procardia; Afeditab; Nifediac), nimodipine (Nimotop), nitrendipine (not available in the United States), and nisoldipine (Sular). The only example of the diphenylpiperazine class, mibefradil (Posicor), was withdrawn from the market in 1998, and the only example of the diarylaminopropylamine class, bepridil (Vascor), was withdrawn in 2003.[5,6] Each class has a different affinity for the L-type calcium channels found in arterial smooth muscle and cardiac tissue.

While there is no published data on the frequency of CCB toxicity in veterinary medicine, the ASPCA Animal Poison Control Center (APCC) has consulted on 3701 cases of CCB exposure between 2000 and 2010 (ASPCA APCC Database, unpublished data, 2011). Overdose from CCBs can result in severe, life-threatening effects on cardiac conduction and blood pressure. In addition, there may also be effects on the digestive tract, pulmonary function, the nervous system, and pancreas. Treatment may involve gastrointestinal decontamination (induction of emesis and administration of activated charcoal), stabilizing the cardiovascular system through blood pressure

The authors have nothing to disclose.
ASPCA Animal Poison Control Center, 1717 South Philo Road, Suite 36, Urbana, IL 61802, USA
* Corresponding author.
E-mail address: cristine.hayes@aspca.org

and cardiac rhythm regulation, and supportive care as needed to address other clinical signs.

PATHOPHYSIOLOGY

Calcium channels play a significant role in a number of cellular functions, particularly in the sinoatrial (SA) and atrioventricular (AV) nodes, myocardium, and arterial smooth muscle myocytes. In the normal physiologic state, there is a large concentration gradient of calcium across the cellular membrane, with high extracellular and low intracellular calcium concentrations.[1,3,4] Since calcium is unable to diffuse freely across the cellular membrane, this large concentration gradient is maintained by limiting calcium influx into the cell through specific calcium channels, sequestration of free intracellular calcium in the sarcoplasmic reticulum of myocytes, and maintaining an adenosine triphosphate (ATP)-driven calcium export pump.[1,3,4] When activated, the various calcium channels will allow an intracellular influx of calcium, triggering a variety of responses depending on the tissue involved.[1,3,4,7]

There are a number of calcium channel types, including receptor-operated, stretch-operated, second messenger operated, and voltage-sensitive calcium channels.[1,3] The voltage-sensitive calcium channels are of most importance to calcium channel blocker toxicity and are so-called because they open in response to a change in the cell membrane potential.[1,3,4,7] The voltage-sensitive calcium channels include long-lasting (L-type), transient or fast (T-type), Purkinje (P-type), Q-type, R-type, and neuronal (N-type) calcium channels.[1,3,7] The L-type calcium channels are found primarily in the heart, vascular smooth muscle, skeletal muscle, and, to a lesser extent, pancreas, lung, brain, and other tissues.[3,7] T-type calcium channels are found in cardiac nodal and conducting cells, smooth muscle, skeletal muscle, and neuronal tissue.[1,3] P-type, Q-type, and R-type calcium channels are found in Purkinje cells of the cerebellum and cerebellar granule cells.[1] N-type calcium channels are found in neurons throughout the brain.[1] Within the L-type calcium channel, there are at least 4 subclasses.[7] The various CCBs currently available act on the α_{1c} subunit of the L-type voltage-sensitive calcium channel.[7] The different classes of the CCBs have affinity for the various isoforms of the L-type calcium channel, which may account for the variability in their cardiovascular effects.[3,7]

In the heart, the L-type voltage-sensitive calcium channel plays a key role in conduction of the cardiac rhythm. The pacemaker cells of the SA node and AV node have L-type calcium channels that allow a slow intracellular flow of calcium.[3,4,7] In those cells, the slow calcium influx results in spontaneous depolarization during phase 4 of the action potential.[3,4] Propagation of the electrical impulse through the AV node, Purkinje fibers, and cardiac myocytes is also maintained by the calcium influx through L-type calcium channels, which open during phase 2 depolarization.[3,4] CCBs prevent this calcium influx in the nodal and myocardial cells, resulting in a slower sinus rate in the SA node and reduced AV conduction.[3,4]

The calcium influx through L-type calcium channels is also important in contraction of the myocardium and smooth muscle by facilitating the excitation-contraction coupling. In the cardiac myocytes during phase 2 depolarization, the small calcium influx stimulates the sodium-calcium exchange pump to further increase intracellular calcium and also causes release of calcium from the sarcoplasmic reticulum (known as calcium-induced calcium release, or CICR).[1,3,4] The excess intracellular calcium binds to troponin-C, leading to a conformation change in the troponin–tropomyosin complex that exposes the actin filament, allowing actin-myosin binding. This results in contraction of the myocyte.[1,3,4] For vascular smooth muscle, the excess intracellular calcium binds to calmodulin rather than troponin-C.[1,3,4] This results in phosphorylation of myosin, which allows the myosin-actin interaction, leading to contraction.[1,3,4] CCBs prevent the calcium influx into cardiomyocytes and vascular smooth muscle, resulting in reduced cytosolic calcium and reduced CICR from the sarcoplasmic reticulum, leading to reduced cardiac inotropy and vascular tone.[1,3,4] For vascular beds with high resting tone (coronary and arterial smooth muscle), significant vasodilation will occur with reduced vascular tone.[3,4] For vascular beds with low resting tone (gastrointestinal and venous smooth muscle), little vasodilation occurs.[3,4]

The L-type calcium channels are also important systemically. In the pancreas, the L-type calcium channels influence insulin release from the pancreatic β cells. CCBs block the L-type calcium channels in these cells, resulting in reduced insulin release and hyperglycemia.[1] At the cellular level, the calcium influx through L-type calcium channels results in increased mitochondrial uptake of calcium, affecting intracellular ATP levels.[1,3] CCBs lower mitochondrial calcium levels, resulting in reduced pyruvate dehydrogenase activity, leading to lactate accumulation.[1,3] Platelet aggregation may also be inhibited to some extent with CCBs.[3] Endothelin-mediated vasoconstriction is also dependent on L-type calcium channels. Acute renal failure secondary to endothelin-mediated vasoconstriction may be attenuated by CCBs.[3]

PHARMACOLOGY

Of the 5 classes of CCB that have been developed, only 3 are currently on the US market. The CCBs mibefradil, a diphenylpiperazine, and bepridil, a diarylaminopropylamine, antagonized both the L-type and T-type calcium channel; however, they were withdrawn from the US market in 1998 and 2003, respectively, because of numerous severe drug interactions.[5,6] The remaining classes of CCB vary in the extent to which they affect the L-type calcium channels within vascular and cardiac tissues.

Phenylalkylamines

The representative drug of the phenylalkylamine class of CCB is verapamil. Verapamil is a nonspecific L-type CCB in that it has effects on both vascular and cardiac tissue, resulting in vasodilation, negative inotropy, and SA and AV node suppression.[3,4]

The pharmacokinetics for verapamil have been studied in dogs and humans (**Table 1**); however, little information regarding cats has been published. Verapamil is rapidly absorbed but has low bioavailability because of extensive first-pass metabolism; bioavailability is lower in the dog (10%–23%) compared to 20% to 35% in healthy humans and approximately 50% in human liver patients.[8,9] In humans, 60% to 80% of the absorbed verapamil is metabolized in the liver via cytochrome P-450 to active and inactive metabolites, with norverapamil being the major metabolite.[9] Norverapamil has a cardiovascular potency 20% that of verapamil.[9] In dogs, verapamil is also metabolized to several active and inactive metabolites.[8] In humans, verapamil reaches the cerebrospinal fluid poorly, crosses the placenta, and passes into the milk.[9] Elimination of verapamil varies between dogs and humans, with biliary excretion as the primary route in dogs and renal excretion as the primary route of elimination of verapamil in humans.[8,9] With intravenous (IV) dose-escalation studies in humans, drug clearance becomes nonlinear due to saturation of hepatic metabolism.[9] The onset of pharmacologic action and time to peak plasma concentration depend on the route of administration and formulation, with IV dosing fastest (1–5 minutes) and oral controlled-onset extended-release (COER) preparations longest at 11 hours in humans.[9]

Table 1
Pharmacokinetics of the different classes of CCB

Class	Phenylalklamine	Benzothiazepine	Dihydropyridine					
Representative Drug	Verapamil	Diltiazem	Amlodipine	Felodipine	Nifedipine	Nicardipine	Nisoldipine	Isradipine
Absorption	Dog: 90% Human: 90%	Dog: rapid Human: 98%	60%–65%	10%–25%	30%–60% (IR) 30%–50% (ER)	35%	87%	15%–24%
% Bioavailability	Dog: 10–23 Human: 20–35	Dog: 17–24 Cat[a]: 71 (IR) 36 (ER)	Dog: 90 Human: 64–90	13–20 (ER)	30–60 (IR) 30–50 (ER)	35	4–8	14–24
Time to Cmax (h) (oral)	1–2 (IR) 7–11 (ER)[b]	Dog: 0.5 Cat[a]: 0.75 (IR) 5.7 (ER) Human: 2–4 (IR) 4–18 (ER)[b]	Dog: 6 Human: 6–12	2–6 (ER)	0.2–0.75 (IR) 6 (ER)	0.5–2 (IR) 1–4 (ER)	1–1.5 (IR) 4–13 (ER)	1.5 (IR) 7–18 (ER)
Time to onset (h) (oral)	0.5–1.5 (IR) 4–5 (ER)	0.25–1 (IR)		1 (IR) 5 (ER)	0.2 (IR) 0.5–1 (ER)	0.2	1–3 (IR)	1 (IR) 2 (ER)
Effect of food	None	None	None	Increases rate of absorption	Variable	Reduced absorption	Slows absorption	?
Metabolism Site	Liver	Liver	Dog: liver Human: liver	Liver	Liver, gut wall	Liver	Liver, gut wall	Liver
Active metabolites?	Dog: yes Human: yes	Yes	Yes	No	No	No	Yes	No

Excretion	Dog: mostly bile Human: kidney 70% Bile/feces 9%–16%	Bile/feces 65% Kidney 35%	Dog: feces 45% kidney 45% as metabolites Human: kidney 70% as metabolites, 10% unchanged bile/feces 20%–25%	Kidney 70%–80% Bile/feces <15%	Kidney 60% Bile/feces 35%	Kidney 60% Bile/feces 35%	Kidney 60%–80% Bile/feces 6%–12%	Kidney 60%–65% Bile/feces 30%
Elimination T½ (h)	Dog: 1.8–3.8 Human: 8–12	Dog: 2–4 Cat[a]: 1.8 (IR) 6.8 (XR) Human: 3–6.6 (IR) 4–10 (ER)	30–60	11–16 (IR) 27–33 (ER)	2–5	8.6	9–17	8

Note: There may be significant variability in pharmacokinetic data between species, and many of the listed medications have only been extensively studied in humans.

Abbreviations: C_{max}, peak plasma concentration; ER, non-immediate-release preparation (including extended-release, sustained-release, controlled-release, long-acting, and controlled-onset extended-release); IR, conventional immediate-release preparation; T½, half-life

[a] Cardizem IR and Cardizem CD have been studied in cats.[12]

[b] The time to peak plasma concentration (oral route) varies with the different extended-release preparations. The time listed is the range including all extended-release, sustained-release, controlled-release, long-acting, and controlled-onset extended-release preparations.

Data are for humans, unless otherwise specified; from Refs.[3,8,9,11–21]

Benzothiazepines

Diltiazem is the most commonly used drug of the benzothiazepine CCB class. Compared to verapamil, diltiazem has less significant effects on arterial vascular smooth muscle, cardiac contractility, and AV node suppression, although the SA node suppression is approximately the same between the 2 drugs.[3,4]

Diltiazem is formulated as a conventional immediate-release tablet or as a COER preparation. There are several different COER preparations available. Cardizem CD is a dual-release capsule that holds 2 types of beads containing the drug; the beads differ in the thickness of the surrounding membranes, with 40% of the beads meant to dissolve within the first 12 hours after oral administration and the remaining 60% formulated to dissolve over a second 12-hour period of time.[10] Dilacor XR is an extended-release capsule that contains several 60-mg tablets contained in a matrix core that swells and slowly releases the drug over a 24-hour period of time in humans.[11] The individual tablets are generally removed from the capsule and sectioned in order to dose small animals.[11]

The pharmacokinetics for diltiazem have been studied in cats, dogs, and humans (see **Table 1**).[3,8,12–15] In dogs and humans, systemic bioavailability is low due to a high first-pass effect; however, in cats bioavailability is much higher.[3,12,13] This difference is hypothesized to be related to a reduced hepatic first-pass effect in the cat.[12] Diltiazem is widely distributed through most tissues.[13] It can cross the placenta and can be found in milk as well, with one report suggesting that concentrations in human breast milk may approximate serum levels.[13] Diltiazem is metabolized in the liver through both deacetylation and demethylation in dogs and primarily through deacetylation in humans.[3,13,14] Deacetyldiltiazem is the major active metabolite in humans and is 25% to 50% as potent a coronary vasodilator as the parent compound.[13] Diltiazem also undergoes enterohepatic recirculation in dogs and humans, with the second plasma peak in humans occurring 3 to 4 hours after ingestion.[3] Elimination of diltiazem in dogs and humans is blood flow dependent, while in cats it is suggested to be independent of blood flow.[12] It is primarily eliminated in the feces, although renal excretion accounts for approximately one-third of elimination in humans.[13] The terminal half-life is dependent on the formulation, with immediate-release preparations eliminated faster compared to extended-release formulations.[13] The time to reach the maximal plasma concentration for oral immediate-release/conventional diltiazem is 30 minutes in dogs and 45 minutes in cats, to an average of 5.7 hours following oral administration of the extended-release capsule Cardizem CD in cats.[11,12]

Dihydropyridines

There are a number of drugs that fall within the dihydropyridine CCB class, including amlodipine, felodipine, isradipine, nicardipine, nifedipine, nimodipine, nitrendipine, and nisoldipine.[7] Of these, the one most commonly involved in exposures reported to the ASPCA APCC is amlodipine, which accounted for 76% of all dihydropyridine cases from 2000 to 2010 (ASPCA APCC Database, unpublished data, 2011). The dihydropyridines are most noted for their effects on vascular smooth muscle while having relatively little effect on cardiac contractility or conduction.[3,4]

Dog and cat pharmacokinetic data are lacking for most of the drugs in the dihydropyridine class of CCB (with the exception of amlodipine in dogs); however, there is a significant amount of pharmacokinetic data in humans (see **Table 1**).[15–21] In general, the absorption, bioavailability, volume of distribution, and terminal elimination half-life of the dihydropyridines vary between drugs. Amlodipine has the highest

Table 2
Therapeutic doses of selected CCB commonly used in veterinary medicine

	Verapamil	Diltiazem	Amlodipine
Dog	IV: 0.05 mg/kg to a maximum cumulative dose of 0.15 mg/kg PO: 0.5–5.0 mg/kg q8h	IV: 0.05–0.35 mg/kg to a maximum cumulative dose of 0.75 mg/kg PO: 0.5–2.0 mg/kg	PO: 0.05–0.4 mg/kg q12h
Cat	IV: 0.025 mg/kg to a maximum cumulative dose of 0.15–0.2 mg/kg PO: 0.5–1.0 mg/kg q8h	IV: 0.125–0.35 mg/kg to a maximum cumulative dose of 0.75 mg/kg PO: 0.5–1.5 mg/kg q8h up to 10 mg/kg daily	PO: 0.625–1.25 mg daily
Human (pediatric)	PO: 3–5 mg/kg daily in 3 divided doses	PO: 1.5–2 mg/kg daily in 3–4 divided doses to a maximum cumulative dose of 3.5 mg/kg daily	PO: 0.1 mg/kg q12–24h to a maximum of 0.6 mg/kg/day or 20 mg/day

Data from Refs.[9,13,16,22–24]

bioavailability and volume of distribution.[15,16] All of the dihydropyridines are highly protein bound, extensively metabolized by the liver, and eliminated primarily through the kidneys.[15–21] The onset of action and time to peak plasma concentrations depend on the formulation, with immediate-release preparations being the shortest and COER preparations being the longest.[15–21]

CLINICAL SIGNS

The minimum oral toxic dose of each CCB has not been established in humans or animals. Signs of toxicity have been noted at therapeutic doses of verapamil, diltiazem, amlodipine, and nifedipine in some dog and cat cases (**Table 2**) (ASPCA APCC Database, unpublished data, 2011).[22–24] The diltiazem oral dose resulting in death of 50% of exposed patients (LD_{50}) in dogs has been reported as somewhere beyond 50 mg/kg but has not been reliably established.[23]

While the various classes of CCBs have distinct differences in their specificity for either the vascular smooth muscle or heart at therapeutic doses, in overdoses the tissue specificity may be lost.[3,4,25–27] Typically, the clinical signs seen are the result of an exaggeration of the normal pharmacologic activity of CCBs.[3,4,25–27] With verapamil and diltiazem toxicity, clinical signs include sinus bradycardia and/or bradyarrhythmias (all degrees of heart block, QT interval prolongation, or junctional rhythms) due to slowed cardiac conduction and also hypotension due to vasodilation and reduced cardiac inotropy (ASPCA APCC Database, unpublished data, 2011).[25–28] Sinus tachycardia likely due to carotid sinus reflex stimulation is possible as well.[25–28] With the dihydropyridines, common clinical signs include profound hypotension due to vasodilation and reflex sinus tachycardia (ASPCA APCC Database, unpublished data, 2011).[25–27]

Additional clinical signs associated with all CCBs include digestive upset, hypothermia (presumably due to hypotension), central nervous system depression due to hypotension and/or bradycardia, noncardiogenic pulmonary edema, hyperglycemia due to inhibition of insulin release, hypokalemia, metabolic acidosis due to tissue hypoperfusion and increased lactate production, and, rarely, stimulatory signs such as seizures, agitation, or tremors (ASPCA APCC Database, unpublished data,

2011).[1,25–27,29] The exact mechanism of pulmonary edema is unknown; however, several mechanisms have been proposed. The development of pulmonary edema is thought to be secondary to aggressive fluid therapy combined with either increased pulmonary capillary permeability, drug-induced changes to alveolar membrane permeability, or selective precapillary vasodilation from CCBs.[30,31]

DIAGNOSIS

The diagnosis of CCB toxicity in veterinary patients is largely based on clinical signs consistent with CCB toxicity and the history of a possible exposure. Serum drug levels for CCBs are not routinely evaluated on presentation because the tests are not widely available and drug levels for specific agents do not necessarily correspond with the degree of clinical signs seen.[1,29] Signs of toxicity can occur at therapeutic drug levels in humans.[1,29] When tests are available, they could be used to confirm an exposure.[1]

The clinical presentation of a patient with hypotension and bradycardia or tachycardia can be consistent with other etiologies as well. Differential diagnoses may include toxicity from digoxin, cardiac glycoside containing plants, β-adrenergic antagonists, α_2-adrenergic agonists, organophosphates, type 1a antiarrhythmic agents such as procainamide or quinidine, bufadienolides, and nontoxic causes such as myocardial infarction or other cardiac disease.[32]

TREATMENT

Treatment for CCB toxicity focuses on the reducing the absorption of the drug, providing supportive care based on the clinical signs seen, and augmenting myocardial function. There is no specific antidote for treatment of CCB toxicity due to the number of mechanisms contributing to clinical signs; however, there are a number of therapies available that can counteract some of the CCB effects.

Decontamination

For the asymptomatic patient with a recent exposure of less than 2 hours, gastric decontamination is recommended.[26] This may be accomplished by inducing emesis, gastric lavage and/or administration of activated charcoal (Toxiban; UAA Gel). In the symptomatic patient, gastric decontamination should only be attempted once the patient's condition is stable. Inducing emesis is contraindicated for a symptomatic patient; however, gastric lavage or activated charcoal administered via a stomach tube could be considered, particularly with large ingestions or ingestion of sustained-release preparations.[25]

Emesis can be accomplished in the asymptomatic patient using a few different methods. For dogs, apomorphine (Apokyn) or hydrogen peroxide 3% can be used as emetics, while in cats xylazine (AnaSed; X-Ject; Xyla-Ject; Sedazine; TranquiVed) can be used.[33–35] Dopaminergic receptors in the chemoreceptor trigger zone are stimulated by apomorphine, resulting in emesis in the dog.[33] The apomorphine dose recommended in dogs is 0.03 to 0.04 mg/kg IV, intramuscularly (IM) or in the subconjunctival sac.[33,34] If given in the subconjunctival sac, the sac can be flushed with saline once emesis has occurred.[33] Common adverse effects associated with apomorphine use include sedation and when given IV or IM protracted vomiting.[34] In dogs, hydrogen peroxide 3% can also be given an alternative to apomorphine. Hydrogen peroxide 3% causes local irritation in the stomach to stimulate emesis, and is used at a dose of 1 to 2 mL/kg PO up to a maximum of 50 mL/patient.[33] In cats, xylazine (1.1 mg/kg IM or subcutaneously [SQ]) causes emesis through stimulation of the α_2-adrenergic receptors in the emetic center.[35] Common adverse effects associated with xylazine include sedation, hypotension, bradycardia, and respiratory depression, although these effects can be reversed with atipamazole (0.2 mg/kg IV) or yohimbine (0.1 mg/kg IV).[33,35] For patients where emesis is contraindicated, gastric lavage performed under anesthesia may be considered.[33]

Activated charcoal can also be used for gastrointestinal decontamination. It is effective for both immediate and extended-release preparations of CCBs.[36] In a human study evaluating the effectiveness of activated charcoal for verapamil exposures, activated charcoal was effective in reducing the absorption of immediate-release verapamil when administered immediately following ingestion but not 2 hours after ingestion.[36] Activated charcoal was effective in reducing absorption of sustained-release verapamil 4 hours after ingestion (the longest time evaluated in the study).[36] Activated charcoal is used in dogs and cats at a dose of 1 to 3 g/kg PO with a cathartic such as sorbitol.[33,37] Activated charcoal can be repeated every 4 to 6 hours for 2 to 4 doses if a high dose of a sustained-release preparation is ingested.[33,37] Adverse effects associated with activated charcoal include aspiration pneumonia or hypernatremia.[37] If the patient is symptomatic, airway protection is critical and the risk versus the benefits of activated charcoal should be considered. For the ingestion of sustained-release preparations, a warm water enema at a rate of 2.5 to 5 mL/kg could also be considered to facilitate evacuation of the intestinal contents.

Extracorporeal decontamination (hemodialysis) is not expected to be of benefit in CCB toxicity. CCBs are highly protein bound, which minimizes the benefit of hemodialysis.[1]

Monitoring

When there has been a possible exposure to a CCB, close monitoring of the cardiovascular system, respiratory system, nervous system, and blood chemistries should be implemented for 12 to 24 hours or longer following exposure.[25] The blood pressure, heart rate, and cardiac rhythm should be monitored frequently. An electrocardiogram (ECG) should be used to monitor the cardiac rhythm. Respiratory system monitoring can involve auscultation, pulse oximetry, or arterial blood gas. The nervous system should also be monitored for depression or seizures. The serum glucose, acid-base status, and electrolytes should be monitored for the development of hyperglycemia, lactic acidosis, hypokalemia, hypophosphatemia, or hypomagnesemia.

As noted previously, plasma CCB levels can be performed to determine if an exposure has occurred; however, monitoring CCB levels is not expected to be beneficial during the course of treatment since reference ranges have not been established in animals and since clinical signs can occur at therapeutic doses of CCBs.[1,22–25,29]

Supportive Care

In the symptomatic patient, stabilization and supportive care should be provided. Fluid therapy using a balanced isotonic crystalloid fluid should be administered for cardiovascular support and to help maintain hydration. Persistent hypotension despite crystalloid therapy should be treated with a colloid-containing fluid such as hetastarch (Hespan). Hetastarch is used in dogs at an initial dose of 5 mL/kg IV bolus over 15 to 30 minutes followed by an IV continuous rate infusion (CRI) of 12 mL/kg/d, and in cats, 10 mL/kg/d IV CRI.[25,26,38] Aggressive fluid therapy should be used with care to minimize fluid overload and the development of pulmonary edema.[25,26,30,31]

An antiemetic such as maropitant (Cerenia) (1 mg/kg SQ q24h), metoclopramide (Reglan) (0.1–0.5 mg/kg SQ or IM or 0.01–0.02 mg/kg/hr IV CRI), ondansetron (Zofran) (0.1–1 mg/kg IV q12–24h), or dolasetron (Anzimet) (0.5–1 mg/kg IV q24h) may be used to manage any vomiting.[39–42] If seizures develop, diazepam (Valium; Diastat) (0.5–1 mg/kg IV) or a barbiturate such as pentobarbital (Nembutal) (3–15 mg/kg IV) or phenobarbital (Tubex; Carpujects; Luminal Sodium) (2–20 mg/kg IV) may be used.[43–45] Potassium should be supplemented in the fluids when the serum potassium is below 2.5 mEq/L. If pulmonary edema develops, oxygen support should be provided.

Specific Therapies

Most conventional therapies specific for CCB toxicity aim to increase transmembrane calcium flow by increasing extracellular calcium concentrations (calcium gluconate or calcium chloride) or increasing intracellular cyclic-adenosine monophosphate (cAMP) concentrations (glucagon [GlucoGen] or inamrinone [Inocor]), increase cardiac inotropy and chronotropy (sympathomimetics, temporary pacemaker), increase peripheral vascular tone (sympathomimetics), and increase glucose or free fatty acid utilization (insulin-glucose, lipid emulsion (Liposyn). Atropine sulfate (0.02 mg/kg) IV can be used for persistent bradycardia. Repeat atropine if and as needed.

Calcium

After attempting cardiovascular stabilization, calcium is commonly administered for persistent hypotension and/or bradycardia.[1,25,26] The increased extracellular calcium available to cells may increase the intracellular calcium influx.[1,25,26] Increased calcium may also increase calcium release from the sarcoplasmic reticulum, enhancing contractility.[1,25,26] Calcium gluconate or calcium chloride may be used, although calcium chloride will provide a higher concentration of calcium ion per milliliter compared to calcium gluconate (13.6 mEq vs 4.5 mEq in 10 mL of a 10% solution).[26] Calcium gluconate 10% can be used at a dose of 0.5 to 1.5 mL/kg IV slowly over 5 minutes while monitoring the ECG closely or as a CRI of 0.05 mL/kg/h.[46] Calcium chloride 10% is used at a dose of 0.1 to 0.5 mL/kg IV slowly over 5 minutes or as a CRI of 0.01 mL/kg/h.[46] If bradycardia develops or worsens during use, discontinue the calcium supplementation.[46] Adverse effects include hypercalcemia and local tissue irritation or necrosis if given extravascularly.[46]

Glucagon

Glucagon is a cardiac inotrope and chronotrope.[1,26] In addition to stimulating hepatic glycogenolysis, thus increasing blood glucose, it also acts on cardiac G protein–coupled receptors, stimulating an increase in intracellular cAMP and thus increasing the myocardial calcium influx.[1,26] The increased intracellular calcium results in increased contractility and enhances impulse generation.[1,26] Glucagon may benefit patients with either hypotension or bradycardia, although it is expensive and may not be readily available. In case reports describing its use for verapamil toxicity in dogs, it was only transiently effective.[28,47] It can be used at an initial dose of 50 nanograms/kilogram body weight (ng/kg) IV bolus followed by a CRI of 10 to 15 ng/kg/min up to 40 ng/kg/min.[48]

Inamrinone

As a phosphodiesterase III inhibitor, inamrinone prevents degradation of cAMP in vascular and cardiac muscle, resulting in increased intracellular cAMP.[1,25,29] Increased cAMP leads to an increase in the myocardial calcium influx, resulting in improved contractility and increased impulse generation.[1,25,29] It can cause peripheral vasodilation, thus worsening hypotension if present.[29] It can be used at an initial dose of 1 to 3 mg/kg IV bolus followed by 10 to 100 μg/kg/min IV CRI.[49]

Sympathomimetics

Refractory hypotension or bradycardia may respond to sympathomimetic drugs, although no one agent has been proved to be consistently effective.[26] Dopamine hydrochloride (Inotropin) (10–20 mcg/kg/min IV), dobutamine hydrochloride (Dobutrex) (2–20 μg/kg/min IV), isoproterenol (Isuprel) (0.04–0.08 μg/kg/min IV), epinephrine (Adrenalin) (0.05–0.4 μg/kg/min IV), or phenylephrine hydrochloride (Neo-Synephrine) (0.5–3 μg/kg/min IV) may be used.[1,26,50–54]

Insulin-glucose

Hyperglycemia is commonly associated with CCB toxicity due to the inhibitory effects CCBs have on insulin release from the pancreatic β cells.[1,25,26] In cardiac myocytes stressed from hypoperfusion, there is a shift from free fatty acid to glucose utilization as the energy substrate.[1,26,47,55–57] Hypoinsulinemia and insulin resistance leading to reduced glucose delivery to cardiac tissue combined with an increase in glucose utilization by the myocardium can have negative cardiac inotropic effects.[26,47,56,57] High-dose insulin therapy with dextrose administered to maintain euglycemia (HIE) enhances glucose uptake by the myocytes to increase energy substrate utilization.[1,26,55–58] HIE also suppresses phosphodiesterase III activity, thus increasing cAMP, resulting in increased intracellular calcium influx.[1,57] In addition, HIE also enhances the intracellular potassium influx resulting in hypokalemia, which can prolong phase 2 depolarization, increasing the intracellular calcium influx.[1] The end result is increased cardiac inotropy.[1,26,29,55–57] HIE will also decrease capillary vascular resistance through increased nitric oxide synthase activity, leading to a reduction in acidosis.[57]

HIE can be used, but the ideal dose in companion animals has not been established. In a study of verapamil toxicity in anesthetized dogs, regular insulin was used at a dose of 4 U/min with 20% dextrose.[47,55] In human medicine, the dose typically used is the IV administration of 1 U/kg bolus followed by 0.1 to 1 U/kg/hr IV CRI along with 10% to 20% dextrose administration.[29,57] In many of the studies, effects were seen after 30 to 45 minutes, and it appears the most benefit was seen earlier in the course of CCB toxicity; if treatment with HIE is delayed, the benefits are reduced.[29,56] If using HIE, the serum glucose and potassium levels should be monitored closely to minimize the risk for hypoglycemia, hyperglycemia and hypokalemia.[1,26,29,56,57] When administering 10% to 20% dextrose, a central catheter should be used to minimize the risk for phlebitis.[26]

Lipid emulsion

Treatment with an intravenous lipid emulsion (ILE) commonly used in total parenteral nutrition has been investigated as an adjunctive therapy for various toxicities, particularly toxicity due to local anesthetics, verapamil, or diltiazem, and has been proposed as a therapy for toxicity due to other substances with high lipid solubility.[59] Although the exact mechanism by which ILE therapy works in toxicity is unknown, a few mechanisms have been suggested. One theory suggests that ILE sequesters lipophilic drug in an expanded plasma lipid phase, reducing the available free drug and promoting clearance of the compound through metabolism of drug-containing chylomicrons ("lipid sink" theory).[59,60] Another theory for ILE benefit when used in treatment of cardiotoxic drugs suggests that the increased availability of free fatty acids provided by ILE may prevent the myocardium from switching to glucose as its preferred energy substrate.[59,61] In addition, the long chain fatty acids in ILE may also activate myocyte calcium channels, resulting in increased calcium influx.[29,59] ILE may also increase nitric oxide and β-ketoacids, which stimulate insulin release.[29]

As with HIE, the ideal dose of ILE in companion animals has not been established. The most commonly suggested dose of ILE has been 1.5 mL/kg IV slow bolus of intralipid 20% followed by 0.25 mL/kg/min for 1 hour.[59,62] This therapy may be repeated in 3 to 4 hours if the serum is not lipemic. Adverse reactions may include hyperlipidemia, fat overload syndrome (fat embolism, hepatomegaly, thrombocytopenia, hemolysis, increased clotting times, or neurologic deficits), or pancreatitis.[59]

Miscellaneous

Severe heart block may require the placement of a temporary cardiac pacemaker.[28] This therapy can improve cardiac output by increasing the heart rate; however, it will not have effects on the peripheral arterial vascular tone or cardiac contractility.[28] Another treatment using 4-aminopyridine (Ampyra) has been described in experimental studies.[63,64] 4-Aminopyridine is a potassium channel blocker; blockade of potassium channels leads to an increased intracellular calcium influx. At high doses it can also increase muscle contractility.[64] In an experimental cat study using anesthetized and manually ventilated cats, 4-aminopyridine was used effectively to treat verapamil toxicity at a dose of 0.5 mg/kg IV twice, 5 minutes apart.[63] This drug can have significant side effects in animals, including seizure activity, and the dose effective for CCB toxicity has not been definitively established.[25,26,64] At this time, 4-aminopyridine should be considered an experimental treatment and could be considered if all other treatments have failed.

SUMMARY

The prognosis of a patient exposed to a CCB depends on the amount ingested, severity of signs, and response to treatment. CCB exposure can be life threatening, with the onset of signs potentially delayed by many hours depending on the individual medication and formulation. The predominant signs include hypotension, cardiac rhythm changes, and hyperglycemia. Treatment can involve decontamination and cardiovascular stabilization with a variety of modalities. The most effective treatment regimen has not been established in companion animals.

REFERENCES

1. Brent J. Calcium channel-blocking agents. In: Brent J, Wallace KL, Burkhart KK, et al, editors. Critical care toxicology: diagnosis and management of the critically poisoned patient. Philadelphia: Elsevier Mosby; 2005. p. 413–26.
2. Johnson JT. Conversion of atrial fibrillation in two dogs using verapamil and supportive therapy. J Am Anim Hosp Assoc 1985;21:429–34.
3. Cooke KL, Snyder PS. Calcium channel blockers in veterinary medicine. J Vet Intern Med 1998;12:123–31.
4. Pion PD, Brown WA. Calcium channel blocking agents. Compend Cont Ed 1995;17: 123–31.
5. Mibefradil. In: DRUGDEX® System [intranet database]. Version 5.1. Greenwood Village (CO): Thomson Reuters (Healthcare) Inc.
6. Bepridil. In: DRUGDEX® System [intranet database]. Version 5.1. Greenwood Village (CO):Thomson Reuters (Healthcare) Inc.
7. Triggle DJ. L-type calcium channels. Curr Pharm Des 2006;12:443–57.

8. Kittleson MD, Kienle RD. Drugs used to treat cardiac arrhythmias. In: Small animal cardiovascular medicine. St Louis (MO): Mosby; 1998. p. 517–8.
9. Verapamil. In: DRUGDEX® System [intranet database]. Version 5.1. Greenwood Village (CO): Thomson Reuters (Healthcare) Inc.
10. Cardizem CD [package insert]. Bridgewater (NJ): Biovail Corporation; 2009.
11. Kittleson MD. Drugs used in the management of heart failure and cardiac arrhythmias. In: Maddison JE, Page SW, Church D, editors. Small animal clinical pharmacology. London: WB Saunders; 2002. p. 371–2, 407–9.
12. Johnson LM, Atkins CE, Keene BW, et al. Pharmacokinetic and pharmacodynamic properties of conventional and CD-formulated diltiazem in cats. J Vet Intern Med 1996;10:316–20.
13. Diltiazem. In: DRUGDEX® System [intranet database]. Version 5.1. Greenwood Village (CO): Thomson Reuters (Healthcare) Inc.
14. Yabana H, Nagao T, Sato M. Cardiovascular effects of the metabolites of diltiazem in dogs. J Cardiovasc Pharmacol 1985;7:152–7.
15. Stopher DA, Beresford AP, Macrae PV, et al. The metabolism and pharmacokinetics of amlodipine in humans and animals. J Cardiovasc Pharmcol 1988;12(Suppl 7): S55–9.
16. Amlodipine. In: DRUGDEX® System [intranet database]. Version 5.1. Greenwood Village (CO): Thomson Reuters (Healthcare) Inc.
17. Felodipine. In: DRUGDEX® System [intranet database]. Version 5.1. Greenwood Village (CO): Thomson Reuters (Healthcare) Inc.
18. Nifedipine. In: DRUGDEX® System [intranet database]. Version 5.1. Greenwood Village (CO): Thomson Reuters (Healthcare) Inc.
19. Nicardipine. In: DRUGDEX® System [intranet database]. Version 5.1. Greenwood Village (CO): Thomson Reuters (Healthcare) Inc.
20. Nisoldipine. In: DRUGDEX® System [intranet database]. Version 5.1. Greenwood Village (CO): Thomson Reuters (Healthcare) Inc.
21. Isradipine. In: DRUGDEX® System [intranet database]. Version 5.1. Greenwood Village (CO): Thomson Reuters (Healthcare) Inc.
22. Plumb D. Verapamil. In: Veterinary drug handbook. 6th edition. St Louis (MO): Blackwell; 2008. p. 1236–9.
23. Plumb D. Diltiazem. In: Veterinary drug handbook. 6th edition. St Louis (MO): Blackwell; 2008. p. 396–8.
24. Plumb D. Amlodipine. In: Veterinary drug handbook. 6th edition. St Louis (MO): Blackwell; 2008. p. 59–61.
25. Holder T. Calcium channel blocker toxicosis. Vet Med 2000;95:912–5.
26. Costello M, Syring RS. Calcium channel blocker toxicity. J Vet Emerg Crit Care 2008;18:54–60.
27. Shepherd G. Treatment of poisoning caused by β-adrenergic and calcium-channel blockers. Am J Health Syst Pharm 2006;63:1828–35.
28. Syring RS, Costello MF. Temporary transvenous pacing in a dog with diltiazem intoxication. J Vet Emerg Crit Care 2008;18:75–80.
29. Arroyo AM, Kao, LW. Calcium channel blocker toxicity. Pediatr Emerg Care 2009;25: 532–8.
30. Humbert VHJ, Munn NJ, Hawkins RF. Noncardiogenic pulmonary edema complicating massive diltiazem overdose. Chest 1991;99:258–9.
31. Brass BJ, Winchester-Penny S, Lipper BL. Massive verapamil overdose complicated by noncardiogenic pulmonary edema. Am J Emerg Med 1996;14:459–61.
32. Hayes C. Calcium channel blocker drug toxicosis. In: Côté E, editor. Clinical veterinary advisor: dogs and cats. 2nd edition. St Louis (MO): Elsevier Mosby; 2011. p.170–2.

33. Poppenga R. Treatment. In: Plumlee KH, editor. Clinical veterinary toxicology. St Louis (MO): Mosby; 2004. p.13–21.
34. Plumb D. Apomorphine. In: Veterinary drug handbook. 6th edition. St Louis (MO): Blackwell; 2008. p. 91–3.
35. Plumb D. Xylazine. In: Veterinary drug handbook. 6th edition. St Louis (MO): Blackwell; 2008. p. 1253–6.
36. Laine K, Kivisto KT, Neuvonen PJ. Effect of delayed administration of activated charcoal on the absorption of conventional and slow-release verapamil. Clin Toxicol 1997;37:263–8.
37. Plumb D. Charcoal, activated. In: Veterinary drug handbook. 6th edition. St Louis (MO): Blackwell; 2008. p. 233–5.
38. Plumb D. Hetastarch. In: Veterinary drug handbook. 6th edition. St Louis (MO): Blackwell; 2008. p. 604–5.
39. Plumb D. Maropitant. In: Veterinary drug handbook. 6th edition. St Louis (MO): Blackwell; 2008. p. 751–3.
40. Plumb D. Metoclopramide. In: Veterinary drug handbook. 6th edition. St Louis (MO): Blackwell; 2008. p. 814–6.
41. Plumb D. Ondansetron. In: Veterinary drug handbook. 6th edition. St Louis (MO): Blackwell; 2008. p. 899–900.
42. Plumb D. Dolasetron. In: Veterinary drug handbook. 6th edition. St Louis (MO): Blackwell; 2008. p. 426–8.
43. Plumb D. Diazepam. In: Veterinary drug handbook. 6th edition. St Louis (MO): Blackwell; 2008. p. 368–72.
44. Plumb D. Pentobarbital. In: Veterinary drug handbook. 6th edition. St Louis (MO): Blackwell; 2008. p. 953–56.
45. Plumb D. Phenobarbital. In: Veterinary drug handbook. 6th edition. St Louis (MO): Blackwell; 2008. p. 962–67.
46. Plumb D. Calcium salts. In: Veterinary drug handbook. 6th edition. St Louis (MO): Blackwell; 2008. p. 168–73.
47. Kline JA, Tomaszewski CA, Schroeder JD, et al. Insulin is a superior antidote for cardiovascular toxicity induced by verapamil in the anesthetized canine. J Pharmacol Exp Ther 1993;267:744–50.
48. Plumb D. Glucagon. In: Veterinary drug handbook. 6th edition. St Louis (MO): Blackwell; 2008. p. 570–1.
49. Plumb D. Inamrinone lactate. In: Veterinary drug handbook. 6th edition. St Louis (MO): Blackwell; 2008. p. 641–2.
50. Plumb D. Dopamine hydrochloride. In: Veterinary drug handbook. 6th edition. St Louis (MO): Blackwell; 2008. p. 430–2.
51. Plumb D. Dobutamine hydrochloride. In: Veterinary drug handbook. 6th edition. St Louis (MO): Blackwell; 2008. p. 422–4.
52. Plumb D. Isoproterenol. In: Veterinary drug handbook. 6th edition. St Louis (MO): Blackwell; 2008. p. 670–2.
53. Plumb D. Epinephrine. In: Veterinary drug handbook. 6th edition. St Louis (MO): Blackwell; 2008. p. 464–7.
54. Plumb D. Phenylephrine. In: Veterinary drug handbook. 6th edition. St Louis (MO): Blackwell; 2008. p. 973–5.
55. Kline JA, Leonova E, Raymond RM. Beneficial myocardial metabolic effects of insulin during verapamil toxicity in the anesthetized canine. Crit Care Med 1995;23:1251–63.
56. Lheureux PER, Zahir S, Gris M, et al. Bench to bedside review: hyperinsulinaemia/euglycaemia therapy in the management of overdose of calcium-channel blockers. Crit Care 2006;10:212.

57. Engebretsen KM, Kaczmarek KM, Morgan J, et al. High-dose insulin therapy in beta-blocker and calcium channel blocker poisoning. Clin Toxicol 2011;49:277–83.
58. Yuan TH, Kerns WP, Tomaszewski CA, et al. Insulin-glucose as adjunctive therapy for severe calcium channel antagonist poisoning. Clin Toxicol 1999;37:463–74.
59. Fernandez AL, Lee JA, Rahilly L, et al. The use of intravenous lipid emulsion as an antidote in veterinary toxicology. J Vet Emerg Crit Care 2011;21:309–20.
60. Weinberg GL, VadeBoncouer T, Ramaraju GA, et al. Lipid emulsion infusion rescues dogs from bupivicaine-induced cardiac toxicity. Reg Anesth Pain Med 2003;28:198–202.
61. Bania TC, Chu J, Perez E, et al. Hemodynamic effects of intravenous fat emulsion in an animal model of severe verapamil toxicity resuscitated with atropine, calcium, and saline. Acad Emerg Med 2007;14:105–11.
62. Crandell DE, Weinberg GL. Moxidectin toxicosis in a puppy successfully treated with intravenous lipids. J Vet Emerg Crit Care 2009;19:181–6.
63. Agoston S, Maestrone E, van Hezik EJ, et al. Effective treatment of verapamil intoxication with 4-aminopyridine in the cat. J Clin Invest 1984;73:1291–6.
64. Kline JA. Calcium channel antagonists. In: Ford MD, Delaney KA, Ling LJ, et al, editors. Clinical toxicology. Philadelphia: WB Saunders; 2001. p. 370–7.

Management of Attention-Deficit Disorder and Attention-Deficit/Hyperactivity Disorder Drug Intoxication in Dogs and Cats

Laura A. Stern, DVM*, Mary Schell, DVM

KEYWORDS
- ADHD • ADD • Drug intoxication • Dog • Cat
- Amphetamines • Atomoxetine

Attention-deficit/hyperactivity disorder (ADD/ADHD) is defined as "a neurodevelopmental behavioral disorder resulting in a pattern of inattention and/or hyperactivity that causes impairment in social, emotional, cognitive, behavioral, and academic functioning,"[1] and it is treated with a variety of stimulants, in both immediate-release and extended-release formulations. The purpose of using the stimulant drugs is to improve brain levels of serotonin and norepinephrine.

Specific drugs prescribed for the management of ADHD include both amphetamine class stimulants and nonstimulants such as atomoxetine (Strattera) (**Table 1**).[1] When these drugs are ingested by dogs and cats, although the drugs differ in rate of absorption and time to onset of clinical signs, those signs are very similar and can be managed similarly. Key to the treatment of dogs and cats is to manage signs as they develop and not delay treatment while the ingested agent is identified.

Second-line therapy may include the use of antidepressant class medications such as imipramine, bupropion, or nortriptyline for patients who do not respond adequately to the first line stimulants or who have coexisting mood disorders. This article does not address these nonstimulant agents beyond noting that they may be included in the general grouping of "ADHD drugs" in the case of ingestion by a household pet.[1]

The authors have nothing to disclose.
ASPCA National Animal Poison Control Center, 1717 South Philo Road, Suite 36, Urbana, IL 61802, USA
* Corresponding author.
E-mail address: laurastern@aspca.org

Table 1
Amphetamine class ADHD drugs

Trade Name	Generic Name	Available Formulations
Adderall	amphetamine	5-, 7.5-, 10-, 12.5-, 15-, 20-, and 30-mg tablet
Adderall XR	amphetamine (extended release)	5-, 10-, 15-, 20-, 25-, and 30-mg capsule
Concerta	methylphenidate (long acting)	18-, 27-, 36-, and 54-mg tablets
Daytrana	methylphenidate patch	10, 15, 20, and 30 mg/9-h patch
Desoxyn	methamphetamine hydrochloride	2.5-, 5-, 10-, and 15-mg tablets; 5-, 10-, and 15-mg SR tablets
Dexedrine	dextroamphetamine	5-, 10-, and 15-mg Spansule XR
Dextrostat	dextroamphetamine	5- and 10-mg tablets
Focalin	dexmethylphenidate	2.5-, 5-, and 10-mg tablets
Focalin XR	dexmethylphenidate (extended release)	5-, 10-, 15-, 20-, 30-, and 40-mg XR capsules
Metadate ER	methylphenidate (extended release)	20-mg extended-release tablet
Metadate CD	methylphenidate (extended release)	10-, 20-, 30-, 40-, 50-, and 60-mg XR capsules
Methylin	methylphenidate (oral solution and chewable tablets)	2.5-, 5-, and 10-mg chewable tablets; 5-, 10-, and 20-mg tablets; 5 and 10 mg/tsp solution; 10- and 20-mg XR tablets
Ritalin	methylphenidate	5-, 10-, and 20-mg tablets
Ritalin SR	methylphenidate	20-mg SR tablet
Ritalin LA	methylphenidate (long acting)	10-, 20-, 30-, and 40-mg XR capsules
Strattera	atomoxetine	10-, 18-, 25-, 40-, 60-, 80-, and 100-mg capsules
Vyvanse	lisdexamfetamine dimesylate	20-, 30-, 40-, 50-, 60-, and 70-mg capsules

Abbreviations: SR, sustained release; XR, extended release.

AMPHETAMINE SALTS AND OTHER SIMILAR AGENTS
Use in Veterinary Medicine

Amphetamines were used in veterinary medicine to increase the respiratory rate and depth in animals undergoing anesthesia with barbiturates, due to its stimulatory effects on the medulla oblongata.[2] Methylphenidate has also been used for the treatment of narcolepsy in dogs, although it has been only partially effective when used as the sole treatment.[3] Amphetamine use was placed under strict control by the 1970 Controlled Substances Act. Amphetamines are no longer available for veterinary use in the United States.

Mechanism of Toxicity

Amphetamines cause release of catecholamines, resulting in the stimulation of the cerebrospinal axis, especially the brain stem, cerebral cortex, medullary respiratory center, and reticular activating system.[2,4] Amphetamines cause marked increased in the release of norephinephirine, dopamine, and serotonin from presynaptic terminals.[5,6] Monoamine oxidase is also inhibited, which is one of the metabolic pathways of catecholamine metabolism.[6] This increase in catecholamine release and inhibition of reuptake cause both α and β stimulation. This results in vasoconstriction with sequelae of hypertension, tachycardia, cardiac dysrhythmias, and central nervous system (CNS) stimulatory signs. Cardiac output is generally not appreciably affected, due to reflex bradycardia.[7] Methylphenidate is a CNS stimulant that is structurally related to amphetamines.[8] Methylphenidate is "thought to block the reuptake of norepinephrine and dopamine into the presynaptic neuron and increase the release of these monoamines into the extraneuronal space."[9]

Pharmackokinetics, Toxicity, and Metabolism

The LD_{50} for orally administered amphetamine sulfate in dogs is 20 to 27 mg/kg.[10] Generally, the LD_{50} for most amphetamines is between 10 and 23 mg/kg.[11] The LD_{50} for methylphenidate has not been established. Experimentally, healthy beagle dogs survived dosage regimens of greater than 20 mg/kg/day for 90 days.[12]

Following rapid absorption from the gastrointestinal tract, amphetamines enter the cerebrospinal fluid at up to 80% of plasma concentrations.[13] Amphetamines are primarily excreted in the urine without any biotransformation. However, in vivo research shows that amphetamines do undergo oxidative deamination and aromatic hydroxylation in the liver of dogs.[14] Deaminated metabolites are oxidized to benzoic acid and excreted in the urine as the glycine conjugate of huppuric acid. Amphetamines are weak bases and urinary excretion is pH dependent.[13] Because the metabolism varies widely between species that were studied, these data cannot be extended to cats.

Clinical Signs

Clinical signs commonly seen with amphetamine intoxication are cardiovascular signs, including significant hypertension, tachycardia, occasionally reflex bradycardia secondary to hypertension, and tachyarrhythmias; CNS stimulatory signs are common, including hyperactivity, agitation, mydriasis, circling, head bobbing, apprehension, and tremors. Seizures can occur but are rare. Lethargy, depression, and coma have been reported later in the course of intoxication. Gastrointestinal upset can also be seen, as well as anorexia. Animals may be hyperthermic secondary to stimulatory signs. Disseminated intravascular coagulopathy (DIC) can be seen as sequelae to the hyperthermia.

Diagnosis

Diagnosis is supported by history of exposure or recovery of pills or capsules in the vomitus. One study group took a human on-site urine multidrug test and evaluated it for the use in dogs; it was found to be sensitive and specific for the detection of amphetamines. It has not been validated for use in cats.[15] Thin layer chromatography is commonly used, and immunologic assays can also be used for urine and plasma. Gas chromatography–mass spectrometry can also be used for detecting amphetamines in urine or plasma samples, especially in legal cases.[10] Necropsy findings in experimental dogs showed subendocardial and epicardial hemorrhage and myocardial necrosis.[10]

Differential Diagnoses

Differential diagnoses include pseudoephedrine, cocaine, methamphetamine, phenylpropanolamine, methylxanthines (caffeine, theobromine, theophylline), ma huang, and serotonergic medication intoxications.

ASPCA Animal Poison Control Center's Experience

A review of the ASPCA Animal Poison Control Center's (APCC) toxicology database from 2006 to 2011 found amphetamine salt and methylphenidate toxicity cases involving 202 dogs and 176 cats.[16] These cases involved exposure to one agent (an amphetamine or methylphenidate) only and were assessed as medium or high suspect cases (history of exposure and clinical signs were consistent with amphetamine or methylphenidate toxicosis). These cases were not confirmed via analytical methods.

Of the canine cases, full recovery was noted in 13 cases and follow-up was not available on 189 cases. The most commonly reported clinical signs (incidence over 5%) were hyperactivity in 78 (38.6%) of 202, agitation in 61 (30.2%) of 202, hyperthermia in 52 (25.7%) of 202, tachycardia in 49 (24.2%) of 202, panting in 31 (15.3%) of 202, disorientation in 25 (12.3%) of 202, restlessness in 25 (12.3%) of 202, mydriasis in 24 (11.9%) of 202, head bobbing in 20 (9.9%) of 202, pacing in 17 (8.4%) of 202, hypertension in 15 (7.4%) of 202, circling in 14 (6.9%) of 202, anxiety in 13 (6.4%) of 202, hypersalivation in 13 (6.4%) of 202, behavior change in 12 (5.9%) of 202, vomiting in 11 (5.4%) of 202, and lethargy in 10 (5.0%) of 202.

With the 176 feline cases, 17 made a full recovery, 2 were continuing to show signs at the time of the follow-up, and for 157, follow-up was not available. The most commonly reported clinical signs (incidence over 5%) were mydriasis in 72 (40.9%) of 157, tachycardia in 53 (30.1%) of 157, agitation in 47 (26.7%) of 157, disorientation in 27 (15.3%) of 157, vocalization in 27 (15.3%) of 157, hyperactivity in 26 (14.8%) of 157, hyperthermia in 22 (12.5%) of 157, tachypnea in 21 (11.9%) of 157, panting in 19 (10.7%) of 157, pacing in 18 (10.2%) of 157, lethargy in 16 (10.1%) of 157, restlessness in 13 (7.6%) of 157, hypertension in 13 (7.6%) of 157, circling in 12 (6.8%) of 157, hyperesthesia in 12 (6.8%) of 157, hypersalivation in 12 (6.8%) of 157, anorexia in 11 (6.3%) of 157, and 9 of (5.1%) 157 for each of vomiting, head bobbing, anxiety, and ataxia.

Clinical signs with amphetamine salt medications started at 0.09 mg/kg with hyperactivity, agitation and restlessness. Tachycardia, hyperthermia, mydriasis, tachypnea, head bobbing, pacing, disorientation, vocalizing, tachypnea, anxiety, hypersalivation, staring, and hiding were seen starting at dosages from 0.15 to 0.2 mg/kg. Circling and hyperesthesia were seen at dosages starting at 0.21 to 0.3 mg/kg, and tremors and seizures were seen starting at 0.3 to 0.5 mg/kg.

Clinical signs with methylphenidate started at slightly higher doses than with amphetamines. Tachycardia and hyperthermia were seen starting at 0.26 mg/kg, hyperactivity at 0.56 mg/kg, anxiety and vomiting at 0.6 mg/kg, head bobbing at 0.7 mg/kg, tachypnea at 0.78 mg/kg, vocalizing at 0.97 mg/kg, hypertension at 1.3 mg/kg, circling at 1.6 mg/kg, and seizures at 13.7 mg/kg.

A case report involving a dog ingesting 19 mg/kg amphetamine (Adderall) in the literature showed increased alanine aminotransferase (ALT), alkaline phosphatase (ALP), and metarubricytosis. The dog was also mildly hypoglycemic. The metarubricytosis was attributed to pyrexia with ensuing damage to the bone marrow sinusoidal epithelium and vacular endothelium. The increased ALT may have occurred due to direct thermal damage to hepatocytes or secondary to hypoprofusion. The increased ALP was attributed to release of endogenous corticosteroids.[17] The blood work abnormalities resolved without treatment. No such bone marrow abnormalities were found in the APCC database.

Treatment Recommendations

There is no specific antidote for amphetamine toxicosis. When a pet is suspected to have ingested a stimulant medication, the immediate response depends on whether there are clinical signs on presentation for evaluation, the potential dose, and the formulation.

The goal of treatment is to prevent absorption of the medication, control the stimulatory signs, treat hyperthermia, treat cardiovascular effects, and protect the kidneys.

Emesis can be induced with apomorphine or hydrogen peroxide, if the exposure to a prompt release product was very recent (<30 minutes). Animals ingesting an extended-release product may benefit from emesis for up to 2 hours postexposure, if clinical signs are not yet being shown. Animals that are showing stimulatory signs, such as hyperactivity, pacing, or tremoring, are at risk for aspiration, and emesis should not be induced. Activated charcoal can be given. With extended-release products, a second half-dose can be given 8 hours after the first dose if stimulatory signs are still observed, but the pet should be monitored for signs of hypernatremia. With very high doses, gastric lavage can be performed under anesthesia with a cuffed endotracheal tube in place, if emesis cannot be safely induced. Activated charcoal can then be instilled via the orogastric tube before anesthesia is discontinued.

Phenothiazines should be considered the mainstay of controlling stimulatory signs with amphetamine intoxication. Phenothiazine tranquilizers are effective due to their effects on dopamine. They inhibit its release, block postsynaptic binding, and increase the turnover of dopamine in the CNS. Additionally, they also help to block the α-adrenergic activity induced by amphetamines.[18] Acepromazine can initially be given at 0.05 mg/kg IV and titrated to effect for stimulatory signs. The dose can be gradually increased to 0.1 to 1.0 mg/kg if clinical signs do not resolve with lower doses. Blood pressure should be monitored at higher doses to ensure that hypotension does not occur. Chlorpromazine can be used as an alternative treatment and is given at 0.5 mg/kg IV initially, and it may also be titrated up as needed to control stimulatory signs. Large doses of phenothiazines may be needed to control the clinical signs. Chlorpromazine has also been shown to have antiarrhythmic effects because it protects the heart from β_1 simulation due to an excess of epinephrine and norepinephrine, which can help alleviate tachycardia and tachyarrhythmias. Phenothiazines can also cause hypotensive and hypothermic effects, both of which are helpful in the treatment of amphetamine intoxication, due to the potential for hypertension and hyperthermia.[19]

Another important part of amphetamine toxicosis involves treatment for cardiac arrhythmias, although they often resolve with the treatment of the CNS stimulatory signs.[10] If the pet has been treated with phenothiazines and is resting quietly but still showing significant tachycardia, propranolol at 0.02 to 0.06 mg/kg slowly IV can be used. The total dosage is based on the clinical response of the tachycardia; monitoring an electrocardiogram (ECG) may be needed while giving propranolol, so it can be titrated to the target heart rate. Do not use this in hypertensive animals, as administration of propranolol can further worsen the hypertension. Treatment of tachycardia with propranolol has not been shown to improve survival in amphetamine intoxication cases.[11] Esmolol, which is a specific β_1-blocking agent, can be used if propranolol is not helping to resolve the tachycardia (25 to 200 μg/kg/min constant rate infusion).

Intravenous fluids should be instituted to help maintain normal hydration status, enhance renal excretion of the medication, and help protect the kidneys, should myoglobinuria occur. If giving fluids above the maintenance rate to a hypertensive animal, the lungs should be monitored for pulmonary edema.

Animals should be kept in a dark and quiet area of the hospital to decrease stimulation, especially in hyperesthetic animals. Thermoregulation in the form of fans and cool towels should help to cool hyperthermic animals. Control of stimulatory signs will usually also help prevent the worsening of hyperthermia.

The use of diazepam is generally avoided in patients showing stimulatory signs as its use can increase the chances of paradoxical hyperactivity and dysphoria.[10] If seizures are seen, they should be controlled with barbiturates. Phenobarbital can be dosed at 3 to 4 mg/kg IV. Gas anesthesia or proprofol can be used for seizures that are refractory to barbiturates. Diazepam, though not generally used with patients showing stimulatory signs can also be used with seizing patients. Antiepileptics will stop the physical signs of the seizures until levels of the amphetamines in the brain drop and the seizures are controlled in the brain. Tremors can be controlled with methocarbamol 50 to 220 mg/kg IV, given slowly to effect. The rate of infusion should not exceeded 2 mL/min.

Urine acidification may be helpful, as amphetamine elimination in the urine is enhanced at a pH between 4.5 and 5.5. This can be achieved with ammonium chloride administration at 100 to 200 mg/kg/day PO divided 4 times daily or ascorbic acid 20 to 30 mg/kg PO, SQ, IM, or IV. Urinary acidification should not be attempted if the pet is acidotic, if acid-base status cannot be monitored, or if rhabdomyolosis or evidence of acute renal failure is present.[11]

Monitoring of the Patient

Pet should have blood pressure and heart rate monitored closely. An ECG should be instituted in all pets with noted tachycardia or reflex bradycardia. Pets should be monitored for hyperactivity and CNS stimulation signs.

Urinalysis can be performed to watch for myoglobinuria. Pets with poorly controlled signs or pets that were significantly hyperthermic may need to have complete blood count and coagulation profile monitored to detect DIC.

Pets may require hospitalization, monitoring, and treatment for up to 72 hours depending on the dosage and whether the medication is a prompt- or extended-release product.

Prognosis

Prognosis is generally good, as long as CNS stimulation and CV signs can be controlled. Seizures and seizure-like activity and cardiac failure pose the highest risk to the pet. Pets with underlying cardiac disease may be at increased risk of developing life-threatening arrhythmias and may be more susceptible to severe signs.[10] Cause of death in amphetamine toxicity is generally attributed to DIC secondary to hyperthermia and respiratory failure.[20] No long-term effects are expected in animals making a full recovery.

ATOMOXETINE

Very little information has been published about the toxicity, mechanism of action, or treatment of atomoxetine in dogs and cats; therefore, information is generally limited to clinical experience in the treatment of atomoxetine intoxication and human data. Atomoxetine is a selective norepinephrine reuptake inhibitor that is used to treat ADHD. The exact mechanism by which produces its therapeutic effects in ADHD is unknown.[21]

Pharmacokinetics and Metabolism

Atomoxetine was well absorbed from the gastrointestinal tracts of dogs. Atomoxetine is highly protein bound at 97% in dogs. The bioavailability in the dog was about 74%.

This appears to have great variability between species and cannot be extrapolated to the cat. Atomoxetine is highly metabolized in the liver of dogs by N-demethylation, aromatic ring hydroxylation, benzylic ring hydroxylation, glucoronidation, and sulfonation. Atomoxetine and its metabolites were excreted 48% in the urine and 42% in the feces of dogs. The fecal excretion appears to be due to biliary elimination and not due to unabsorbed drug. In fact, very little atomoxetine was eliminated intact.[20]

Mechanism of Action

Atomoxetine is a methylphenoxy-benzene propanamine derivative with antidepressant activity. Atomoxetine purportedly enhances noradrenergic function via selective inhibition of the presynaptic norepinephrine transporter. The mechanism of action by which produces its therapeutic effects in ADHD is unknown.[16]

ASPCA Animal Poison Control Center's Experience

A review of the APCC toxicology database from 2006 to 2011 found atomoxetine toxicity cases involving 32 dogs and 14 cats.[16] These cases involved exposure to one agent (atomoxetine) only and were assessed as medium or high suspect cases (history of exposure and clinical signs were consistent with atomoxetine toxicosis). In the 32 canine cases, 2 dogs had a full recovery, but in 30 cases follow-up was not available. Signs were seen at doses starting at 1.2 mg/kg. The signs that were most commonly seen were mydriasis in 7 (21.9%) of 32 cases, agitation in 6 (18.8%) of 32, hyperactivity in 6 (18.8%) of 32, vomiting in 6 (18.8%) of 32, tachycardia in 5 (15.6%) of 32, hypersalivation in 4 (12.5%) of 32, lethargy in 4 (12.5%) of 32, and tremors, polydipsia, ataxia, and disorientation were all seen occasionally in 2 (6.3%) of 32. Finally, the following signs were rarely seen (in 1 [3.1%] of 32): anorexia, anxiety, apprehension, fasciculations, head bobbing, hesitancy to move, hyperesthesia, hypertension, hyperthermia, nystagmus, pacing, panting, paranoia, premature ventricular contractions, pruritis, seizure, staring, subdued, and trembling. In the 14 feline cases, 1 case was followed up successfully and that pet made a full recovery. The signs that were most commonly seen were hypersalivation in 4 (28.6%) of 14, mydriasis in 4 (28.6%) of 14, tremors in 2 (14.3%) of 14, vomiting in 2 (14.3%) of 14, shaking or trembling in 2 (14.3%) of 14, agitation in 1 (7.1%) of 14, anxiety in 1 (7.1%) of 14, hyperactivity in 1 (7.1%) of 14, hypertension in 1 (7.1%) of 14, lethargy in 1 (7.1%) of 14, and tachypnea in 1 (7.1%) of 14. No deaths were reported in these cases. With the feline and canine cases, lethargy and hypersalivation were seen starting at 1.2 mg/kg, ataxia was seen starting at 1.9 mg/kg, hypertension at 2.0 mg/kg, hyperactivity and agitation at 3.5 mg/kg, vomiting at 4.0 mg/kg, mydriasis and tachycardia at 4.4 mg/kg, head bobbing at 8.8 mg/kg, and tremors starting at 24 mg/kg.

Diagnosis

Diagnosis is based on history and recovery of pills or capsules in the vomitus. There is no on-site test for this medication. Serum levels may be available at a human hospital.

Differential Diagnoses

This includes methylxanthines (caffeine, theobromine, theophylline) and serotonergic medication intoxications.

Monitoring

The onset of clinical signs is generally 30 minutes to 2 hours. The duration of signs is between 12 and 24 hours. Pets should have heart rate, blood pressure, and CNS status monitored. Electrolytes and hydration status should be monitored in pets with significant vomiting.

Treatment

Treatment is based largely on providing good supportive care to patients exhibiting clinical signs, as there are little published data about the treatment of atomoxetine toxicity in dogs and cats.

Emesis can be induced in asymptomatic animals (as discussed in the section on amphetamine treatment). Activated charcoal can be given following emesis, but the animals should be monitored for hypernatremia. If a high dosage has been ingested, gastric lavage can be performed with the animal under anesthesia with a cuffed endotracheal tube in place, if emesis cannot be safely induced. Activated charcoal can then be instilled via the orogastric tube before anesthesia is discontinued.

Vomiting can be managed symptomatically with antiemetic medications. Intravenous fluids should be given to help support the pet's cardiovascular system and to help prevent dehydration secondary to gastrointestinal upset.

Diazepam at 0.1 to 0.5 mg/kg IV to effect or methocarbamol 50 to 220 mg/kg IV to effect can be used to treat tremors. Nitroprusside 0.5 to 10 μg/kg/min in D5W titrated to effect can be used to treat hypertension. Diphenhydramine 2 mg/kg IM can be used for atomoxetine-induced dystonia (involuntary muscle spasms and contractions).

Affected animals should be kept in a dark and quiet area in order to decrease stimulation, if the animal is hyperesthetic. Thermoregulation in the form of fans and cool towels should help to cool hyperthermic animals. Control of stimulatory signs will also help prevent the worsening of hyperthermia.

Prognosis

Prognosis should be considered good and animals generally respond well to treatment. Animals with underlying liver disease, hypertension, tachycardia, or other cardiovascular or cerebrovascular disease may be more sensitive to this medication.[22] No long-term effects are expected.

SUMMARY

In summary, amphetamines or similar stimulants and the non-amphetamine atomoxetine are commonly used in the treatment of ADD/ADHD in humans. Because these medications are often found in homes, dog and cat exposure to these medications is a fairly common intoxication. Amphetamine intoxication can cause life-threatening CNS and CV stimulation, even when small amounts are ingested. This medication is quickly and well absorbed orally and the onset of clinical signs is generally 30 minutes to 2 hours with immediate release products. Treatment is aimed at preventing absorption, controlling the stimulatory signs, and protecting the kidneys. Prognosis is generally good, and treatment is very rewarding with control of the stimulatory signs.

Atomoxetine also has a fast onset of action with development of clinical signs within 30 minutes to 2 hours. Stimulatory signs, such as hyperactivity and tachycardia are often seen with atomoxetine toxicosis. Treatment is aimed at providing symptomatic and supportive care to patients showing clinical signs. Prognosis is generally good with animals receiving prompt and appropriate treatment.

REFERENCES

1. DRUGDEX System [intranet database]. Version 5.1. Greenwood Village (CO): Thomson Reuters (Healthcare) Inc.
2. Adams HR. Adrenergic agonists and antagonists. In: Riviere JE, Papch MG, editors. Veterinary pharmacology and therapeutics. Ames (IO): Wiley-Blackwell; 2009. p. 141–2.
3. Mitler MM, Soave O, Dement WC. Narcolepsy in seven dogs. J Am Vet Med Assoc 1976;168:1036–8.
4. Beasley VR, Dorman DC, Fikes JD, et al. A systems affected approach to veterinary toxicology. Urbana: University of Illinois; 1999. p. 133–4.
5. Volmer P. Human drugs of abuse. In: Bonaguara JD, Twedt DC, editors. Kirk's current veterinary therapy XIV. St Louis (MO): Elsevier; 2009. p. 144–5.
6. Diniz PP, Sousa MG, Gerardi DG, et al. Amphetamine poisoning in a dog: case report, literature review and veterinary medicine perspectives. Vet Hum Toxicol 2003;45:315–7.
7. Amphetamines. DRUGDEX System [intranet database]. Version 5.1. Greenwood Village (CO): Thomson Reuters (Healthcare) Inc.
8. Genovese DW, Gwaltney-Brant SM. Methylphenidate toxicosis in dogs: 128 cases (2001-2008). JAVMA 2010;12:1438–43.
9. Methylphenidate. In: POISINDEX® System (electronic version). Greenwood Village (CO): Thomson Reuters (Healthcare) Inc.; 2011. Available at: http://www.thomsonhc.com. Accessed January 12, 2012.
10. Bischoff K. Toxicity of drugs of abuse. In: Gupta R, editor. Veterinary toxicology: basic and clinical principles. Amsterdam: Elsevier; 2007. p. 401–3.
11. Wismer T. Amphetamines. In: Osweiler GD, Howvda, LR, Brutlag AG, et al, editors. Clinical companion: small animal toxicology. Ames (IO): Wiley-Blackwell; 2011. p. 125–30.
12. Teo SK, Stirling DI, Thomas SD, et al. A 90 day oral gavage toxicity study of D-methylphenidate and D,L methylphenidate in beagle dogs. Int J Toxicol 2003;22:215–26.
13. Kissebereth WC, Trammel HL. Toxicology of selected pesticides, drugs, and chemicals. Illicit and abused drugs. Vet Clin North Am Small Anim Pract 1990;20(2):405–18.
14. Green CE, LeValley SE, Tyson CA. Comparison of amphetamine metabolism using isolated hepatocytes from five species including human. Am Soc Pharmacol Exp Ther 1986;237:931–6.
15. Teitler J. Evaluation of a human on-site urine multidrug test for emergency use with dogs. J Am Anim Hosp Assoc 2009;45:59–66.
16. ANTOX: ASPCA Animal Poison Control Center's toxicology database. Urbana (IL): 2003–2011.
17. Wilcox A, Russell KE. Hematologic changes associate with Adderall toxicity in a dog. Vet Clin Pathol 2008;37:184–9.
18. Mensching D, Volmer PA. Neurotoxicity. In: Gupta R, editor. Veterinary toxicology: basic and clinical principles. Amsterdam: Elsevier; 2007. p. 135.
19. Gross ME, Booth NH. Tranquilizers. In: Adams HR, editor. Veterinary pharmacology and therapeutics. Ames (IO): Iowa State University Press; 1995.
20. Atomoxetine. In: POISINDEX® System (electronic version). Greenwood Village (CO): Thomson Reuters (Healthcare) Inc.; 2010. Available at: http://www.thomsonhc.com. Accessed January 12, 2012.
21. Mattuiz EL, Ponsler GD, Barbuch RJ, et al. Disposition and metabolic fate of atomoxetine hydrochloide: pharmacokinetics, metabolism, and excretion in the fischer 344 rat and beagle dog. Am Soc Pharmacol Exp Ther 2003;31:88–97.
22. Atomoxetine protocol. Urbana (IL): ASPCA Animal Poison Control Center.

Toxicology of Frequently Encountered Nonsteroidal Anti-Inflammatory Drugs in Dogs and Cats

Safdar A. Khan, DVM, MS, PhD*, Mary Kay McLean, MS

KEYWORDS

• Toxicology • NSAIDs • Incidents • Dogs • Cats

The nonsteroidal anti-inflammatory drugs (NSAIDs) are a group of heterogeneous compounds other than steroids that suppresses one or more substances produced during inflammatory reactions. NSAIDs are extensively used in both human and veterinary medicine for their antipyretic, anti-inflammation, and analgesic properties. Chemically, most NSAIDs are substituted organic acids. Although most NSAIDs consist of a wide range of pharmacologically active agents with diverse chemical structures and properties, they have similar therapeutic and adverse effects associated with their use. Each year the ASPCA Animal Poison Control Center (APCC) receives hundreds of cases involving acute accidental ingestion of human and veterinary approved NSAIDs in dogs and cats. The purpose of this article is provide a brief overview on the classification, mechanism of action, and pharmacologic and toxicologic properties of most commonly encountered human and veterinary NSAIDs in dogs and cats. For this purpose, the top 10 most frequently reported NSAIDs, as reported to the APCC in dogs and cats from 2005 to 2010, were selected. The article discusses general information about NSAIDs—classification, uses, pharmacokinetics, mechanisms of actions, and treatment followed by specific toxicity information involving the top 10 NSAIDs reported to the APCC.

GENERAL USES AND CLASSIFICATION

NSAIDs are used to treat a variety of conditions, including headaches and migraines, rheumatoid arthritis, osteoarthritis, inflammatory arthropathies, acute gout, dysmenorrheal, metastatic bone pain, postoperative pain, mild-to-moderate pain due to inflammation and tissue injury, pyrexia, ileus, and renal colic. In dogs, NSAIDs are approved for osteoarthritis and postoperative pain. Along with their benefits, NSAIDs

The authors have nothing to disclose.

ASPCA Animal Poison Control Center, 1717 South Philo Road, Suite 36, Urbana, IL 61802, USA

* Corresponding author.

E-mail address: safdar.khan@aspca.org

also have some undesirable effects that can be seen both with therapeutic use and in overdose situations.

The first NSAID discovered in 1897 was acetylsalicylic acid, or aspirin. In 1961, ibuprofen was discovered after scientists had been searching for an option that had less risk for adverse gastrointestinal (GI) effects compared to aspirin. Ibuprofen became available on an over-the-counter basis in the United States in 1984. In 1999, in a continued attempt to discover an NSAID with even less risk for side effects, the first selective cyclooxygenase (COX)-2 inhibitor was approved by the Food and Drug Administration (FDA). Most NSAIDs are substituted organic acids classified into 3 main groups: carboxylic acids, enolic acids, and the newer COX-2 inhibitors (**Table 1**). The carboxylic acids can be further divided into salicylic acids, acetic acids, propionic acid, and fenamic acid. The enolic acid group can be further divided into pyazolones and oxicams. NSAIDs are placed in each of these groups based on their mechanism of action or chemical structure if the mechanism of action is not, or was not, known at the time of classification. Some veterinary approved NSAIDs (approved by the FDA) for use in dogs include Etogesic (etodolac), Rimadyl (carprofen), Metacam (meloxicam), Deramaxx (deracoxib), Previcox (firocoxib), and Zubrin (tepoxalin). Meloxicam is also approved for postoperative pain relief in cats (0.3 mg/kg SC once).

INCIDENT DATA

The widespread availability of NSAIDs has resulted in a marked increase in the number of overdose cases in humans. During 1985 to 1988, 55,800 cases of ibuprofen exposure were reported to the American Association of Poison Control Centers (AAPCC). In 1994 alone, the total number of NSAID exposures was 50,154, of which 35,703 were related to ibuprofen exposure. Despite their widespread use, the adverse effects associated with NSAID use are relatively few. One report suggests the incidence of adverse drug reactions associated with NSAID use is 24.4 per 1 million prescriptions. The fatal adverse reactions are estimated at 1.1 per 1 million prescriptions.[1] According to more recent information compiled by the AAPCC from 2003 to 2007, approximately 4% of all human incidents reported to AAPCC involved exposure to an NSAID. This translates to about 90,000 to 100,000 calls annually. The fatality review board of the AAPCC in their annual report during 2006 and 2007 assigned 5 fatalities and 107 life-threatening manifestations to NSAID exposures.[2]

Although there are several case reports that discuss toxicity reactions resulting from exposure to different NSAIDs in dogs and cats, the total incidence of adverse effects resulting from NSAID ingestion in dogs and cats is not known. Data from the ASPCA Animal Poison Control Center (APCC) electronic medical record database involving exposure to different NSAIDs (human and veterinary approved NSAID) was reviewed from 2005 to 2010. This review included information retrieved from the APCC public database. During this time period, the APCC received 22,206 reports of animals exposed to different types of NSAIDs in dogs and cats. These cases accounted for approximately 3% of the total cases called into the APCC. Of 22,206 incidents, 17,193 involved exposure to one agent only (1 NSAID). The dog was the most commonly reported species (15,823 dogs), followed by the cat (1244 cats). The other animals exposed to NSAIDs included birds, horses, ferrets, and pigs. The most common NSAID involved was ibuprofen (10,763 incidents) followed by aspirin (4170 incidents), naproxen (2690 incidents), deracoxib (1683 incidents), meloxicam (609 incidents), diclofenac (506 incidents), piroxicam (217 incidents), indomethacin (201 incidents), nabumetone (134 incidents), and etodolac (93 incidents). Of the 3 classes of NSAIDs, exposures to carboxylic acid–derivative was most commonly reported, with ibuprofen being the most commonly reported ingredient, followed by aspirin and naproxen.

Table 1		
Classification scheme of commonly available NSAIDs		
Carboxylic Acid	**Enolic Acid**	**COX-2 Inhibitors**
Salicylic acids • Aspirin • Diflunisal • Salsalate	Pyazolones • Oxyphenbutazone • Phenylbutazone • Azapropazone • Feprazone • Ampyrone • Clofezone • Kebuzone • Metamizole • Mofebutazone • Phenazone • Sulfinpyrazone	• Celecoxib • Deracoxib • Etoricoxib • Firocoxib • Lumiracoxib • Parecoxib • Rofecoxib • Valdecoxib
Acetic acids • Diclofenac • Alclofenac • Fenclofenac • Indomethacin • Sulindac • Tolmectin • Etodolac • Ketorolac • Nabumetone	Oxicam • Piroxicam • Sudoxicam • Isoxicam • Droxicam • Lornoxicam • Meloxicam • Tenoxicam • Amiroxicam	
Propionic acid • Ibuprofen • Naproxen • Flurbiprofen • Fenbufen • Benoxaprofen • Fenoprofen • Indoprofen • Ketoprofen • Pirprofen • Suprofen • Tiaprofenic acid • Oxaprozin • Loxoprofen		
Fenamic acid • Flufenamic acid • Mefenamic acid • Meclofenamic acid • Niflumic acid • Tolfenamic acid		

GENERAL INFORMATION REGARDING ABSORPTION, DISTRIBUTION, METABOLISM, AND EXCRETION

Most NSAIDs are absorbed rapidly and almost completely following oral administration. Peak plasma concentration is usually achieved within 2 to 4 hours after oral administration. Absorption occurs mainly in the stomach and upper small intestine and is influenced by pH. Since NSAIDs are weak acids, they are un-ionized in the highly acidic gastric environment. In this state, NSAIDs are lipid soluble and easily diffuse into gastric cells, whereas the pH is higher and the drug dissociates. In this manner, NSAIDs become "ion-trapped" within the gastric cells. These high local concentrations contribute to the GI side effects of NSAIDs.[3]

Concurrent administration of aluminum or magnesium antacids or presence of food may delay absorption of NSAIDs. Although presence of antacids may delay absorption, the total amount of drug absorbed is unaffected. A larger fraction of the NSAID dose is absorbed in the small intestine under these circumstances. Rectal administration of NSAIDs does not provide any advantage because absorption is erratic and incomplete.[3]

All NSAIDs are highly protein bound (98%–99%), mainly to albumin, only the unbound drug is biologically active. NSAIDs are metabolized in the liver and metabolites are mainly excreted in the urine. The major mechanism of conjugation is with glucuronic acid, which in some cases, is preceded by oxidation and hydroxylation.[1] In general, less than 10% of a dose is excreted unchanged by the kidneys; however, larger amounts of indomethacin, flurbiprofen, tolmectin, and piroxicam are eliminated by this route.[1,3,4] The high degree of protein binding restricts these drugs to the plasma compartment, accounting for small volumes of distribution. Most NSAIDs bind only to albumin. The concentration of free drug rapidly increases after the albumin binding sites are saturated, leading to rapid efficacy of most NSAIDs. The kidney rapidly excretes the unbound drug, so that accumulation is prevented. Because the NSAIDs are strongly protein bound, they can be displaced from binding sites or can displace other protein-bound drugs (for example corticosteroids), potentiating the effects of these drugs.[3]

Elimination half-lives of NSAIDs vary considerably ranging from 1 to 1.5 hours for tolmectin, ketoprofen, and diclofenac and 25 to 50 hours for oxaprozin and piroxicam.[1,3,4] In neonates and patients with renal or hepatic disease, half-lives of NSAIDs are usually increased. Many NSAIDs such as naproxen, sulindac, indomethacin, diclofenac, flufenamic acid, ibuprofen, phenylbutazone, and piroxicam undergo significant enterohepatic recirculation.[3] Naproxen in dogs is known to have much longer half-life (74 hours) compared to other NSAIDs.

GENERAL MECHANISMS OF ACTIONS

Salicylates inhibit the enzyme cyclooxygenase (COX) that enables the synthesis of prostaglandins (PGs), which mediate inflammation and fever. All members of the salicylate class have similar properties because the parent compound is first metabolized to salicylic acid. Salicylic acid is then further metabolized to the primary metabolite salicyluric acid by glycine, and then to the more minor metabolites phenolic glucuronide, acylglucuronide, and gentisic acid by glucruonide and oxidation. Salicylic acid is also eliminated unchanged in the urine. Alkaline urine allows for a greater percentage to be eliminated unchanged than acidic urine.

The 2 forms or isoenzymes of COX are COX-1 and COX-2.[5,6] COX-1 appears to be present naturally in the body and is involved in important physiologic functions such as autoregulation of renal blood flow. It is mainly found in the stomach, kidney, endothelium, and platelets. COX-2, which is an inducible form of COX, is believed to be responsible for production of inflammatory mediators.[5] COX-2 is mainly produced by monocytes, fibroblasts, synoviocytes, and chondrocytes in association with inflammation. It has been suggested that inhibition of COX-2 helps decrease inflammation and that inhibition of COX-1 may lead to adverse effects associated with the use of NSAIDs such as GI ulceration and kidney damage.[5] Thus, the NSAIDs that act mainly against COX-1 are more likely to result in GI tract injury compared to NSAIDs that act mostly against COX-2.

Other NSAIDs including carboxylic acids, enolic acids, and COX-2 selective inhibitors all share the ability to inhibit PG synthesis by inhibiting COX just like salicylates. Lipo-oxygenase (LOX) also aids in the synthesis of PG, and most NSAIDs are unable to directly affect the LOX enzyme.

PROSTAGLANDINS

PGs are unsaturated fatty acid compounds derived from 20-carbon essential fatty acids found in tissue membranes, primarily phospholipids.[3,7] PGs are synthesized from the dietary essential fatty acids linoleic acid and linolenic acid. The most important precursor to PG synthesis is arachidonic acid (AA). PG synthesis is started within the cell by cleavage of AA from the membrane phospholipids through the action of cellular phospholipase. Synthesis is stimulated due to membrane damage from any mechanisms such as trauma, infection, fever, or platelet aggregation. The phospholipase causes phospholipids in the membrane to release AA into the cytoplasm. AA is then available for use in the COX or LOX pathways.[7] The COX pathway leads to production of PG (PGH_2, PGI_2, PGE_2, $PGF_{2\alpha}$), prostacyclin, and thromboxane (TX)A_2, and the LOX cascade results in the production of leukotrienes (**Fig. 1**).[5] Collectively, PGs, TXs, and leukotrienes are known as eicosanoids. TXs is primarily produced by platelets and is a potent vasoconstrictor and inducer of platelet aggregation.[5] PGs are known as local hormones since they have an effect on target cells in the immediate vicinity of their site of synthesis. PGs are produced in small quantities, have a short half-life (seconds to minutes), are not stored in appreciable quantities, and are present throughout the body.

PGs are involved in a number of activities including inflammation, protection of the GI mucosa against injury, and regulation of renal blood flow.[6] Decreased acid production, increased gastric mucus production, increased gastric mucosal cytoprotection, and enhancement of renal blood flow during times of reduced renal perfusion are some of the beneficial effects of PGs.[8] PGI_2 is the main PG produced in the renal cortex, whereas PGE_2 is the primary PG produced in the renal medulla.[5] PGE_2 and prostacyclin are potent vasodilators and hyperalgesic. They presumably contribute to erythema, swelling, and pain during inflammation.[6]

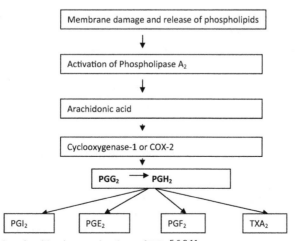

Fig. 1. Pathway involved in the production of PGs.[5,6,8,11]

GI tract abnormalities and renal toxicity are the most common adverse effects associated with NSAID use.[5,9] It has long been recognized that some NSAIDs are associated with a greater risk of GI toxicosis than others. The reason for this has been partly explained recently with the identification of different forms of COX. The 2 forms or isoenzymes of COX are COX-1 and COX-2.[5,6] COX-1 appears to be present naturally in the body and is involved in important physiologic functions such as autoregulation of renal blood flow. It is mainly found in the stomach, kidney, endothelium, and platelets. COX-2, which is an inducible form of COX, is believed to be responsible for production of inflammatory mediators.[5] COX-2 is mainly produced by monocytes, fibroblasts, synoviocytes, and chondrocytes in association with inflammation. It has been suggested that inhibition of COX-2 helps decrease inflammation and inhibition of COX-1 may lead to adverse effects associated with the use of NSAIDs such as GI ulceration and kidney damage.[5] Thus, the NSAIDs that act mainly against COX-1 are more likely to result in GI tract injury compared to NSAIDs that act mostly against COX-2.

Role of PGs in Gastropathies Associated with NSAID Use

There are a number of defense mechanisms that play a role in preventing gastric ulceration resulting from normal insults to the GI tract. It is believed that endogenous PGs play an integral part in these defense mechanisms. The most superficial barrier to gastric ulceration is a protective mucous gel layer that provides a defense against gastric acid. This layer contains a bicarbonate-rich fluid secreted by the gastric epithelium. Bicarbonate mixes with the gel to produce a gradient that forms an effective barrier to acid penetration. The gel also contains phospholipids that make it hydrophobic and prevent back-diffusion of acid from the gastric lumen to the epithelial cells. The second defense mechanism is due to the ability of surface epithelial cells to rapidly migrate and divide to repair small defects. Moreover, the vasculature of the stomach is designed so that bicarbonate can be rapidly transported from parietal cells to the surface epithelium to replenish used bicarbonate. Adequate mucosal blood flow allows the epithelium to tolerate a wide array of insults, whereas reduced mucosal blood flow may result in severe muscosal injury.[6,9]

It is generally believed that NSAIDs can induce gastric damage through both local and systemic effects. Local effects are associated with the physical properties of NSAIDs. Most NSAIDs are slightly acidic and may become concentrated in the gastric mucosa through a process known as ion trapping. This can lead to direct cellular injury. Aspirin is especially known to cause these local toxic effects. Systemic effects are thought to be associated with the inhibition of endogenous PG production. Decreased PG production can result in decreased mucin quality and bicarbonate content of the mucous gel layer, making the mucosa more vulnerable to acid-induced injury. NSAIDs are also thought to decrease mucosal proliferation, although it has been suggested recently that alterations in gastric cellular proliferation may not play a significant role in the development of NSAID-induced gastropathy. NSAIDs may also cause areas of reduced blood flow within the mucosa by inhibiting endogenous prostanoids that have a vasodilatory effect.[6,8 9] Adherence of neutrophils to vascular endothelium contributes to gastric mucosal injury as a result of activation of neutrophils and release of oxygen-derived free radicals and other enzymes.[6] The NSAID-induced gastropathy can be reduced in dogs by administering exogenous PGs. Misoprostol, a synthetic PGE_1 analogue, has been shown to reduce aspirin-induced gastropathy in clinical studies in dogs.[10]

Role of PGs in Renal Toxicosis Associated with NSAID Use

PGE_2 and PGI_2 function as vasodilatory agents to regulate renal blood flow. During a period of decreased renal perfusion, PGE_2 and PGI_2 cause afferent arteriolar dilation, which in turn help maintain renal blood flow, counteracting the effect of systemic vasoconstrictors such as vasopressin, angiotensin, and norepinephrine.[5,11] Clinically, important adverse renal effects of NSAIDs are primarily the result of decreased PG production. Usually, short-term use of NSAIDs by healthy individuals has little effect on renal hemodynamics and function. During periods of hemodynamic compromise such as dehydration, hemorrhage, anesthesia, heart failure, or liver or kidney disease, circulating vasoconstrictors are released to maintain vascular resistance and blood pressure at the expense of organ blood flow. Under these conditions, the kidney becomes increasingly dependent on the vasodilatory effects of PG to maintain renal blood flow and glomerular filtration rate. The use of NSAIDs during hemodynamic compromise may result in ischemic injury of the kidneys, which may progress to acute renal failure.[5,6] NSAID-induced nephropathy is characterized by papillary necrosis and interstitial nephritis. This condition has been associated with the use of several different types of NSAIDs.

GENERAL TREATMENT RECOMMENDATIONS FOR ACUTE NSAID OVERDOSE

The goals of treatment of acute NSAID overdose in dogs and cats consist of aggressive decontamination, supportive care, GI protection, and monitoring of renal functions. In clinically normal patients within few hours of exposure with no clinical signs of toxicosis present, emesis should be induced with 3% hydrogen peroxide or apomophine in dogs. In cats, emesis can be tried with xylazine with varying degrees of success. Gastric lavage or eneterogastric lavage should be considered in animals in which emesis cannot be induced due to the presence of neurologic signs such as coma, ataxia, or seizures. Induction of emesis should be followed with administration of activated charcoal (1–3 g/kg PO; use labeled dose for commercial products). Since many NSAIDs are known to undergo enterohepatic recirculation, multiple doses (2–6 doses) of activated charcoal every 6 to 8 hours may be needed. Patients receiving activated charcoal need to be watched for signs of hypernatremia (ataxia, tremors, seizures) and aspiration.[12,13] GI irritation and ulceration can be treated with GI protectants such as H2 blockers (cimetidine, famotidine, ranitidine) or proton pump inhibitors (omeprazole, esomeprazole, pantoprazole) and sucralfate. Misoprostol (Cytotec), a synthetic PG analogue, has been successfully used to prevent GI ulcers when used concurrently with some NSAIDs; however, its usefulness in acute NSAID overdose is not known. Treatment with GI protectants may be needed for 7 to 10 days or more depending on the dose of the NSAID and severity of the clinical signs present. Control vomiting with antiemetics like maropitant (Cerenia) or metoclopramide (Reglan). Broad-spectrum antibiotics and surgical repair may be needed for perforated ulcers and associated peritonitis.

Animals ingesting nephrotoxic doses of NSAIDs often require intravenous fluids at twice the maintenance rate for 48 to 96 hours depending on the dose and the type of NSAID involved. The use of dopamine (2.5 μg/kg/min) may increase renal perfusion and minimize degree of renal impairment. The use of sodium bicarbonate (1–3 mEq/kg) in salicylate poisoning may increase excretion of parent compound and its metabolites in alkaline urine. With nephrotoxic dose ingestion, monitoring of renal functions (blood urea nitrogen [BUN], serum creatinine, phosphorous) on presentation and then daily for 3 to 5 days and serial urinalysis analysis with monitoring of specific gravity are often needed. Large NSAID overdoses can also result in increase in liver enzymes along with signs of renal damage. For such patients, monitor liver-specific enzymes (alanine transaminase, aspartate aminotransferase, alkaline phosphatases, gamma-glutamyl transferase) for few days. SAMe (S-adenosylmethionine) may be helpful for patients showing signs of increased liver enzymes.

Control seizures with diazepam or barbiturates as needed. Repeated doses (2–3 doses within 5–10 minutes) of naloxone (0.01–0.02 mg/kg IV) can be tried in comatose and severely depressed dogs, as are seen with large doses of ibuprofen (>400 mg/kg). Provide respiratory support and treat hypothermia and acidosis as needed. Treat any other associated clinical signs symptomatically.

SPECIFIC TOXICITY INFORMATION REGARDING THE TOP 10 MOST FREQUENTLY REPORTED NSAIDs IN DOGS AND CATS
Ibuprofen

Ibuprofen [2-(4-isobutylphenyl)propionic acid] is an NSAID with anti-inflammatory, antipyretic, and analgesic properties in animals and humans. Ibuprofen has similar pharmacologic actions to other NSAIDs such as aspirin, phenylbutazone, and indomethacin.[14]

Ibuprofen is commonly used to treat acute and chronic rheumatoid arthritis and osteoarthritis as well as headaches and fever and various joint, musculoskeletal, and gynecologic disorders.[15] It is available over the counter in 50-, 100-, and 200-mg tablets and 100 mg/5 mL suspension. Prescription strengths are available at 400, 600, and 800 mg. Ibuprofen is also available in combination with decongestant products.[14,16]

Before the availability of veterinary approved NSAID, ibuprofen was recommended in dogs at a dose of 5 mg/kg.[15,17,18] However, Ibuprofen may cause gastric ulcers and perforations in dogs at this dose and is generally not recommended for prolonged use anymore.[17,18] GI irritation, GI hemorrhages, and renal damage are the most commonly reported toxic effects of ibuprofen ingestion in dogs.[14–16,19–21] In addition, CNS depression, hypotension, ataxia, cardiac effects, and seizures can be seen. Ibuprofen has a narrow margin of safety in dogs.[18] Dogs dosed with ibuprofen orally at 8 mg/kg/d or 16 mg/kg/d for 30 days showed gastric ulceration or erosions along with clinical signs of GI disturbances.[22] According to one report, acute single ingestion of ibuprofen in dogs at 100 to 125 mg/kg can lead to clinical signs of vomiting, diahrrea, nausea, abdominal pain, and anorexia.[19] Renal failure can be seen with 175 to 300 mg/kg. Central nervous system (CNS) effects (seizure, ataxia, depression, and coma) along with renal and GI signs can be seen when dosage is greater than 400 mg/kg. Greater than 600 mg/kg is considered a lethal dose in the dog.[13,19,23]

Cats are susceptible to ibuprofen toxicosis at approximately half the doses required to cause toxicosis in dogs although no experimental data are available to confirm this observation.[19] Cats are especially sensitive to NSAID toxicosis because they have a limited glucuronyl-conjugating capacity.[24,25] Clinical signs of ibuprofen toxicosis in ferrets are more severe than those expected at similar doses in dogs. Typical toxic effects of ibuprofen in ferrets include CNS and GI and renal system effects.[26,27]

Aspirin

Aspirin (acetylsalicylic acid or ASA), the salicylate ester of acetic acid, is the prototype of salicylate drugs. It is a weak acid derived from phenol.[14,28] Aspirin is available as plain, film-coated, buffered, time-release, and enteric-coated tablets, suppositories, and capsules.[29] Oral bioavailability of aspirin may vary due to difference in drug formulation. Aspirin reduces PG and TX synthesis by inhibition of COX. Salicylates also uncouple mitochondrial oxidative phosphorylation and inhibit specific dehydrogenases.[14,28,30] Platelets are incapable of synthesizing new COX. This fact causes an effect on platelet aggregation.[14,30] Salicylates also inhibit the formation and release of kinins, stabilize lysosomes, and remove energy needed for inflammation by uncoupled oxidative phosphorylation.[29]

Aspirin is recommended at 10 to 20 mg/kg twice daily in dogs and 10 to 20 mg/kg every 48 hours in cats.[30] Aspirin has a relatively good margin of safety in most species. Aspirin toxicosis is usually characterized by depression, fever, hyperpnea, seizures, respiratory alkalosis, metabolic acidosis, coma, gastric irritation or ulceration, liver necrosis, or increased bleeding time.[28,29] Ataxia and seizures may occur as a consequence of aspirin intoxication, although the exact etiology is unknown.

Aspirin is a phenol compound and cats have poor ability to glucuronide it. Cats are deficient in glucuronyl transferase and have prolonged excretion of aspirin (half-life in cats is 37.5 hours). Half-life of salicylates can increase with dose. In one study, no clinical signs of toxicosis occurred when cats were dosed with 25 mg/kg of aspirin every 48 hours for up to 4 weeks. Doses of 5 grains (325 mg) twice a day were lethal to cats. Erosive gastritis has been seen after a single 5-grain dose in dogs.[28]

Dogs can tolerate aspirin better than can cats. Doses of 25 mg/kg 3 times daily of regular aspirin caused mucosal erosions in 50% of dogs in 2 days, while there was minimal damage seen in animals receiving buffered and enteric-coated aspirin.[29] Gastric ulcers were induced in 4 of 6 dogs at 35 mg/kg of aspirin given orally 3 times a day on day 30 of dosing.[6,10] Similarly, gastric ulcers were seen in 3 of 7 dogs following aspirin administration at 50 mg/kg orally twice after 5 to 6 weeks of dosing.[19] In dogs, toxicity has been noted at doses of 100 to 300 mg/kg/day PO for 1 to 4 weeks.[29] Acute ingestion at 450 to 500 mg/kg can cause signs of GI disturbances, hyperthermia, panting, seizure, or coma.[19] Alkalosis due to stimulation of respiratory center can occur in the early course of intoxication. Metabolic acidosis with an elevated anion gap usually develops later.[19]

Naproxen

Naproxen, a propionic acid derivative, is an NSAID available over the counter as acid or the sodium salt. Structurally and pharmacologically, naproxen is similar to carprofen and ibuprofen. In humans and the dog, it has been used for its anti-inflammatory, analgesic, and antipyretic properties. It is generally better tolerated than aspirin or indomethacin at therapeutic doses.[31,32] Because of its relatively long plasma half-life (12–15 hours) in humans, it can be conveniently administered twice daily. The half-life of naproxen in dogs is very long at 74 hours.[30]

Several cases of naproxen toxicity have been described in dogs. In one case report, naproxen was administered to a dog at 11.11 mg/kg PO for 3 days and resulted in melena, frequent vomiting, and abdominal pain. Abdominal radiograph revealed generalized gastric wall thickening. Further investigation with barium sulfate suspension (barium meal) confirmed presence of a perforating duodenal ulcer. Due to perforating nature of the ulcer, bacteria- and barium sulfate–induced peritonitis was also diagnosed. Surgical resection of the ulcer along with supportive care (antibiotics, fluids, cimetidine, sucralfate, B-complex) resulted in complete recovery. The authors concluded that due to lack of efficacy and safety information of naproxen, this drug should not be used in dogs at doses comparable to those for humans.[33]

Similarly, a 34-kg dog developed vomiting, progressive weakness, and stumbling following naproxen administration by the owner at 5.6 mg/kg/d for 7 days. Feces were tarry, and dog had paled mucous membranes. On radiography, hepatomegaly and prostatomegaly were observed. Blood work showed regenerative anemia, neutrophilia with a left shift, high BUN (66 mg/dL) and creatinine (2.1 mg/dL), and lower total protein (4 g/dL), albumin (2.1 g/dL), potassium (3.1 mEq/L), and total CO_2 (15 mm/L). Treatment with fluids, antacids, and antihistamines along with multi-vitamins resulted in recovery in 11 days.[34]

A 13-year-old Basenji dog was given naproxen 250 mg twice a day for 7 days by the owner for the treatment of rheumatoid arthritis. The dog showed signs of anorexia, weight loss, and lethargy over a period of 2 weeks. Physical examination showed pale mucous membranes, moderate abdominal pain, and melena. Blood work showed left-shift regenerative anemia. Abdominal radiography revealed mild splenomegaly and prostatomegaly. Urinalysis also indicated the presence of increased granular and hyaline casts. Dog recovered with supportive care in 3 weeks.[35]

Toxicity of naproxen from a single oral dose of 35 mg/kg (250-mg tablet in a 7-kg dachshund) resulted in clinical signs of listlessness, vomiting, diarrhea, abdominal pain, and profound depression within the first 24 hours of administration followed by profuse hematemesis and melena and low plasma proteins. The dog recovered with supportive care over the next 3 days.[36] The same author reported another case of naproxen toxicosis in which naproxen was administered twice, approximately 48 hours apart, to an aged Labrador at 14.2 mg/kg. Within 12 hours after the last dose, the dog developed severe hemorrhagic dysentery. Due to his age and the severity of illness, the dog was euthanized. On post-mortem, gastric mucosa was erythematous and hemorrhagic. Similar but more severe lesions were found in small intestinal and colonic mucosae.[36]

There are several other reports of naproxen toxicosis in the dog described in the literature.[37–42]

Deracoxib

Deracoxib is a coxib, COX-2 inhibitor used in veterinary medicine to treat osteoarthritis in dogs. Deracoxib is available in chewable tablets that have beef flavoring to make them more palatable. Tablets are either 25, 75, or 100 mg and are sold under the trade name Deramaxx. It is not approved or recommended for use in cats.[43] For control of pain and inflammation, the recommended dose is 1 to 2 mg/kg once daily or 3 to 4 mg/kg/d as needed for postoperative pain, not to exceed 7 days of therapy.[43]

Deracoxib is a coxib-class NSAID. In vitro studies have shown that deracoxib predominantly inhibits COX-2 and spares COX-1 at therapeutic dosages.[43,44] This, theoretically, would inhibit production of the PGs that contribute to pain and inflammation (COX-2) and spare those that maintain normal GI and renal function (COX-1).

After oral administration to dogs, bioavailability is greater than 90%; the time to peak serum concentration occurs at approximately 2 hours.[43] The presence of food in the gut can enhance bioavailability. Terminal elimination half-life in the dog is dependent on dose and is about 3 hours after dosages up to 8 mg/kg. The half-life at a dose of 20 mg/kg is approximately 19 hours.[43] Drug accumulation can occur with higher dosages, leading to increased toxic effects as increased COX-1 inhibition can occur at higher concentrations.

After administering 1-mg of deracoxib in cats orally, peak levels (0.28 mcg/mL) occurred about 3.6 hours after administration. Elimination half-life was about 8 hours.

There are little data available regarding this drug's acute toxicity. A 14-day study in dogs demonstrated no clinically observable adverse effects in the dogs that received 10 mg/kg. Dogs that received 25, 50, or 100 mg/kg/d for 10 to 11 days survived but showed vomiting and melena; no hepatic or renal lesions were demonstrated in these dogs.[43]

Because nonlinear elimination occurs in dogs at dosages of 10 mg/kg and above, dogs acutely ingesting dosages above this amount should be observed for GI[45] erosion or ulceration and treated symptomatically for vomiting and GI bleeding. Aggressive decontamination and fluid therapy to prevent renal damage should be considered for dogs ingesting acute dosages greater than 20 mg/kg.

Meloxicam

Meloxicam has analgesic and fever-reducing effects. It is approved for both human and veterinary use. Veterinary formulations are available as both an oral suspension at 1.5 mg/mL and an injectable solution of 5 mg/mL. Meloxicam is principally used for treatment of osteoarthritis in dogs; however, single-dose injectable use is also approved for use in cats to control postoperative pain and inflammation associated with orthopedic surgery, ovariohysterectomy, and castration when administered prior to surgery. Dogs should receive 0.2 mg/kg initially PO, IV, or SC on the first day of treatment with subsequent doses of 0.1 mg/kg PO once daily.[30] Cats should receive 0.3 mg/kg SC once.[30,45]

Like other NSAIDs, meloxicam exhibits analgesic, antiinflammatory, and antipyretic activity probably through its inhibition of COX, of phospholipase A_2, and of PG synthesis. It is considered COX-2 preferential (not COX-2 specific) because at higher dosages, its COX-2 specificity is diminished.

In dogs, meloxicam is well absorbed after oral administration. Food does not appear to alter absorption. Peak blood levels occur in about 7 to 8 hours after administration.[30,45] Meloxicam is extensively metabolized in the liver, and a majority of the metabolites (and unchanged drug) are eliminated in the feces. A significant amount of enterohepatic recirculation occurs. The elimination half-life in dogs averages 24 hours (range, 12–36 hours). In cats, subcutaneous injection is nearly completely absorbed. Peak levels occur about 1.5 hours after injection. Meloxicam is relatively highly bound to feline plasma proteins (97%). After a single dose, total systemic clearance is approximately 130 mL/hr/kg and elimination half-life is approximately 15 hours.[30,45]

In a 6-month target animal safety study, meloxicam was administered orally at 1, 3, and 5 times ($\times$) the recommended dose with no significant clinical adverse reactions.[46] All animals in all dose groups (controls and 1$\times$, 3$\times$, and 5$\times$ the recommended dose) exhibited some GI distress (diarrhea and vomiting). Treatment-related changes seen in hematology and chemistry included decreased red blood cell counts in 7 of 24 dogs (4 dogs at the 3$\times$ dose and 3 dogs at the 5$\times$ dose); decreased hematocrit in 18 of 24 dogs (including 3 control dogs); dose-related neutrophilia in 1 dog at the 1$\times$ dose, 2 dogs at the 3$\times$ dose, and 3 dogs at the 5$\times$ dose; and evidence of regenerative anemia in 2 dogs at the 3$\times$ dose and 1 dog at the 5$\times$ dose. Also noted were increased BUN in 2 dogs at the 5$\times$ dose and decreased albumin in 1 dog at the 5$\times$ dose. Endoscopic changes consisted of reddening of the gastric mucosal surface covering less than 25% of the surface area. This was seen in 3 dogs at the recommended dose, 3 dogs at the 3$\times$ dose, and 2 dogs at the 5$\times$ dose. Two control dogs exhibited reddening in conjunction with ulceration of the mucosa covering less than 25% of the surface area. Gross GI necropsy results observed included mild discoloration of the stomach or duodenum in 1 dog at the 3$\times$ dose and 1 dog at the 5$\times$ dose. Multifocal pinpoint red foci were observed in the gastric fundic mucosa in 1 dog at the recommended dose and in 1 dog at the 5$\times$ dose. No macroscopic or microscopic renal changes were observed in any dogs receiving meloxicam in this

6-month study. Microscopic GI findings were limited to 1 dog at the recommended dose and 2 dogs at the 3× dose. Mild inflammatory mucosal infiltrate was observed in the duodenum of 1 dog at the recommended dose. Mild congestion of the fundic mucosa and mild myositis of the outer mural musculature of the stomach were observed in 2 dogs receiving the 3× dose.

There have been anecdotal reports of acute renal failure and death associated with the use of meloxicam in cats.

Nabumetone

Nabumetone is an effective naphthylalkanone-derivative NSAID that is available in 500- and 750-mg tablets.[47,48] It is available only by prescription. This drug differs from other NSAIDs in that it is neutral as opposed to acidic.[4(pp572,573)] This drug is widely used in humans for its anti-inflammatory effects as it is believed to have comparatively fewer GI side effects than most standard NSAIDs.[48,49] As terminal plasma half-life of nabumetone is 24 hours, once-daily dosing is recommended.[50] In animal models, peak plasma concentrations were noted 2 hours after oral dosing.[48]

Nabumetone is absorbed orally in animals, mainly intact from the intestine. However, the drug is extensively metabolized in the liver.[50] The absorption rate is increased when given with food, but the bioavailability of the drug remains unchanged.[51] The parent molecule, as previously stated, is nonacidic and inactive.[48] Nabumetone is metabolized by oxidation in intact liver cells into its main circulating active metabolite in rats, mice, dogs, rabbits, rhesus monkeys, and humans—6-methoxy-2-naphthylacetic acid (6-MNA).[50] This metabolism takes place only in the liver, not in other tissues.[48] Due to its nonacidic nature, PG synthesis does not appear to be inhibited by nabumetone as it is in other NSAIDs. Therefore, the risk of GI irritation in all studied species is thought to be reduced.[50] 6-MNA is not secreted in the bile; therefore, no GI irritation via enterohepatic recirculation is seen.[48] Nabumetone is primarily excreted in the urine by most species; however, in one study when 20 mg/kg of nabumetone was administered to 8- to 10-kg beagles, only 27% of the dose was found in the urine.[49]

Toxicity studies have been performed mainly in rats and mice. The LD_{50} in rats is greater than 2 g/kg, which makes nabumetone significantly less acutely toxic than either indomethacin (LD_{50} 12 mg/kg) or naproxen (LD_{50} 543 mg/kg). With high-dose levels (>300 mg/kg), the lower GI tract and the kidneys were the organ systems that showed the most effects in long-term studies in rats, mice, rabbits, and rhesus monkeys.[51] The mouse had the least renal involvement, and the rhesus monkey had minimal renal effects as well. There was very little impact on the GI systems of all species.[50]

Piroxicam

Piroxicam is an oxicam derivative and a prototypical NSAID labeled for use in humans. Structurally it is unrelated to other NSAIDs and, like naproxen, is chondroprotective. Available by prescription only, it is supplied in either 10- or 20-mg capsules under the trade name of Feldene.[30]

In humans, it is used for its anti-inflammatory and analgesic properties. Piroxicam has been used in dogs and cats as an adjunctive therapy in the treatment of transitional cell carcinoma of the bladder. The ability to reduce tumor size may due to immunomodulation and/or reduction of inflammation at the tumor site.[52]

The recommended off-label dosage for dogs and cats is 0.3 mg/kg PO every other day.[30]

The pharmacokinetics of piroxicam have been studied in the dog. After oral administration, piroxicam is rapidly absorbed (t_{max} 1.4 hours) with 100% bioavailability.[52,53] Food decreases the rate of absorption but not the amount absorbed. Antacids do not appear to affect absorption. In one study the half-life of the drug in beagle dogs after oral and intravenous administration of 0.3 mg/kg was found to be 40 hours.[53,54] In humans, the average half-life is reported by the manufacturer to be 50 hours.[55] Piroxicam is highly protein bound.

Piroxicam is extensively metabolized. In humans, it is metabolized primarily by hydroxylation followed by conjugation. These metabolites do not possess anti-inflammatory activity. Excretion of the metabolites occurs in both the urine and feces; urinary excretion is approximately twice the fecal excretion. Less than 5% of the parent compound is excreted unchanged in the urine and feces.[55] In dogs, the drug undergoes extensive enterohepatic recirculation, which may account for the reported long half-life.[53] Maternal milk concentrations of the drug reach approximately 1% of maternal serum concentrations.[30]

The LD_{50} of piroxicam in the dog is greater than 700 mg/kg.[52] In dogs, the therapeutic index of piroxicam is reported to be greater than that of aspirin.[53] In a blinded study, endoscopic examination of dogs treated orally with 0.3 mg/kg daily for 28 days failed to reveal a difference in gastroduodenal lesion development between control and treated dogs.[56] Piroxicam given to dogs orally at 0.3 mg/kg daily for many months resulted in GI toxicity in 18% of the patients.[56]

In a toxicity study, dogs receiving 1 mg/kg/d for 12 to 18 months developed renal papillary necrosis. An 8-year-old female dog treated with 0.8 mg/kg every 48 hours for 10 days developed life-threatening gastric ulceration and hemorrhage.[57]

Based on this information, it is apparent that piroxicam has the potential to cause significant adverse effects. It should be used cautiously and accompanied by diligent patient monitoring.

Diclofenac

Diclofenac is a phenylacetic acid–derivative NSAID. It structurally related to meclofenamate sodium and mefenamic acid, but unlike these anthranilic acid (2-aminobenzoic acid) derivatives, diclofenac is a 2-aminobenzeneacetic acid derivative. Diclofenac is commercially available as diclofenac sodium delayed-release and extended-release tablets and as diclofenac potassium conventional tablets. Diclofenac is also available as a fixed combination of diclofenac sodium in an enteric-coated core with an outer shell of misoprostol. The primary uses of diclofenac in human medicine are for inflammatory diseases, pain, and dysmenorrhea. The usual initial dosage of diclofenac sodium in adults is 75 mg twice daily or 50 mg 3 times daily but can be increased to 200 mg daily if needed. Dosages of diclofenac greater than 225 mg/d is not recommended by the manufacturer due to the increased risk of adverse effects. The usual adult dosage of diclofenac potassium is 100 to 200 mg daily.[58]

Diclofenac sodium and diclofenac potassium are rapidly and almost completely absorbed from the GI tract in humans but undergo extensive first-pass metabolism in the liver. Only about 50% to 60% of a dose of diclofenac reaches the systemic circulation as unchanged drug. After oral administration, peak plasma concentrations of diclofenac generally occur within 1 hour for diclofenac potassium conventional tablets and 2 to 3 hours for delayed-release diclofenac sodium tablets. Food decreases the rate of absorption of diclofenac tablets, resulting in delayed and decreased peak plasma concentrations. Significant accumulation of diclofenac during repeated dosing reportedly does not occur, although the degree of accumulation of metabolites is unknown. Following intravenous administration of diclofenac in rats, it is widely distributed, with highest concentrations achieved in bile, liver, blood, heart, lungs, and kidneys and lower concentrations in adrenals, thyroid glands, salivary glands, pancreas, spleen, muscles, brain, and spinal cord. Like other NSAIDs, diclofenac is also distributed into synovial fluid. Diclofenac is 99% to 99.8% but reversibly protein bound, mainly to albumin. Along with its metabolites, diclofenac has been shown to cross the placenta in mice and rats. The exact metabolic fate of diclofenac is unknown, but it is rapidly and extensively metabolized in the liver via hydroxylation and then conjugation with glucuronic acid, taurine amide, sulfuric acid, and other biogenic ligands. Diclofenac is excreted in urine (50%–70%) and feces (30%–35%), with only minimal amounts eliminated as unchanged drug (<1%). Although there is some evidence that diclofenac undergoes enterohepatic recirculation, this appears to be minimal in humans. Following oral administration of delayed-release diclofenac sodium tablets, the elimination half-life is approximately 1.2 to 2 hours but may by prolonged in individuals with severe renal impairment.[58]

After a single injection of 1 mg/kg of diclofenac sodium in the dog, 35% to 40% is excreted in the urine.[59] In the dog, the major metabolite of diclofenac found in urine is the taurine conjugate of unchanged diclofenac. In the urine of rats, baboons, and humans, conjugates of the hydroxylated metabolites predominate.[60] The dog does not oxidize diclofenac. An unstable ester glucuronide of diclofenac found in dog bile has also been found in rat bile. It is presumed to hydrolyze in the duodenum, releasing diclofenac that then undergoes enterohepatic recirculation.[59]

The oral LD_{50} of diclofenac sodium is 55 to 240 mg/kg in rats, 500 mg/kg in dogs, and 3200 mg/kg in monkeys. Another source reported the LD_{50} in dogs to be 59 mg/kg.[61] Hydroxylated metabolites exhibited less toxic potential than did the unchanged drug in LD_{50} studies in rats.[58]

Indomethacin

Indomethacin, an indoleacetic acid derivative, is commercially available as the base and as the sodium trihydrate salt. Available forms of indomethacin include conventional capsules, extended-release capsules, rectal suppositories, and suspension; indomethacin sodium trihydrate is supplied for intravenous use only. Oral and rectal forms of indomethacin are administered 2 to 4 times daily in divided doses. Intravenous indomethacin sodium trihydrate is given for the treatment of patent ductus arterisus in premature human neonates, at the initial dose of 0.2 mg/kg. The drug is structurally and pharmacologically related to sulindac.[62]

Following oral administration of indomethacin, the bioavailability is virtually 100%, with 90% of a single oral dose being absorbed within 4 hours. The extended-release capsules are 90% absorbed within 12 hours. The bioavailability of indomethacin following rectal administration is generally reported as comparable to or slightly less than that following oral administration. When taken with food or antacids, peak plasma concentrations of indomethacin may be slightly decreased or delayed, although the clinical significance of this is unknown. Although the relationship between plasma indomethacin concentrations and its anti-inflammatory effects has not been precisely determined, a therapeutic range of 0.5 to 3 $\mu g/mL$ has been suggested. At therapeutic concentrations, indomethacin is approximately 99% protein bound. Indomethacin crosses the blood-brain barrier in small amounts, is distributed into milk, and appears to freely cross the placenta. Clearance of indomethacin from plasma appears to be biphasic in humans, an initial half-life of approximately 1 hour, and a half-life of 2.6 to 11.2 hours in the second phase. Indomethacin is metabolized in the liver to its glucuronide conjugate and to desmethyl, desbenzoyl, and desmethyl-desbenzoyl metabolites and their glucuronides. These metabolites do not appear to have antiinflammatory activity. Indomethacin and its conjugates undergo enterohepatic recirculation. About 33% of a 25-mg oral dose of indomethacin is excreted in feces, primarily as unconjugated metabolites, and 60% is excreted in urine (30% as indomethacin and its glucuronide) within 48 hours.[62]

Based on 14-day mortality studies, the oral LD_{50} of indomethacin is 50 mg/kg in mice and 12 mg/kg in rats.[62]

Etodolac

Etodolac is an indole acetic acid derivative, used for pain relief, osteoarthritis, and rheumatoid arthritis in human medicine. Human preparations are available as 200- and 300-mg capsules, 400- and 500-mg film-coated tablets, and 400-, 500-, and 600-mg extended-release, film-coated tablets. The usual human dosage is up to 1 g daily, divided into 1 to 4 doses depending on the condition being treated.[63] Etodolac is approved in the United States for use in dogs to manage pain and inflammation associated with osteoarthritis[64] and is available as 150- and 300-mg scored tablets.[30] The suggested canine dosage is 10 to 15 mg/kg.[64] Safe use of etodolac in dogs that are less than 12 months of age, breeding, pregnant, or lactating has not been determined.[30]

While the extent of GI absorption and time to peak concentration of etodolac do not seem to be significantly affected by administration with food or antacids in humans, peak concentrations may be reduced.[63] Etodolac appears to be well absorbed following oral administration in dogs, with maximum blood concentrations and onset of action reported to occur as quickly as 30 to 60 minutes after ingestion.[64] The mechanism of action of etodolac is believed to be associated with inhibition of COX activity and macrophage chemotaxis.[65] Etodolac is highly bound to serum proteins and primarily excreted via bile into feces. Glucuronide conjugates of etodolac have been detected in bile but not urine. Elimination half-life in dogs varies depending on the presence of food in the GI tract, which probably affects the rate of enterohepatic recirculation of the drug. Elimination half-lives in dogs vary from 8 hours for fasted animals to 12 hours for nonfasted animals.[30]

In clinical trials, the primary adverse effect reported in association with etodolac administration was vomiting/regurgitation in about 5% of dogs tested. Diarrhea, lethargy, and hypoproteinemia were also reported in a small number of dogs. Less than 1% of treated dogs exhibited urticaria, behavioral changes, and inappetance.[30] GI effects of etodolac were evaluated with gastroduodenal endoscopy in dogs receiving an average of 12.8 (range 11.7–13.8) mg/kg orally every 24 hours for 28 days. Only minor gastric lesions were observed, with no significant difference among dogs receiving carprofen, etodolac, or placebo.[66] In safety studies in dogs, 40 mg/kg/d was associated with GI ulcers, weight loss, emesis, and local occult blood; 80 mg/kg/d caused 6 of 8 dogs to die or become moribund due to GI ulceration.[30] Gastroduodenal erosions have been reported in dogs after 28 days of etodolac administration.[64]

REFERENCES

1. Donovan JW. Nonsteroidal anti-inflammatory drugs and colchicine. In: Haddad LM, Shannon MW, Winchester JF, editors. Clinical management of poisoning and drug overdose. 3rd edition. Philadelphia: WB Saunders; 1998. p. 687–99.
2. Holubek W. Nonsteroidal anti-inflammatory drugs. In: Nelson LS, Hoffman RS, Lewin NA, editor. Goldfrank's toxicologic emergencies. 9th edition. New York: McGraw-Hill; 2011. p. 528–36.
3. Bryson PD. Nonsteroidal anti-inflammatory agents. In: Comprehensive review in toxicology for emergency clinicians. 3rd edition. Washington, DC: Taylor and Francis; 1996. p. 565–75.

4. Ellenhorn MJ. Nonsteroidal antiinflammatory drugs. In: Ellenhorn's medical toxicology: diagnosis and treatment of human poisoning. 2nd edition. Baltimore: Williams & Wilkins; 1997. p. 196–206.

5. Forrester SD, Troy GC. Renal effects of nonsteroidal antiinflammatory drugs. Compend Cont Educ 1999;21:910–9.

6. Johnston SA, Fox SM. Mechanisms of action of anti-inflammatory medications used for the treatment of osteoarthritis. JAVMA 1997;210:1486–92.

7. Lees P, May SA, McKeller QA. Pharmacology and therapeutics of non-steroidal anti-inflammatory drugs in the dog and cat: I. General pharmacology. J Small Anim Pract 1991;32:183–93.

8. MacAllister CG. Nonsteroidal anti-inflammatory drugs: their mechanism of action and clinical uses in horses. Vet Med 1994;March:237–40.

9. Wolfe MM. NSAIDs and the gastrointestinal mucosa. Hosp Pract 1996;December 15:37–48.

10. Bowersox TS, Lipowitz AJ, Hardy RM, et al. The use of a synthetic prostaglandin E_1 analog as a gastric protectant against aspirin-induced hemorrhage in the dog. J Am Anim Hosp Assoc 1996;32:401–7.

11. Rubin SI. Nonsteroidal antiinflammatory drugs, prostaglandins, and the kidney. JAVMA 1986;188:1065–8.

12. Kore AM. Toxicology of nonsteroidal anti-inflammatory drugs. Vet Clin N Am Small Anim Pract 1990;20:419–30.

13. Dunayer E. Ibuprofen toxicosis in dogs, cats, and ferrets. Vet Med 2004;July:580–5.

14. McEvoy GK, editor. Ibuprofen. In: American Hospital Formulary Service drug information. Bethesda (MD): American Society of Healthsystem Pharmacists Inc.; 2000. p. 1815.

15. Kore AM. Toxicology of nonsteroidal anti-inflammatory drugs. Vet Clin North Am Small Anim Pract 1990;20:419–28.

16. Rumack BH, et al, editors. Ibuprofen (toxicologic managements). Poisindex System Vol 100. Englewood (CO): Micromedex. Expires 9/2000.

17. Roush JK. Diseases of joints and ligaments. In: Morgan RV, editor. The handbook of small animal practice. 3rd edition. New York: Churchill Livingstone; 1997. p. 813–29.

18. Osweiler G, Carson TL. Household drugs. In: Morgan RV, editor. The handbook of small animal practice. 3rd edition. New York: Churchill Livingstone; 1997. p. 1279–83.

19. Villar D, Buck WB. Ibuprofen, aspirin, and acetaminophen toxicosis and treatment in dogs and cats. Vet Hum Toxicol 1998;40:156–62.

20. Smith KJ, Taylor DH. Another case of gastric perforation associated with administration of ibuprofen in a dog. JAVMA 1993;202:706.

21. Spyridakis LK, Bacia JJ, Barsanti JA, et al. Ibuprofen toxicosis in a dog. JAVMA 1986;188:918–9.

22. Adams SS, Bough RG, Cliffe EE, et al. Absorption, distribution and toxicity of ibuprofen. Toxicol Appl Pharmacol 1969;15:310–30.

23. Richardson JA. Management of acetaminophen and ibuprofen toxicoses in dogs and cats. Vet Emerg Crit Care 2000;10:285–91.

24. Rumbeiha WK. Nephrotoxins. In: Bonagura JD, editor. Kirk's current veterinary therapy XIII. Small animal practice. Philadelphia: W.B. Saunders Co; 2000. p. 212–7.

25. Owens-Clark J, Dorman DC. Toxicity from newer over the counter drugs. In: Bonagura JD, editor. Kirk's current veterinary therapy XIII. Small animal practice. Philadelphia: W.B. Saunders Co; 2000. p. 227–31.

26. Richardson JA, Balabuszko RA. Ibuprofen ingestion in ferrets: 43 cases (January 1996–March 2000). J Vet Emerg Crit Care 2001;11:53–9.

27. Cathers TE. Acute ibuprofen toxicosis in a ferret. JAVMA 2000;216:1426–8.
28. Rumack BH, editor. Aspirin (toxicologic managements). Poisindex System Vol 100. Englewood (CO): Micromedex. Expires 9/2000.
29. Booth DM. The analgesic-antipyretic-antiinflammatory drugs. In: Richard AH, editor. Veterinary and pharmacology and therapeutics. 7th edition. Ames (IA): Iowa State University Press; 1995. p. 432–9.
30. Plumb DC. Veterinary drug handbook. 3rd edition. Ames (IA): Iowa State University Press; 1999. p. 56–8, 221, 434, 462, 518–9, 562, 583.
31. Brogden RN, Heel RC, Speight TM, et al. Naproxen up to date: a review of its pharmacological properties and therapeutic efficacy and use in rheumatic diseases and pain states. Drugs 1979;18:241–77.
32. Brogden RN, Pinder RM, Sawer PR, et al. Naproxen: a review of its pharmacological properties and therapeutic efficacy and use. Drugs 1975;9:326–63.
33. Gfeller RW, Sandors AD. Naproxen-associated duodenal ulcer complicated by perforation and bacteria- and barium sulfate-induced peritonitis in a dog. JAVMA 1991; 198:644–6.
34. Gilmour MA, Walshaw R. Naproxen-induced toxicosis in a dog. JAVMA 1987;191: 1431–2.
35. Roudebush P, Morse GE. Naproxen toxicosis in a dog. JAVMA 1981;179:805–6.
36. Steel RJS. Suspected naproxen toxicity in dogs. Aust Vet J 1981;57:100–1.
37. Hallesy D, Shott L, Hill R. Comparative toxicology of naproxen. Scand J Rheumatol Suppl 1973;2:20–8.
38. Dye TL. Naproxen toxicosis in a puppy. Vet Hum Toxicol 1997;39:157–9.
39. Daehler MH. Transmural pyloric perforation associated with naproxen administration in a dog. JAVMA 1986;189:694–5.
40. Dean SP, Reid JFS. Use of naproxen [letter]. Vet Rec 1985;116:479.
41. Smith RE. Naproxen toxicosis [letter]. JAVMA 1982;180:107.
42. Shiltz RA. Naproxen in dogs and cats [letter]. JAVMA 1982;180:1397.
43. Deramaxx (Decracoxib) package insert. Greensboro (NC): Novartis Animal Health, US Inc.; 2011. NADA # 141-203, approved by FDA. Available at: http://valleyvet.naccvp. com/index.php?m=product_view_basic&u=country&p=msds&id=1131012. Accessed January 10, 2012.
44. Anti-inflammatory agents. In: Kahn Cynthia M, editor. The Merck veterinary manual. 10th edition. New Jersey: Merck & Co; 2010. p. 2313–28.
45. Plumb DC. Veterinary drug handbook. 5th edition. Ames (IA): Blackwell Publishing; 2005. p. 222.
46. Boehringer Ingelheim Vetmedica, Inc. Freedom of information summary new animal drug application Metacam® (meloxicam) 0.5 mg/mL and 1.5 mg/mL oral suspension. 2003. NADA 141–219. Available at: http://www.fda.gov/downloads/animalveterinary/ products/approvedanimaldrugproducts/foiadrugsummaries/ucm118026.pdf. Accessed January 10, 2012.
47. Kirchner T, Argentieri A, et al. Evaluation of the anti-inflammatory activity of a duel cyclooxygenase-2 selective/5-lipoxygenaxe inhibitor, RWJ 63556, in a canine model of inflammation. J Pharmacol Exp Ther 1997;282:1094–101.
48. Blower P. Nabumetone: the science – equivalent efficacy and diminished risk. Eur J Rheumatol Inflamm 1991;11:29–37.
49. Haddock RE, Jeffery DJ, Lloyd JA, et al. Metabolism of nabumetone by various species including man. Xenobiotica 1984;14:327–37.
50. Mangan F, Flack J, Jackson D. Preclinical overview of nabumetone: pharmacology, bioavailability, metabolism, and toxicology. Am J Med 1987;83:6–10.

51. Jackson D, Hardy T, Langley P, et al. Pharmacokinetic, toxicological, and metabolic studies with nabumetone. Proc. Symp. Held by BPUK Madera, 1983/R Soc. Med. Int. Congr. Symp. Ser. 1985 (69).

52. Adams HR. Veterinary pharmacology and therapeutics. 7th edition. Ames (IA): Iowa State University Press; 1995. p. 443.

53. McKellar QA, Lees P, May SA. Pharmacology and therapeutics of non-steroidal anti-inflammatory drugs in the dog and cat: 2 individual agents. J Small Anim Pract 1991;32:225–35.

54. Boothe D. Analgesia/anti-inflammatories. CVMA 1997;June:13–20.

55. McEvoy GK, editor. Piroxicam. In: American Hospital Formulary Service drug information. Bethesda (MD): American Society of Healthsystem Pharmacists Inc.; 2000. p. 1815.

56. Galbraith EA, McKellar QA. Pharmacokinetics and pharmacodynamics of piroxicam in dogs. Vet Rec 1991;128:561–5.

57. Thomas NW. Piroxicam-associated gastric ulceration in a dog. Compend Small Anim Pract 1987;9:1028–30.

58. McEvoy GK, editor. Diclofenac. In: American Hospital Formulary Service drug information. Bethesda (MD): American Society of Healthsystem Pharmacists Inc.; 2000. p. 1800.

59. Stierlin H, Faigle JW. Biotransformation of diclofenac sodium (Voltaren in animals and man: II. Quantitative determination of the unchanged drug and principal phenolic metabolites, in urine and bile. Xenobiotics 1979;9:611–21.

60. Stierlin H, Faigle JW, et al. Biotransformation of diclofenac sodium (Voltaren) in animals and in man: I. Isolation and identification of principal metabolites. Xenobiotics 1979;9:601–10.

61. Diclofenac. In: RTECS: Registry of Toxic Effects of Chemical Substances. Cincinnati (OH): National Institute for Occupational Safety and Health. CD-ROM. MICROMEDEX, Greenwood Village (CO). Expires 7/02.

62. McEvoy GK, editor. Indomethacin. In: American Hospital Formulary Service drug information. Bethesda (MD): American Society of Healthsystem Pharmacists Inc.; 2001. p. 1924–34.

63. McEvoy GK, editor. Etodolac. In: American Hospital Formulary Service drug information. Bethesda (MD): American Society of Healthsystem Pharmacists Inc.; 2001. p. 1913–4.

64. Mathews KA. Nonsteroidal anti-inflammatory analgesics: indications and contraindications for pain management in dogs and cats. Vet Clin N Am Sm Anim Pract 2000;30:783–804.

65. Budsberg SC, Johnston SA, et al. Efficacy of etodolac for the treatment of osteoarthritis of the hip joints in dogs. JAVMA 1999;214:206–10.

66. Reimer ME, Johnston SA, et al. The gastroduodenal effects of buffered aspirin, carprofen, and etodolac in healthy dogs. J Vet Intern Med 1999;13:472–7.

Xylitol Toxicosis in Dogs

Lisa A. Murphy, VMD[a],*, Adrienne E. Coleman, DVM[b]

KEYWORDS

- Xylitol • Hypoglycemia • Liver failure • Coagulopathy

The 5-carbon sugar alcohol xylitol is used as a sweetener in many products including gums, candies, and baked goods. In recent years the use of xylitol has increased due to the popularity of low-carbohydrate diets and low–glycemic index foods.[1] Xylitol also prevents oral bacteria from producing acids that damage the surfaces of teeth, leading to its inclusion in toothpaste and other oral care products.[1,2] While xylitol is considered safe in humans, canine ingestions have resulted in severe and life-threatening signs associated with increased insulin secretion leading to hypoglycemia. Acute death due to severe hypoglycemia if untreated is possible, and liver failure may develop 1 to 3 days after xylitol ingestion.

SOURCES

Initially xylitol was used as a sugar substitute during World War II, when sucrose availability was low. During that time, xylitol was derived from birch and other hardwoods.[3] More recently, the sweetener has been used as a sugar substitute for human diabetics. It has a similar sweetness to sucrose and the same number of calories.[4] It has also been eagerly embraced by dental care professionals and the general public due to its anticariogenic properties.[5] Its presence in gum, mints, and candies including gumballs, lollypops, and taffy has been fairly well known for years; however, recently several additional, lesser known products are now also made with xylitol. Veterinarians and pet owners should be aware that this sugar substitute may be found in several common household products, both edible and nonedible, and even in some prescription drugs.

Based on a 2001–2011 search of the ASPCA Animal Poison Control Center's (APCC) product database, xylitol was found to be present in several vitamins (ie, iron, vitamin D, calcium chews, multivitamin tablets, gummy vitamins) and nutritional supplements (coenzyme Q10, 5-hydroxytryptophan, caffeine). Xylitol can also be found in chocolate, baked goods, puddings, syrup, fruit preserves, jellies, nutritional/diet bars, and drink powders. It is also available in its pure form as a sugar substitute

The authors have nothing to disclose.

[a] Department of Pathobiology, University of Pennsylvania School of Veterinary Medicine, New Bolton Center Toxicology Laboratory, 382 West Street Road, Kennett Square, PA 19348, USA
[b] ASPCA Animal Poison Control Center, 1717 South Philo Road, Suite 36, Urbana, IL 61802, USA
* Corresponding author.
E-mail address: murphylp@vet.upenn.edu

under several different brand names. Xylitol is also used as an ingredient in toothpaste, tooth wipes and towelettes for babies, oral lozenges, moisturizing mouth sprays and gels, and mouthwash because of its ability to prevent cavity formation. It can additionally be found in exfoliating facial wipes, personal lubricants, deodorants, and night creams.

Xylitol is used in medicinal products, most notably both brand-name and generic nicotine gums. It is also found in oral drug suspensions, cold remedies, some sublingual tablets, and nasal sprays.

If an exposure to any of these substances has occurred, the ingestion of xylitol should be considered. It may be listed on product labels using a number of possible synonyms, including Eutrit, Kannit, Klinit, Newtol, xylite, Torch, or Xyliton.[6]

Xylitol is also an ingredient in drinking water additives for dogs and cats. Exposures have been reported to the APCC; however, no evidence of associated xylitol toxicity has been documented to date (ASPCA APCC, unpublished data, 2011). A study involving dogs that received 5 times the recommended xylitol drinking water dose also failed to demonstrate any toxic effects.[7]

TOXICOKINETICS

Xylitol is quickly absorbed from the canine gastrointestinal tract, with peak plasma levels occurring within 30 minutes of ingestion.[8] And 80% of xylitol metabolism occurs in the liver where it is rapidly oxidized to D-xylulose, then metabolized to glucose, glycogen, and lactate via the pentose-phosphate pathway.[9]

Xylitol ingestion in dogs causes a dose-related insulin release that is greater than the response to an equal dose of glucose.[10,11] Peak serum insulin concentrations have been observed to be 6-fold greater following ingestion of xylitol compared to glucose[8] and so may lead to severe hypoglycemia. Xylitol does not cause similar insulin release or blood glucose changes in humans, rats, and horses, although increased insulin releases have been documented in cows, goats, and rabbits.[12] Dogs experimentally dosed with 1 or 4 g of xylitol per kilogram of body weight orally showed sharp increases in plasma insulin concentrations within 20 minutes, peaking at 40 minutes.[13] Another study indicates that xylitol directly stimulates secretion of insulin by pancreatic islet β cells.[8]

The mechanism of action for liver damage in dogs is not fully understood; however, it is thought to be related to either ATP depletion during the metabolism of xylitol leading to hepatic necrosis or the production of hepatocyte-damaging reactive oxygen species.[14] Histopathologic changes observed in 3 dogs with known xylitol toxicosis included severe acute periacinar and midzonal hepatic necrosis with periportal vacuolar degeneration, diffuse hepatic necrosis, and moderate to marked subacute centrilobular hepatocyte loss and atrophy with lobular collapse and disorganization.[14]

TOXICITY

Oral xylitol has a wide margin of safety in most species. The estimated oral LD_{50} of xylitol in rabbits is 4 to 6 g per kilogram of body weight.[15] People consuming more than 130 g of xylitol per day may develop diarrhea but no other abnormalities.[16] Xylitol toxicity has not been reported in cats. Anecdotal reports indicate ferrets have shown evidence of hypoglycemia following ingestion but this has not been confirmed. In fact, the 3 cases of xylitol exposure received by the APCC did not show evidence of hypoglycemia or other adverse effects as reported in dogs.

Based on canine xylitol ingestions reported to the ASPCA APCC, only mild clinical signs of hypoglycemia would be expected with ingestions of less than 100 mg of xylitol per kilogram of body weight (100 mg/kg), although exposures greater than 50 mg/kg may at least warrant decontamination and blood glucose monitoring. Ingestions involving greater than 500 mg/kg of xylitol in dogs can be associated with hepatic failure.[3]

CLINICAL SIGNS AND LABORATORY CHANGES

A 2001–2011 search of canine xylitol ingestions in the APCC database was performed, limited to cases where the xylitol concentration of the product involved was known and no other potentially toxic exposures were known to have occurred. While ingestions involving mints and 100% xylitol products appear to develop clinical signs quickly (often within 30 minutes potentially due to quick disintegration and release of xylitol from these products), this most recent database search supports previously reported observations that dogs ingesting xylitol-containing gums may not develop clinical signs of hypoglycemia until 12 hours later.[3] These variations in the onset of clinical signs may be related to the formulation-specific product involved and the amount of mastication (chewing) that may have occurred during consumption. When dogs ingest xylitol-containing gums, they usually do not chew/masticate it. This may be the main reason for a delay in onset time of hypoglycemia. Increased mastication of chewing gum would cause an increased likelihood of developing clinical signs relatively more quickly due to an increased release of the product's total available xylitol.[17]

Clinical signs most commonly noted in dogs in the APCC database include vomiting, lethargy, and weakness. Vomiting was most commonly reported with gum ingestions (especially those containing xylitol in the outer coating), mints, and 100% xylitol products, typically within 30 minutes and up to several hours post-exposure. In many of these cases the dogs at least partially self-decontaminated and the xylitol-containing product could be seen in the vomitus.

In cases where lethargy and weakness were reported by the owners, dogs were generally also hypoglycemic on presentation to the veterinary clinic. However, not all animals exhibited hypoglycemia on presentation for veterinary care and sometimes appeared clinically normal on initial examination. Dogs that were presented either nonresponsive or with seizure activity were often hypoglycemic, although in some cases, blood glucose levels performed postictally showed levels within the normal limits. Of the cases reviewed, ingestions involving less than 100 mg of xylitol per kilogram of body weight usually resulted in mild signs. Hyperglycemia has sometimes been reported following xylitol ingestion and may be a result of the Somogyi phenomenon (rebound hyperglycemia) that occurs with insulin overdose.[3]

Some dogs in the APCC database developed mild to moderate hypokalemia or an initial hypophosphatemia, typically within 12 hours of the initial exposure, and appeared to respond well to supplementation. Hyperphosphatemia was instead associated with subsequent hepatic damage and is considered a poor prognostic indicator.

The time at which liver enzyme elevations were first detected generally varied from 4 to 24 hours, but in some cases alanine aminotransferase became elevated in less than 4 hours post-exposure. This early development of mild liver enzyme elevations is consistent with a recent research study performed in China.[13] Dogs in the APCC database that developed hypoglycemia did not always develop evidence of liver damage. Additionally, there were several cases of dogs that developed liver enzyme elevations but not hypoglycemia. Many dogs with elevated liver enzymes did eventually recover, even in some cases where coagulopathies (prolonged prothrombin and activated partial thromboplastin times) were noted (ASPCA APCC, unpublished data, 2011).

TREATMENT AND MONITORING

On arrival to the veterinary clinic, a baseline blood glucose level should be measured. Emesis should be induced if the dog has not vomited prior to presentation (either by induction or self-decontamination) and no contraindications are indicated by the patient's history or physical examination findings. Apomorphine can be administered either injectably (0.03 mg/kg IV or 0.04 mg/kg IM) or by subconjunctival administration (a crushed ¼ of a 6-mg tablet).[18] If excessive sedation occurs, naloxone can be used as a reversal agent, but the depression associated with apomorphine is generally mild. If the apomorphine is applied to the conjunctiva, a thorough ocular flushing should occur once vomiting has been initiated in order to avoid excessive ocular irritation and retching. As an alternative to apomorphine for the induction of emesis, 3% active hydrogen peroxide can be orally administered at a dosage of 1 to 2.2 mL/kg (generally not exceeding 45 mL as a total dose). If vomiting does not occur after the first dose, it can be repeated once.[19] Additional doses could result in gastric irritation. Vomitus should be thoroughly evaluated for the presence of the ingested xylitol product(s) in order to determine if decontamination was successful.

Emesis is not recommended in patients that have ingested 100% xylitol products more than 30 minutes prior to presentation. Due to the rapid absorption of this form of xylitol, an insulin peak plasma effect can occur within 40 minutes, meaning that clinical signs of hypoglycemia (ataxia, disorientation, and seizures) may develop before or during decontamination.[13] If significant clinical signs and weakness associated with xylitol toxicosis develop during emesis, aspiration may occur.

Activated charcoal is not typically recommended because xylitol is so readily absorbed from the gastrointestinal tract. Also, in vitro studies suggest that activated charcoal binds poorly to xylitol.[20]

Initial blood work should include electrolytes (including potassium), blood glucose, a baseline liver profile, a baseline complete blood count, and a serum phosphorus level. The electrolytes can be repeated in 8 to 12 hours post exposure in several affected animals, and hypokalemia should be corrected as needed. Blood glucose should be evaluated every 2 hours for the first 12 hours and checked more frequently in severely affected patients. Monitoring of blood glucose levels for more than 12 hours may be necessary if hypoglycemia continues to be an issue. Baseline liver enzymes should be reevaluated at 12, 24, and 48 hours later. If liver enzymes become elevated, the patient's coagulation times should be monitored[3] and the complete blood count should be examined for evidence of mild to moderate thrombocytopenia.[14] Serum phosphorus should be evaluated once daily.

An intravenous catheter should be placed in dogs exposed to doses suspected to result in hypoglycemia. If hypoglycemia is identified, an IV dextrose bolus should be administered, followed by parenteral fluids containing 2.5% to 5% dextrose.[3] The dextrose may prevent hypoglycemia in mild intoxications and can be hepatoprotective in patients at risk for hepatic necrosis. S-Adenosyl-L-methionine (SAMe) or Denosyl (20 mg/kg per day) and Marin (per label instructions) or milk thistle (50 mg/kg per day) may also be used,[18] although the efficacy of these hepatoprotectants for xylitol toxicosis has not been established. There may also be some benefit for using N-acetylcysteine (140 mg/kg PO initially at a 5% concentration, then 70 mg/kg PO at a 5% concentration every 6 to 8 hours for an additional 7 treatments).[18] The efficacy of hepatoprotective effects of N-acetylcysteine used in xylitol toxicosis has not been determined. If evidence of hepatic damage develops and the patient's coagulation profile becomes abnormal, vitamin K_1 therapy should be initiated and plasma transfusions may be considered.

Dogs should be hospitalized for a minimum of 12 to 24 hours post-ingestion because of the risk of delayed-onset hypoglycemia, particularly with chewing gum exposures.[3] If symptoms develop, the patient should receive veterinary care and frequent feedings until the blood glucose level has stabilized. The addition of dietary fiber in the diet may be useful for facilitating the elimination of wrapper materials and packaging that may have been concurrently consumed.

Prognosis is generally good with early decontamination and effective management of hypoglycemia, even in cases where mild liver enzyme elevations have develop. The prognosis becomes more guarded for dogs that develop repeated bouts of profound hypoglycemia (often with central nervous system signs), or significant prolonged liver enzyme elevations, with or without coagulopathy, suggestive of hepatic necrosis. Patients that develop hyperphosphatemia tend to have a poor prognosis for survival; however, even some of these severely affected dogs have successfully recovered.

SUMMARY

Xylitol ingestions in dogs may result in severe hypoglycemia followed by acute hepatic failure and associated coagulopathies. Aggressive treatment may be needed, but the prognosis is generally expected to be good for dogs developing uncomplicated hypoglycemia. Due to increased availability of xylitol-containing products in the market, we will continue to see increased exposures and toxicity in dogs.

REFERENCES

1. Gare F. The sweet miracle of xylitol. North Bergen (NJ): Basic Health Publications; 2003.
2. Cronin JR. Xylitol: a sweet for healthy teeth and more. Altern Complement Ther 2003;9:139–41.
3. Dunayer EK. New findings on the effects of xylitol ingestion in dogs. Vet Med 2006;12:791–6.
4. Dills WL. Sugar alcohols as bulk sweeteners. Annu Rev Nutr 1989;9:161–86.
5. Todd JM, Powell LP. Xylitol intoxication associated with fulminant hepatic failure in a dog. J Vet Emerg Crit Care 2007;17:286–9.
6. Budavari S, editor. The Merck index: an encyclopedia of chemicals, drugs, and biologicals. Rahway (NJ): Merck; 1989. p. 9996.
7. Anthony JP, Weber LP, Alkemade S. Blood glucose and liver function in dogs administered a xylitol drinking water additive at zero, one and five times dosage rates. Vet Sci Dev 2011;1:7–9.
8. Kuzuya T, Kanazawa Y, Kosaka K. Stimulation of insulin secretion by xylitol in dogs. Endocrinology 1969;84:200–7.
9. Froesch ER, Jakob A. The metabolism of xylitol. In: Sipple HL, McNutt KW, editors. Sugars in nutrition. New York: Academic Press; 1974. p. 241–58.
10. Kuzuya T, Kanazawa Y, Kosaka K. Plasma insulin response to intravenously administered xylitol in dogs. Metabolism 1966;15:1149–52.
11. Hirata Y, Fujisawa M, Sato H, et al. Blood glucose and plasma insulin responses to xylitol administered intravenously in dogs. Biochem Biophys Res Commun 1966;24:471–5.
12. Kuzuya T, Kanazawa Y, Hayashi M, et al. Species difference in plasma insulin responses to intravenous xylitol in man and several mammals. Endocrinol Jpn 1971;18:309–20.

13. Xia Z, He Y, Yu J. Experimental acute toxicity of xylitol in dogs. J Vet Pharmacol Ther 2009;32:465–9.
14. Dunayer EK, Gwaltney-Brant SM. Acute hepatic failure and coagulopathy associated with xylitol ingestion in eight dogs. J Am Vet Med Assoc 2006;229:1113–7.
15. Wang YM, King SM, Patterson JH, et al. Mechanism of xylitol toxicity in the rabbit. Metabolism 1973;22:885–94.
16. Brin M, Miller ON. The safety of oral xylitol. In: Sipple HL, McNutt KW, editors. Sugars in nutrition. New York: Academic Press; 1974. p. 591–606.
17. Kvist CL, Andersson SB, Berglund J, et al. Equipment for drug release testing of medicated chewing gums. J Pharm Biomed Anal 2000;22:405–11.
18. Plumb DC. Veterinary drug handbook, 6th ed. Stockholm (WI): PharmaVet/Ames (IA): Blackwell; 2005. p. 14–5, 91–2, 1086–7, 1101–2.
19. Poppenga R. Treatment. In: Plumlee KH, editor. Clinical veterinary toxicology. St Louis (MO): Mosby; 2004. p. 15.
20. Cope RB. A screening study of xylitol binding *in vitro* to activated charcoal. Vet Hum Toxicol 2004;46:336–7.

Toxicology of Avermectins and Milbemycins (Macrocylic Lactones) and the Role of P-Glycoprotein in Dogs and Cats

Valentina M. Merola, DVM, MS[a],*, Paul A. Eubig, DVM, MS[b]

KEYWORDS

- Macrocyclic lactones • Ivermectin • Dogs
- Cats • P-glycoprotein

The macrocyclic lactones (MLs) are parasiticides able to kill a wide variety of arthropods and nematodes. They have a high margin of safety for labeled indications, and ivermectin has become the best selling antiparasitic in the world.[1] Dogs of certain breeds and mixtures of those breeds have a defect in the *ABCB1* gene (formerly *MDR1* gene) that results in a lack of functional P-glycoprotein (P-gp), which leads to accumulation of the MLs in the central nervous system (CNS) and a higher risk of adverse effects when exposed. With toxicosis, CNS signs such as ataxia, lethargy, coma, tremors, seizures, mydriasis, and blindness predominate. In general, the MLs have a long half-life and therefore exposure results in a long duration of illness when overdoses occur. There is no specific antidote for ML toxicosis so the most important part of treatment is good supportive care.

CHEMISTRY OF MACROCYCLIC LACTONES

The MLs (macrolides) include 2 groups: avermectins and milbemycins. The avermectins include abamectin, ivermectin, eprinomectin, doramectin, and selamectin. The milbemycins consist of moxidectin, milbemycin, and nemadectin. These structurally similar compounds are derived from natural compounds produced by soil-dwelling fungi from the genus *Streptomyces*.[1] The natural compound avermectin is composed

PAE was supported by National Institute of Environmental Health Sciences grant K08 ES017045. The authors have nothing to disclose.

[a] ASPCA Animal Poison Control Center, 1717 South Philo Road, Suite 36, Urbana, IL 61802, USA
[b] Department of Comparative Biosciences, College of Veterinary Medicine, University of Illinois at Urbana-Champaign, 2001 South Lincoln Avenue, Urbana, IL 61821, USA
* Corresponding author.
E-mail address: valentina.merola@aspca.org

of 8 closely related compounds: 4 A- and B-components (A_1, A_2, B_1, B_2), each of which further contains 2 homologous a- and b-components, for example, B_{1a} and B_{1b}.[1] Abamectin and ivermectin are both composed of avermectin B_1 components, differing only in the absence of a double bond in ivermectin.[1] Further modification of B_1 produces eprinomectin.[1] Doramectin and selamectin are closely related and contain A_1 and B_1 components, respectively.[2] Moxidectin is produced from the *Streptomyces* fermentation product nemadectin.[2] Milbemycin oxime (milbemycin) is composed of 5-oxime derivatives of milbemycins A_4 and A_3.[1]

MECHANISMS OF TOXICITY AND THE ROLE OF P-GLYCOPROTEIN

Avermectins and milbemycins have minor differences in some substituents, but they share the same general structure that confers on them the ability to bind to chloride channel receptors.[1] One main mechanism by which the MLs exert their effect is by binding ligand-gated chloride channels.[2,3] Binding of glutamate-gated chloride channels, which are specific to invertebrates, causes influx of chloride ions into the parasite neurons leading to hyperpolarization, paralysis, and death.[2]

In mammals, MLs bind to gamma-aminobutyric acid type A–gated chloride channels ($GABA_A$ receptors).[4] GABA is the primary inhibitory neurotransmitter in the brain, and postsynaptic binding of GABA to its receptors serves to modulate firing of excitatory neurons, such as glutamatergic neurons. MLs are believed to bind $GABA_A$ receptors at sites different than those where GABA, benzodiazepines, barbiturates, or picrotoxin separately bind.[5] Because $GABA_A$ receptors are only present in the CNS, binding of MLs is prevented by the blood-brain barrier (BBB), as discussed later. However, in overdoses, enough ML permeates the BBB that binding to $GABA_A$ receptors, as well as to glycine- and voltage-gated chloride channels, occurs.[3,6] Subsequent chloride influx causes hyperpolarization and decreased firing of the excitatory neurons that express these chloride receptors and channels, leading to clinical signs. Of interest, avermectins actually may reduce GABA effects at lower concentrations, resulting in signs such as tremoring (excitatory signs), and then start to enhance GABA effects as concentrations at the receptor increase, causing a progression of signs to ataxia and CNS depression (inhibitory effects).[3] So avermectins may have stimulatory CNS effects (tremors) at lower concentrations but inhibitory effects (ataxia, depression) at higher concentrations.

Permeability glycoprotein (P-gp) is a transmembrane efflux protein that influences the pharmacokinetics of many of its substrates, including MLs, by actively transporting absorbed substrates back across a variety of cell membranes in the body.[7] P-gp, which is a member of the ATP-binding cassette (ABC) superfamily of transporters, is found in all mammalian species[8] and is well distributed throughout the tissues of dogs[9] and cats.[10] It is characteristically located along the apical border of cell types that serve a barrier function (eg, enterocytes, bile canalicular cells, renal tubular cells, and endothelial cells), so P-gp can be viewed as having a protective function because it limits entry of substrates into internal compartments.[11]

P-gp is important in limiting the entry of MLs and other xenobiotics into the CNS.[12] The BBB regulates entry of endogenous substances and xenobiotics from the circulation into the brain. Tight junctions between endothelial cells prevent paracellular diffusion of substances into the CNS. Also, endothelial cells in the brain are specialized in that they lack pinocytotic vacuoles and fenestrations in their plasma membranes, thus making the BBB selectively permeable.[13] Substances that enter the brain must either diffuse through the endothelial cells or be actively transported into the endothelial cells by uptake transporters.[14] As substances enter the endothelial cells in the brain, they are potentially subject to being extruded back across the apical

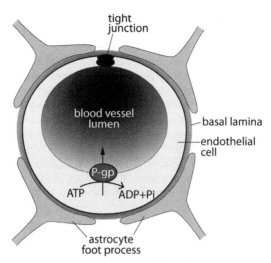

Fig. 1. P-glycoprotein (P-gp) is a component of the blood brain barrier. P-gp actively transports substrates entering CNS endothelial cells back into the systemic circulation, thus preventing entry of substrates, such as ivermectin, into the parenchyma of the brain. Information from Refs.[49,59,82–84] (*Adapted from* Linnet K, Ejsing TB. A review on the impact of P-glycoprotein on the penetration of drugs into the brain. Focus on psychotropic drugs. Eur Neuropsychopharmacol 2008;18:159; with permission.)

membrane by P-gp and other efflux proteins,[13,14] as shown in **Fig. 1**. Further components of the BBB include the basal lamina on the abluminal side of the endothelial cells and the foot processes of the glial astrocytes.[13]

The *ABCB1* gene (formerly called *MDR1*) codes for P-gp in vertebrates[8] and has been sequenced in dogs.[15] In some dog breeds there is a genetic defect in P-gp: a 4–base pair deletion in the *ABCB1* gene (*ABCB1-1Δ*) results in production of an extremely truncated, nonfunctional P-gp.[15] Having the *ABCB1-1Δ* mutation can result in accumulation of P-gp substrates in the brain that would normally be removed by P-gp,[12] so the BBB is compromised and becomes permeable to P-gp substrates, including MLs. In dogs with this defect, treatment with doses of MLs above those used for heartworm prevention may result in accumulation of the drug in the CNS, resulting in neurologic effects. Adverse neurologic effects can also occur in animals without the gene defect when overdoses of MLs are administered, in which case saturation of the transport capacity of P-gp likely occurs. Dogs may be homozygous or heterozygous for the defect, with homozygous dogs being at greater risk of developing toxicosis from ML exposure.[7]

EXPOSURE SOURCES, FORMULATIONS, AND THERAPEUTIC AND TOXIC DOSAGES

Because the MLs are commonly used as parasiticides in many species, they are available in a wide array of formulations.[1] Some of the most common small animal veterinary products include tablets with ivermectin, moxidectin, or milbemycin and topical products with selamectin that are used for heartworm prevention. Ivermectin, moxidectin, milbemycin, and doramectin are also used off-label for various indications including as a heartworm microfilaricide and for treating demodectic and sarcoptic mange as well as other ecto- and endoparasites.[16] Dogs and cats may also be exposed to large animal products either accidentally or by intentional administration. Many formulations intended for large animals are concentrated so it is easy for accidental overdoses to occur.

Signs of intoxication with MLs generally are related to the CNS. Neurologic depression, ataxia, mydriasis, blindness, tremors, and hypersalivation all may be seen and, as signs progress, an animal may become comatose. Seizures may also occur. The blindness is typically temporary and has been associated with retinal edema and electroretinogram abnormalities in the case of ivermectin.[17] The signs seen are similar in both dogs and cats for all the MLs. Depending on the dose and the breed involved and due to the long half-life of these agents, toxicosis may persist for days to weeks.

Formulations, labeled and off-label therapeutic dosage ranges, and documented "safe" versus toxic dosages for specific MLs are discussed next. When possible, distinctions are made between dosages that affect dogs with or without the *ABCB1-1Δ* gene defect. **Table 1** provides a summary of the information in this section.

Ivermectin

Ivermectin is available in numerous forms for large animal applications including injectable liquid, oral bolus, pour-on, paste, and feed pre-mix. It is available as chewable tablets for heartworm prevention in small animals. Ivermectin is also produced as a 3-mg tablet (Stromectrol) for humans indicated for treatment of gastrointestinal (GI) strongyloidiasis in the United States and for onchocerciasis and strongyloidiasis in other countries. Many of the large animal formulations are of relatively high concentration, from 1% to 1.87% (10–18.7 mg/mL), so it is easy for accidental overdose to occur either from miscalculation of a dosage when using these products off-label, from accidental exposure to the remnants in a discarded tube of equine dewormer, or from blobs of dewormer that fall from a horse's mouth during deworming. Exposure to concentrated (eg, ivermectin 1.87%) MLs eliminated in the dung of treated large animals is also a potential source of exposure (ASPCA Animal Poison Control Center [APCC], Urbana, IL, unpublished information, 2011). In one study, ivermectin concentrations in horse dung were monitored after horses were treated with a manufacturer's recommended therapeutic dosage.[18] Peak ivermectin levels of 2.4 mg/kg of dung were measured 2.5 days after exposure. To place this concentration in perspective, a 27.3 kg (60 lb) collie homozygous for *ABCB1-1Δ* would need to ingest 1.1 kg (2.4 lb) of dung to attain a dosage of 0.1 mg/kg of ivermectin, which is mildly toxic in sensitive collies.[19] In contrast, tablets for heartworm prevention range from 0.068 to 0.272 mg of ivermectin per tablet so toxicosis is rare even when small animals ingest several of these pills.

Ivermectin is used for heartworm prevention at dosages of 0.006 to 0.012 mg/kg in dogs and 0.024 mg/kg in cats. It is also used off-label in dogs as a microfilaricide at 0.05 to 0.2 mg/kg and to treat ectoparasites at 0.3 to 0.6 mg/kg.[16]

Clinical signs have been reported in breeds with a history of ivermectin sensitivity at dosages ranging from 0.08 to 0.34 mg/kg.[20–22] However, none of these dogs were tested for the *ABCB1* gene deletion. In breeds considered to be normal in their response to ivermectin, mild clinical signs have been documented at dosages starting from 0.2 mg/kg,[22] with more severe signs developing at dosages of 1 to 2.5 mg/kg or greater.[22,23] Some of the dogs reported to show signs at relatively low ivermectin dosages in one retrospective study[22] were German shepherds. A small percentage of this breed does carry the *ABCB1* gene defect,[24] which might partly explain the presence of signs in "normal" dogs at relatively low dosages. It is important to emphasize that problems are not expected with standard heartworm preventative dosages even in *ABCB1-1Δ* dogs. Ivermectin-sensitive collies were treated with 10

Table 1
Therapeutic, nontoxic, and toxic dosages of macrocyclic lactones in both normal and sensitive dogs and in cats

Agent	Formulations	Therapeutic Dosages (Labeled and Off-Label) (mg/kg)	Acute, Subacute or Chronic Dosages Published as Safe (mg/kg)	Toxic Dosages ML Sensitive Dogs (mg/kg)	Acute Toxic Dosage Normal Dog/Cat (mg/kg)	References
Ivermectin	Tablets, oral liquid, oral paste, feed premix, injectable, topical, otic	0.006–0.6 PO D 0.024 PO C 0.2–0.4 SC D, C	0.5 PO daily × 12 weeks[a] D 0.06 PO Collies 0.2–1.33[a] PO or SC C 0.72 PO C	0.1–0.4[b] PO 0.2–0.25[b] SC	0.2–2.5 PO D 0.3 SC C	16,22,25 26,27,32 69,85,87
Selamectin	Topical	6 topical D, C	6 PO D, C[c] 40 topical Collies 72–114 topical D 236–367 topical C	5 PO[d]	None found	16,88,93
Moxidectin	Tablets, oral drench, injectable, topical	0.003 PO D 0.17 sustained release SC D 2.5 topical D 1 topical C	1.15 PO daily × 1 year D 0.09 PO Collies 0.85 SC D, Collies	1 PO[e]	1.9–2.8 PO D 1 PO C[f]	2,16,28 89,90,94 95,96
Doramectin	Injectable, pour-on	0.6 SC D, C	0.5–1 PO daily × 91 days D 0.2 SC C	0.29–0.7 SC	None found	16,37,38 86,91
Milbemycin	Tablets	0.5–2 PO D 2 PO C	10 PO Collies 10 PO C	5–10[g] PO 0.8 PO × 2 days 1.5 PO × 13 days	None found	16,33,34 92

Abbreviations: C, cat; collies, ivermectin-sensitive collies; D, dog; PO, orally; SC, subcutaneously.
[a] It should be noted that some animals are also reported to have problems at this dosage.
[b] Many of the collies in these reports were not tested for the *ABCB1-1*Δ gene defect.
[c] Cats exhibited drooling and intermittent vomiting with oral dosing.
[d] One collie was ataxic after this dosage in the safety studies, but others tolerated up to 15 mg/kg PO.
[e] Administered as a product containing 2.5% moxidectin and 10% imidacloprid.
[f] Generally only mild signs seen.
[g] Collies at these dosages were not tested for the *ABCB1-1*Δ gene defect.

times the heartworm preventative dosage (0.06 mg/kg) without signs developing.[25] However, when ivermectin is used at higher dosages as a microfilaricide or for demodicosis, problems can easily occur in patients with the *ABCB1* gene deletion, and sometimes even in dogs with normal *ABCB1* genotype. Clinical signs have developed following oral dosages as low as 0.1 mg/kg in ivermectin-sensitive collies.[19] In overdoses, the most frequent clinical signs reported in dogs were lethargy, ataxia, hypersalivation, tremors, mydriasis, blindness, and bradycardia.[22,26] Coma, seizures, and death have been seen in severely affected animals. Similar signs have been seen in cats[27] (ASPCA APCC, unpublished information, 2011), although miosis rather than mydriasis was noted in one case report.[27]

Moxidectin

Moxidectin is available in many forms including injectable, pour-on, and oral drench for ruminants and horses. It is available as a topical preparation, a subcutaneous (SC) injection and a monthly tablet for heartworm prevention in small animals. As with ivermectin, moxidectin products intended for use in horses and ruminants are of relatively high concentration (0.5%–2% or 5–20 mg/mL), so small animals may be exposed to high doses from relatively small amounts of these products. Also similar to ivermectin, horse dung could be another potential source of moxidectin exposure for dogs, with peak moxidectin concentrations of 2.6 mg/kg of horse dung measured 2.5 days after horses were treated with a manufacturer's recommended therapeutic dosage.[18]

Moxidectin is used in dogs for heartworm prevention orally at 0.003 mg/kg monthly and in sustained-release SC injection at 0.17 mg/kg every 6 months. It is also used topically in dogs at 2.5 mg/kg and in cats at 1 mg/kg monthly for heartworm prevention.[16]

At oral dosages of 1.9 to 2.8 mg/kg, adverse effects have been documented in dogs with normal P-gp genotype.[28] Signs in dogs exposed to equine moxidectin dewormers include ataxia, tremors, seizures, hyperthermia, tachycardia, blindness, hypersalivation, bradycardia, coma, and respiratory depression.[28–31]

Selamectin

Selamectin is available as a topical formulation for dogs and cats that is labeled for prevention of heartworm and for killing fleas and ear mites at a minimum dosage of 6 mg/kg, with concentrations of 60 and 120 mg/mL. It is also used at the same dosages to treat sarcoptic mange and tick infestation in dogs and hookworms and ascarids in cats.[16] Because it is not available as a more concentrated form, overdose is less likely. The most common clinical signs following selamectin exposure include vomiting, drooling, retching, licking of lips, lethargy, agitation, anorexia, and ataxia (ASPCA APCC, unpublished information, 2011). Many of these signs likely result from inadvertent oral exposure or administration.

Abamectin (Avermectin B₁)

Abamectin is generally used in products used to control ants, cockroaches, mites, and other insects. Sometimes abamectin products are labeled as containing avermectin B$_1$. These are usually found in the form of plastic traps ("baits") for ants and cockroaches, insect spikes, granules, or liquids intended to be sprayed for outdoor and indoor use. The liquids range in concentration from 0.15% to 2%. Generally, the ant/cockroach traps contain between 0.01% and 0.05% of abamectin. A typical ant "bait" weighs about 1.6 to 2 g, giving a range of 0.16 to 1 mg of abamectin per trap;

thus it is rare to see significant signs with exposure. Subchronic studies in several species (dogs, rats, rabbits, and mice) suggest that abamectin and ivermectin have a similar degree of toxicity and that abamectin is marginally more toxic than ivermectin.[32] Dogs are primarily exposed to these insecticide products because some contain attractants, such as peanut butter, which are intended to lure insects but are also appealing to dogs. The clinical signs most commonly reported to the APCC following abamectin exposure are vomiting, ataxia, hypersalivation, lethargy, mydriasis, and diarrhea (ASPCA APCC, unpublished information, 2011). Many of the clinical signs are also likely related to the inert ingredients that can cause mild GI upset.

Milbemycin

Milbemycin is available as an oral chewable tablet (2.3–27 mg) for heartworm prevention in dogs and cats as well as a 0.1% otic solution for treating ear mites.[16] It is not available in a more concentrated dosage form, so overdoses are relatively rare.

The therapeutic dosages of milbemycin for heartworm prevention are 0.5 mg/kg in dogs and 2 mg/kg in cats. Mild clinical signs of ataxia, hypersalivation, mydriasis, and lethargy have been documented in ivermectin-sensitive dogs dosed at 5 to 10 mg/kg.[33] In a separate report, two ABCB1-defective dogs developed mild signs (ataxia) after being dosed repeatedly with milbemycin for demodicosis; one dog received 0.8 mg/kg 2 days in a row and the other dog received 1.5 mg/kg daily for 13 days before developing signs.[34] Mild clinical signs have been reported to develop in normal dogs at 10 to 20 mg/kg and in both cats and in dogs with suspected ABCB1 gene deletions at greater than 5 to 10 mg/kg (ASPCA APCC, unpublished information, 2011). The most common clinical signs reported include ataxia, tremors, lethargy, vomiting, mydriasis, disorientation, and hypersalivation.

Doramectin, Eprinomectin, and Nemadectin

Doramectin is available as an injectable formulation (10 mg/mL) for ruminants and pigs as well as a pour-on for cattle (5 mg/mL).[2] Doramectin has been used off-label to treat demodicosis in dogs and cats at 0.6 mg/kg SC once weekly.[16] Eprinomectin is available as a pour-on for cattle (5 mg/mL).[2] Eprinomectin has been used experimentally to treat Toxocara canis at 0.1 mg/kg in dogs,[35] while nemadectin has been used at 0.2 to 0.6 mg/kg in dogs to treat GI helminths.[36] Side effects were not seen in either study. Further information about eprinomectin and nemadectin use in small animals could not be located.

Exposure of small animals to these products occurs less frequently than to some of the more common MLs, but these products are of high concentration so it is plausible that accidental exposure could result in toxicosis. Two case reports regarding dogs exposed to doramectin give us an idea of what clinical signs can be seen. One report involved a collie given 0.2 mg/kg of doramectin SC,[37] while the other involved 2 white Swiss shepherds exposed to 0.7 mg/kg doramectin SC.[38] The dogs in the latter report were confirmed to have the ABCB1 gene defect, while the collie was assumed to have the gene defect. Clinical signs included blindness, restlessness, CNS depression, recumbency, hypersalivation, tremors, tachypnea, ataxia, head pressing, disorientation, lack of menace response, and bradycardia. Clinical signs from eprinomectin or nemadectin overdose in animals with normal P-gp are expected to be similar, but it is uncertain at what dosage signs would emerge.

TOXICOKINETICS OF MACROCYCLIC LACTONES AND THE ROLE OF P-GLYCOPROTEIN

In general, the MLs have relatively fast oral absorption but a much more gradual absorption rate after SC injection.[39] They also are all highly fat soluble, have a large volume of distribution, and accumulate in fat tissue resulting in a long elimination half-life.[1,40] The authors were unable to locate specific information about metabolism and amounts of drug or metabolites eliminated in bile and urine in the dog or cat. Data from species where this information is known indicate that generally large percentages of MLs are eliminated in the bile with the degree of metabolism varying among the different compounds.[1] Studies in large animal species[1] and humans[41] suggest that enterohepatic circulation, by which xenobiotics are eliminated in the bile and then reabsorbed from the gut, occurs with MLs. However differences in product formulation can alter pharmacokinetic parameters significantly even for the same agent.[39,42]

In dogs, it takes about 4 hours for orally administered ivermectin to reach maximum plasma levels (t_{max} = 4 hours).[43,44] Subcutaneous absorption is slower, with t_{max} being 32 to 36 hours in dogs[43,45] and about 28 hours in cats.[40] The elimination half-life after oral administration of ivermectin to dogs is 3.3 days,[43,44] while after SC administration, the half-life is 3.2 days in dogs[43] and 3.4 days in cats.[40] One study evaluated the differences in pharmacokinetic parameters after SC injection of the same dosage of 7 different ivermectin preparations in dogs.[45] The maximum plasma concentrations ranged from 26.5 to 49.6 ng/mL and the area under the curve ranged from 2523 to 4956 ng • h/mL. The area under the curve, which reflects bioavailability, is a measure of the amount of free drug that reaches systemic circulation.[45] These significant differences illustrate the influence of formulation on pharmacokinetic parameters.

Moxidectin is absorbed faster than ivermectin following oral administration, with a t_{max} of 2 to 3 hours in dogs.[44,46] Moxidectin is highly bioavailable after oral dosing: about 90% of the drug is absorbed in dogs.[47] Reported elimination half-lives in dogs vary from 13.9 to 25.9 days.[44,46,47] This variability is associated with body condition. More obese dogs had a higher volume of distribution,[46,47] resulting in indirectly prolonged elimination due to distribution of the lipophilic drug into their relatively larger fat compartment.

Selamectin is used in dogs and cats topically. With dermal exposure, peak blood levels are reached in 72 hours in dogs and 15 hours in cats; if given orally, t_{max} is 8 hours in dogs and 7 hours in cats.[48] The elimination half-life in dogs is 11.1 days after dermal exposure and 1.9 days with oral exposure. In cats, the half-life is 8.25 days after dermal exposure and 1.1 days after oral exposure.[48] Selamectin is much more bioavailable in cats than in dogs after dermal applications: 72% bioavailability in cats versus 4.4% in dogs.[48] However, it is not known how much of this difference is due to grooming behavior (and therefore oral absorption) in cats. Oral bioavailability of selamectin was 109% in cats and 62% in dogs,[48] which, especially in cats, suggests enterohepatic circulation of selamectin.

Doramectin reaches peak blood levels in 2 hours after oral dosing and 1.4 days after subcutaneous administration in dogs, while the half-life in dogs is 3 to 3.7 days.[43] Kinetic information in small animals could not be located for eprinomectin and nemadectin.

P-gp potentially both limits drug absorption, by moving substrates out of enterocytes and back into the intestinal tract, as well as enhances drug elimination, by depositing substrates into the bile, intestine, and renal tubules.[7,49] Several factors can affect the ability of P-gp to alter the kinetics of MLs. One factor is the affinities of the

MLs for P-gp, with MLs that have higher affinities being more readily transported at lower concentrations. Ivermectin, abamectin, doramectin, and eprinomectin all have higher affinities for P-gp compared to selamectin and moxidectin.[50]. The concentration of MLs presented to transporters is another potentially important factor. P-gp substrates can often stimulate their own transport at lower concentrations while inhibiting transport at higher concentrations,[51] so as levels of an ML crossing the cellular apical border increase, P-gp may become less able to effectively transport it back across the plasma membrane.

Unfortunately, the ability of P-gp to alter the pharmacokinetics of MLs has not been closely examined. One way to evaluate for this is to compare kinetic parameters of MLs between dogs with and without the *ABCB1-1Δ* gene defect. Ivermectin plasma levels did not differ between normal and ivermectin-sensitive collies administered 0.1 mg/kg ivermectin orally,[52] but 0.1 mg/kg may be too small a dose for pharmacokinetic differences to be evident. It has been demonstrated that dogs with the *ABCB1* defect are impaired in the ability to eliminate P-gp substrates into the bile[53] but do not appear to have enhanced intestinal absorption of P-gp substrates.[54] However, MLs were not evaluated in the latter two studies.

SENSITIVE POPULATIONS
Dogs with the ABCB1-1Δ Gene Defect

The *ABCB1-1Δ* mutation is typically seen in herding type breeds, primarily collies as well as Shetland sheepdogs and Australian shepherds; in addition, it has been detected in longhaired whippets, old English sheepdogs, silken windhounds, white Swiss shepherds, German shepherds, and some mixes of these breeds.[38,55]

Dogs can be easily tested for the gene defect.[7] However, it is difficult to know whether the frequencies of the gene defect in populations of dogs that are tested is representative of the general population since there may be bias in submitting samples (eg, dogs may be more likely to be tested after an ML-related toxicosis develops or if they are related to dogs known to have the *ABCB1* defect). Mealey and colleagues[24] found that of 5368 client-owned dogs, the breeds with the highest frequency of the *ABCB1-1Δ* mutation were collies and Australian shepherds: of 1424 collies tested, 35% were homozygous and 42% were heterozygous, and of 1421 Australian shepherds tested, 10% were homozygous and 37% were heterozygous. In miniature Australian shepherds, silken windhounds, and longhaired whippets, between 30% and 60% of the dogs tested had one or both copies of the gene defect. In border collies, German shepherds, herding breed mixes, old English sheepdogs, Shetland sheepdogs, and other mixed breeds, less than 15% of dogs had one or both copies of the gene defect. They also tested 659 purebred dogs of other breeds with none having the gene defect. In a smaller study of dogs in Australia, higher rates of the gene defect in collies and Australian shepherds were seen compared to rates in the United States.[55] Interestingly, in both of these studies, it was rare (about 1% frequency) to find the *ABCB1* mutation in border collies. However, a recent report of an *ABCB1* mutation that differs from the *ABCB1-1Δ* mutation in an ivermectin-sensitive border collie[56] demonstrates that other gene defects can produce the ivermectin-sensitive phenotype. Thus, just because a dog does not have the *ABCB1-1Δ* genotype does not mean that it is absolutely certain that it will tolerate higher dosages of MLs.

Animals Treated with Other P-Glycoprotein Substrates

Chronic administration of MLs for demodicosis has resulted in toxicosis in dogs of breeds in which the *ABCB1-1Δ* mutation has not been documented[57] (ASPCA APCC, unpublished information, 2011), suggesting that factors other than genetics might play a role in the development of ML toxicosis. These dogs developed signs such as ataxia, lethargy, and tremors after administration of extra-label doses of ivermectin, moxidectin, or milbemycin for periods ranging from days to weeks. Bissonnette and colleagues[57] had 28 of these dogs genotyped and found that 27 were normal while one was heterozygous for the ABCB1-1Δ gene mutation. Of these dogs, 10 were on other medications that also are P-gp substrates. Acquired P-gp dysfunction due to drug interactions may make animals more susceptible to ML toxicosis.[7] It also may be possible that in these dogs there were other, as yet unidentified, mutations that may impair P-gp function.

Mechanisms by which other P-gp substrates can potentially cause elevated levels of MLs in the brain or plasma include competing with MLs for transport by P-gp and inhibiting P-gp function. These effects can be concentration dependent where a substrate can become an inhibitor as its concentrations at the transporter rise.[51] **Table 2** lists several medications that are known P-gp substrates or inhibitors. In many cases it is not known if an interaction between MLs and these drugs will occur, so this list should be taken as a guideline for when caution should be exercised when co-administering avermectins or milbemycins with the listed medications. However, combining a P-gp substrate with a P-gp inhibitor is more likely to be problematic than treating a patient with 2 P-gp substrates. Two commonly used veterinary drugs that are P-gp inhibitors (as well as substrates) and that interact unfavorably with MLs in dogs, as discussed next, illustrate this principle.

The antifungal drug ketoconazole can cause problems when administered concurrently with ivermectin. Hugnet and colleagues[58] reported that administration of ketoconazole to dogs over a period spanning from 5 days before through 5 days after ivermectin administration resulted in higher plasma concentrations and longer residence time of ivermectin than in dogs treated with ivermectin alone. Ketoconazole is an inhibitor of P-gp, which may result in decreased elimination of ivermectin from the CNS as well as decreased biliary excretion of ivermectin.

When ivermectin and the insecticide spinosad were co-administered, signs of ivermectin toxicosis sometimes developed at dosages not typically expected to cause problems.[59] One study determined that ivermectin pharmacokinetics were altered when ivermectin was given with spinosad: maximum plasma concentrations and area under the curve of ivermectin were increased while clearance was decreased compared to dogs given ivermectin alone.[59] It was determined that spinosad is a substrate and inhibitor of human P-gp, prompting the authors to hypothesize that this inhibition is responsible for the increased risk of ivermectin toxicosis when spinosad is co-administered in dogs.[59] A different study assessed the effects of co-administration of spinosad and milbemycin in collies with the ABCB1-1Δ mutation.[60] Up to 10 times the heartworm preventative dose of milbemycin along with spinosad at either 3 or 5 times the labeled therapeutic dose did not result in signs of milbemycin toxicosis. It is interesting to speculate whether milbemycin has a relatively poorer affinity for P-gp, as does moxidectin,[50] compared to ivermectin, which might explain the difference between the 2 studies. However the authors cannot locate information regarding the affinity of milbemycin for P-gp in the literature.

Neonatal and Elderly Dogs and Cats

An important question is whether very young dogs and cats have an immature BBB that would make them more susceptible to ML toxicosis. However, studies that would directly address this question could not be located. Tight junctions between endothelial cells in the brain, which begin forming in conjunction with the development of

P-gp Substrates	P-gp Inhibitors
Table 2	
P-glycoprotein substrates and inhibitors	
Antibiotics	
Erythromycin	Erythromycin
Tetracycline	Clarithromycin
Doxycycline	
Antifungals	
Ketoconazole	Ketoconazole
Itraconazole	Itraconazole
Antidepressants	
Paroxetine	Paroxetine
Venlafaxine	Fluoxetine
Amitriptyline	St. John's wort
Chemotherapeutics	
Vinblastine	
Vincristine	
Doxorubicin	
Actinomycin D	
Mitoxantrone	
Etoposide	
Docetaxel	
Cardiac drugs	
Digoxin	Amiodarone
Diltiazem	Quinidine
Verapamil	Verapamil
	Carvediol
	Nicardipine
Opioids	
Loperamide	Methadone
Morphine	Pentazocine
Steroid hormones	
Dexamethasone	
Triamcinolone	
Hydrocortisone	
Aldosterone	
Methylprenisolone	
Proton pump inhibitors	
	Omeprazole
	Esomeprazole
	Lansoprazole
	Pantoprazole

(continued on next page)

Table 2 (continued)	
P-gp Substrates	**P-gp Inhibitors**
Miscellaneous agents	
Cyclosporine	Cyclosporine
Phenothiazines	Chlorpromazine
Spinosad	Spinosad
Cimetidine	
Fexofenadine	

Data from Refs. [49,59,82–84]

blood vessels in the fetal brain, are vital for sealing the BBB.[61] Evidence suggests that tight junctions exist in the brain prenatally in dogs, with further modifications occurring between 6 days prior to birth and 3 days postpartum.[62] In the authors' opinion, adequate P-gp expression in the endothelial cells is the other important component necessary for the BBB to be able to prevent MLs from accumulating in the brain. Information on P-gp expression in fetal or neonatal dogs or cats could not be located in the literature. In other species, times when there are marked increases in P-gp expression range from, at the earliest, during fetal development in humans[63] to, at the latest, post-natal days 16 to 21 in mice.[64] Given that times for increased P-gp expression are not expected to vary greatly beyond the times seen in other mammalian species, it is best to avoid ML exposure in neonatal dogs and cats. However, the authors speculate that sensitivity to MLs diminishes by weaning, if not sooner, in dogs and cats.

Aging also significantly affects the BBB. Brain P-gp expression is significantly decreased in aged dogs, with a 72% decrease occurring in expression in dogs over 8.3 years of age compared to dogs less than 3 years of age.[65] It is not known if this change is significant in reducing elimination of MLs from the central nervous system, but it does suggest that older patients could be more susceptible to ML toxicosis than adults.

Obese and Malnourished Animals

An animal's nutritional plane and body condition may also impact both the likelihood of ML toxicosis developing and the duration of treatment needed when toxicosis occurs. In moxidectin pharmacokinetic studies, obese dogs, which have a relatively larger volume of distribution, had a significantly longer elimination half-life for moxidectin.[46,47] It is not known if this difference is clinically significant, but it suggests that obese patients may require a longer duration of treatment after overdose due to the longer length of time needed for MLs to redistribute out of the fat compartment. Conversely, obesity could have a protective effect by basically providing more body volume for a given ML dose to distribute into, thus lowering plasma and tissue concentrations. So it is difficult to predict which effect might have more impact in ML toxicosis. A case report describing 3 rottweilers that ingested moxidectin noted that, of the 3, the obese dog received the lowest dose but had the most severe signs.[28] Two of the 3 dogs in the study (including the obese dog) were negative for the *ABCB1-1Δ* gene defect, while the third dog's sample was not adequate for testing.

But what if a patient is malnourished? In vitro binding studies in dogs have shown that ivermectin binds extensively to plasma albumin and lipoproteins.[42] In a severely undernourished or hypoalbuminemic patient, it is possible that a higher free drug concentration could develop resulting in more severe clinical signs. For now, the influence of body condition on ML toxicosis remains speculative, but it should be considered.

TREATMENT

There are no specific antidotes for ML toxicosis. Appropriate decontamination and good supportive care are the cornerstones of treatment. Some patients need to be hospitalized for several days, so it is important that animal owners are advised up front regarding this possibility. However, with commitment to treatment, it is possible for even severely affected animals to make a complete recovery.

Decontamination

Inducing emesis may be considered if oral exposure was recent and the animal is asymptomatic. There are no established criteria for when emesis should be induced or avoided with ML ingestion. Rather, several factors must be considered. Liquid or paste formulations of MLs are anticipated to empty from the stomach rather quickly compared to solid formulations,[66] although mixing with recently ingested food may slow the emptying of nonsolid formulations.[67] Also, inducing emesis will not only delay the administration of activated charcoal, which is likely to be of greater benefit in reducing absorption of MLs than emesis, but will also make it more likely that subsequently administered activated charcoal will be vomited. Additionally, care must be taken to avoid aspiration if neurologic signs have already developed,[68] so emesis should not be induced in patients who are already showing signs such as tremors, seizures, or CNS depression. Ultimately, the decision to induce emesis is best determined on a case-by-case basis, but a rule-of-thumb is to induce emesis if ingestion was within the past 30 to 60 minutes. Emesis could also be considered beyond 1 hour post-ingestion in circumstances such as the consumption of a large meal prior to oral ML exposure.

An initial dose of activated charcoal is likely to be of benefit if given within the first 4 hours of ingestion, given what is known regarding the absorption rate of MLs. Administering repeated doses of activated charcoal as frequently as every 8 hours for 2 days has been advised for ivermectin toxicosis,[22,69] although the efficacy of activated charcoal in treating overdoses of MLs has not been established. Whether a substance undergoes enterohepatic circulation is a key factor in whether repeated doses of activated charcoal are beneficial in enhancing elimination.[67] Since there is evidence that MLs are enterohepatically circulated, it is reasonable to consider repeated doses of activated charcoal in small animal patients regardless of the route of exposure. However, this recommendation caries some caveats. As with emesis, the risk of aspiration can be higher when administering charcoal in a symptomatic patient, especially a comatose patient, so this should not be attempted in a patient with an absent gag reflex. Intubation may offer some degree of airway protection during charcoal administration, but it does not completely remove risk of aspiration.[70] Other complications of activated charcoal administration to consider include hypernatremia and hypermagnesemia, likely due to the loss of free water osmotically drawn into the GI lumen.[67] These electrolyte disturbances are considered infrequent in humans, with an incidence of 6% and 3.1%, respectively, in one study,[71] but the incidence of either has not been reported in small animal patients. An additional consideration is that dogs with the *ABCB1-1Δ* gene defect may have minimal biliary elimination of P-gp substrates due to nonfunctional P-gp.[53] Therefore, repeated doses of activated charcoal may not be of much benefit in these animals, although this has not been proven. Because the amounts of MLs eliminated in bile in canines have not been evaluated, this would be an excellent avenue for further research that would help better answer questions about the role of repeated administration of activated charcoal in both wild-type and P-gp–defective dogs. In summary, decisions on the frequency of administration of activated charcoal are also best decided on a case-by-case basis, with the authors urging caution and moderation. An initial dose of charcoal given within 4 hours of exposure is strongly advised, provided that marked CNS signs are not present. Subsequent doses administered every 8 hours may be of some benefit, more so in animals with a normal *ABCB1* genotype. Risks of hypernatremia and aspiration should always be kept in mind whenever activated charcoal is used.

Supportive and Symptomatic Care

Fluid therapy, good nursing care of the recumbent animal, and thermoregulation are essential for these patients.[72] If respiratory depression develops, patients may require oxygen, intubation, and positive pressure ventilation. Nutritional support may also be needed. If bradycardia develops, a preanesthetic dose of atropine or glycopyrrolate may be given.

Treatment of tremors or seizures resulting from ML toxicosis is a challenging topic, with the uncertainty of which drugs to use being the main question. In clinical case reports, administration of diazepam either seemed to be of no benefit[30] or resulted in improvement of CNS stimulation soon followed by worsening of CNS depression.[26,28,29] This led Hopper and colleagues[26] to suggest that diazepam be avoided in favor of other suitable drugs such as barbiturates or propofol. Yet a progression of signs from tremors or seizures to severe CNS depression describes a typical clinical course as concentrations of MLs rise in the brain. It is likely that an onset of CNS depression would have occurred regardless of whether diazepam was given. While benzodiazepines such as diazepam can potentiate GABAergic effects, so can barbiturates and propofol, which both bind $GABA_A$ receptors, albeit at different sites than benzodiazepines and MLs.[5] Moreover, an experimental study in rodents suggests that ivermectin worsens the CNS effects caused by barbiturates.[6] The present state of knowledge is that there are several different binding sites on $GABA_A$ receptors, each of which binds different types of xenobiotics. The different binding sites interact allosterically, with binding of a compound to one site influencing the likelihood of different compounds binding to other sites—all of which then influence opening of the channel in the receptor and subsequent chloride influx.[4,73] Assessment of allosteric relationships in the $GABA_A$ receptor can be very challenging,[5] and the relationships between MLs and drugs that bind $GABA_A$ receptors have not been well investigated. Until these allosteric relationships are better established, it is the authors' opinion that diazepam, barbiturates, or propfolol may be cautiously used to attempt to control tremors or seizures.

Specific Therapies

Intravenous lipid emulsion therapy has been suggested to be a treatment that may shorten the duration of clinical signs of ML toxicosis. Lipid therapy was used to treat moxidectin intoxication in a 16-week-old Jack Russell terrier.[29] The dog recovered quickly compared to other reported cases of moxidectin toxicosis, but the amount of moxidectin the puppy ingested is unknown, so it is difficult to draw firm conclusions. Lipid therapy has also been successfully used in a border collie that ingested up to 6 mg/kg of ivermectin paste.[74] The authors demonstrated decreasing blood levels of ivermectin and a relatively rapid improvement in clinical signs in this case with use of lipid therapy. The dog in this case report was found to not have the *ABCB1-1Δ* gene mutation, which may be why the therapy appeared effective: the ability of P-gp to clear ivermectin from the CNS and the circulation was intact in this patient. When lipid therapy was administered several hours after ivermectin exposure in 3 dogs homozygous for the P-gp gene defect, lipid therapy failed to improve stupor or coma.[75] Speculatively, these dogs may have had higher CNS levels or been impaired in the elimination of ivermectin due to nonfunctional P-gp, resulting in the lack of efficacy of lipid therapy.[75] The use of intravenous lipid therapy to treat macrocyclic lactone toxicosis has not been reported in feline patients, but lipid therapy has been used to successfully treat lidocaine toxicosis in a cat.[76]

It is hypothesized that the lipids act as a "sink" and draw lipophilic xenobiotics into the plasma lipid phase, thus removing the harmful agent from the target tissues[29] and increasing the likelihood for more rapid elimination. Although moxidectin is likely the best candidate for this therapy due to its very high lipid solubility, all of the MLs are lipophilic so lipid therapy is potentially beneficial in treating toxicity from any of the avermectins or milbemycins. On one hand, it is important to emphasize that effectiveness and safety of this treatment in reducing the duration of clinical signs or improving outcome with acute toxicosis in clinical patients has not been proven in human[77] or veterinary patients. On the other hand, thus far, adverse effects of lipid therapy have not been reported in case reports and experimental studies where lipid emulsions were administered on a short-term basis.[78] Yet the APCC has received several reports of cases where hyperlipemic serum was noted in dogs after receiving lipid emulsion treatment. Two cases of hemolysis were also reported (ASPCA APCC, unpublished data, 2011). Consider intravenous lipid therapy if pronounced CNS signs, such as severe stupor, coma, or seizures, emerge. The APCC recommends using a 20% lipid solution starting with a 1.5 mL/kg bolus followed by a constant rate infusion (CRI) of 0.25 mL/kg/min for 30 to 60 minutes. This may be repeated every 4 hours as long as serum is not lipemic but should be discontinued if a positive response is not seen after 3 treatments. This protocol is based on the human literature where dose ranges include boluses of 1 to 3 mL/kg and CRIs of 0.2 to 0.5 mL/kg/min for up to 6 hours, with a 1.5 mL/kg bolus and a 0.25 to 0.5 mL/kg/min CRI for 30 to 60 minutes being the most commonly used.[77]

Physostigmine can cause short-term improvement in patients severely affected by MLs. Administration of physostigmine resulted in 30 to 90 minutes of improvement in moderate to severe CNS depression resulting from ivermectin-sensitive collies being administered 0.2 mg/kg ivermectin.[19] Physostigmine is a cholinergic drug that causes increased amounts of acetylcholine to accumulate at the synapse. Acetylcholine modulates inhibitory GABAergic and excitatory glutamatergic neuronal firing,[79] the net result of which may result in an improvement of clinical signs. Physostigmine is best used either to give an owner visual reassurance that the patient can still recover or to try to arouse a patient enough to encourage it to eat and drink. Frequent administration is not recommended as the effects are very temporary and significant cholinergic effects including drooling, urination, and diarrhea, as well as tremors and seizures, may be seen.[26]

Flumazenil is a $GABA_A$ antagonist that appeared to reverse the effects of ivermectin in an experimental model of drug interactions in rodents.[6,80] However, the use of flumazenil to treat ML toxicosis has not been evaluated clinically. Flumazenil is an antagonist at the benzodiazepine binding site, rather than at the GABA binding site, on $GABA_A$ receptors,[73] so flumazenil prevents benzodiazepines from binding $GABA_A$

receptors rather than directly influencing the effect of GABA. If flumazenil interacts with ML binding sites in an allosteric manner to reduce the effect of ML binding, then flumazenil would be of benefit, but it is unknown if this occurs. If it were beneficial, then it would serve a similar purpose to physostigmine: to improve clinical signs, but only transiently since flumazenil has a short time of effect.[81] Reported dosages for flumazenil in dogs range from 0.04 to 0.25 mg/kg IV.[81] Starting at the low end of the dosage range is advised, especially since flumazenil can potentially cause seizures at higher dosages through its effect as a benzodiazepine antagonist.[81]

DIAGNOSTICS

Genotyping in dogs to determine if the *ABCB1-1*Δ gene mutation is present can be performed through the Veterinary Clinical Pharmacology Laboratory at Washington State University College of Veterinary Medicine (http://www.vetmed.wsu.edu/depts-VCPL/) using either blood or cells from a cheek swab. Ideally dogs should be tested prior to using any dose of an ML higher than one for heartworm prevention, especially if the dog is a breed or breed mix of those known to carry the gene defect.

Plasma or stomach contents can be submitted to a veterinary diagnostic laboratory to test for levels of MLs in an effort to document exposure. Response to physostigmine can also be suggestive of ML intoxication if exposure is uncertain.[72] For post-mortem testing, samples to submit include frozen brain, liver, and fat.[72]

OUTCOME

The prognosis may be guarded to good depending on the exposure dose and agent involved. Severely affected dogs may require long-term care, which may be a financial burden for some owners. Depending on the dose and half-life of agent involved, recovery can take days to weeks. Reportedly one dog recovered completely after being comatose for 7 weeks.[69] After recovery, long-term sequelae are not expected.[72] Sedation and blindness seem to the longest lasting signs, but even blindness is not expected to be permanent as most dogs seem to recover visual ability (ASPCA APCC, unpublished information, 2011). Two dogs with documented retinal edema did recover well with only residual retinal scarring.[17]

SUMMARY

Drugs in the avermectin and milbemycin classes have a wide margin of safety between therapeutic and toxic dosages when administered to companion animals at their labeled dosages and dosing frequency. Toxicosis becomes more likely when higher, extra-label dosages are administered to dogs with the *ABCB1-1*Δ gene mutation or when companion animals are inadvertently exposed to, or iatrogenically overdosed with, concentrated ML-containing products intended for large animal use. Drug interactions between MLs and other P-gp substrates, such as spinosad or ketoconazole, might also result in ML toxicosis. Once clinical signs develop, recovery can take days to weeks due to extensive distribution of MLs in the body and their slow elimination. Decontamination measures instituted soon after exposure and good supportive care are the aspects of treatment that are most likely to favorably influence outcome. Intravenous lipid emulsion therapy has been suggested to be a beneficial treatment of ML toxicosis. However controlled clinical trials are lacking, and questions remain as to whether dogs with defective P-gp are a subpopulation in which lipid therapy is effective.

REFERENCES

1. Vercruysse J, Rew RS, editors. Macrocyclic lactones in antiparasitic therapy. New York: CABI; 2002.
2. Lanusse CE, Lifschitz AL, Imperiale FA. Macrocyclic lactones: endectocide compounds. In: Riviere JE, Papich MG, editors. Veterinary pharmacology and therapeutics. 9th edition. Ames (IA): Wiley-Blackwell; 2009. p. 1119–44.
3. Bloomquist JR. Chloride channels as tools for developing selective insecticides. Arch Insect Biochem Physiol 2003;54:145–56.
4. Sieghart W. Structure, pharmacology, and function of GABAA receptor subtypes. Adv Pharmacol 2006;54:231–63.
5. Sieghart W. Structure and pharmacology of gamma-aminobutyric acidA receptor subtypes. Pharmacol Rev 1995;47:181–234.
6. Trailovic SM, Nedeljkovic JT. Central and peripheral neurotoxic effects of ivermectin in rats. J Vet Med Sci 2011;73:591–9.
7. Mealey KL. Canine ABCB1 and macrocyclic lactones: heartworm prevention and pharmacogenetics. Vet Parasitol 2008;158:215–22.
8. Dean M, Annilo T. Evolution of the ATP-binding cassette (ABC) transporter superfamily in vertebrates. Annu Rev Genom Hum Genet 2005;6:123–42.
9. Ginn PE. Immunohistochemical detection of P-glycoprotein in formalin-fixed and paraffin-embedded normal and neoplastic canine tissues. Vet Pathol 1996;33:533–41.
10. Van Der Heyden S, Chiers K, Ducatelle R. Tissue distribution of p-glycoprotein in cats. Anat Histol Embryol 2009;38:455–60.
11. Macdonald N, Gledhill A. Potential impact of ABCB1 (p-glycoprotein) polymorphisms on avermectin toxicity in humans. Arch Toxicol 2007;81:553–63.
12. Mealey KL, Greene S, Bagley R, et al. P-glycoprotein contributes to the blood-brain, but not blood-cerebrospinal fluid, barrier in a spontaneous canine p-glycoprotein knockout model. Drug Metab Dispos 2008;36:1073–9.
13. Bernacki J, Dobrowolska A, Nierwinska K, et al. Physiology and pharmacological role of the blood-brain barrier. Pharmacol Rep 2008;60:600–22.
14. Urquhart BL, Kim RB. Blood-brain barrier transporters and response to CNS-active drugs. Eur J Clin Pharmacol 2009;65:1063–70.
15. Mealey KL, Bentjen SA, Gay JM, et al. Ivermectin sensitivity in collies is associated with a deletion mutation of the mdr1 gene. Pharmacogenetics 2001;11:727–33.
16. Plumb DC. Plumb's veterinary drug handbook. 5th edition. Stockholm (WI): PharmaVet; 2005.
17. Kenny PJ, Vernau KM, Puschner B, et al. Retinopathy associated with ivermectin toxicosis in two dogs. J Am Vet Med Assoc 2008;233:279–84.
18. Perez R, Cabezas I, Sutra JF, et al. Faecal excretion profile of moxidectin and ivermectin after oral administration in horses. Vet J 2001;161:85–92.
19. Tranquilli WJ, Paul AJ, Seward RL, et al. Response to physostigmine administration in collie dogs exhibiting ivermectin toxicosis. J Vet Pharmacol Ther 1987;10:96–100.
20. Houston DM, Parent J, Matushek KJ. Ivermectin toxicosis in a dog. J Am Vet Med Assoc 1987;191:78–80.
21. Hadrick MK, Bunch SE, Kornegay JN. Ivermectin toxicosis in two Australian shepherds. J Am Vet Med Assoc 1995;206:1147–50.
22. Merola V, Khan S, Gwaltney-Brant S. Ivermectin toxicosis in dogs: a retrospective study. J Am Anim Hosp Assoc 2009;45:106–11.
23. Hopkins KD, Marcella KL, Strecker AE. Ivermectin toxicosis in a dog. J Am Vet Med Assoc 1990;197:93–4.

24. Mealey KL, Meurs KM. Breed distribution of the ABCB1-1Delta (multidrug sensitivity) polymorphism among dogs undergoing ABCB1 genotyping. J Am Vet Med Assoc 2008;233:921–4.
25. Fassler PE, Tranquilli WJ, Paul AJ, et al. Evaluation of the safety of ivermectin administered in a beef-based formulation to ivermectin-sensitive Collies. J Am Vet Med Assoc 1991;199:457–60.
26. Hopper K, Aldrich J, Haskins SC. Ivermectin toxicity in 17 collies. J Vet Intern Med 2002;16:89–94.
27. Lewis DT, Merchant SR, Neer TM. Ivermectin toxicosis in a kitten. J Am Vet Med Assoc 1994;205:584–6.
28. See AM, McGill SE, Raisis AL, et al. Toxicity in three dogs from accidental oral administration of a topical endectocide containing moxidectin and imidacloprid. Aust Vet J 2009;87:334–7.
29. Crandell DE, Weinberg GL. Moxidectin toxicosis in a puppy successfully treated with intravenous lipids. J Vet Emerg Crit Care (San Antonio) 2009;19:181–6.
30. Snowden NJ, Helyar CV, Platt SR, et al. Clinical presentation and management of moxidectin toxicity in two dogs. J Small Anim Pract 2006;47:620–4.
31. Beal MW, Poppenga RH, Birdsall WJ, et al. Respiratory failure attributable to moxidectin intoxication in a dog. J Am Vet Med Assoc 1999;215:1813–7.
32. Woodward KN; for Joint WHO/FAO Expert Committee on Food Additives. 771. Ivermectin (WHO Food Additives Series 31). 1993. Available at: http://www.inchem.org/documents/jecfa/jecmono/v31je03.htm. Accessed November 20, 2011.
33. Tranquilli WJ, Paul AJ, Todd KS. Assessment of toxicosis induced by high-dose administration of milbemycin oxime in collies. Am J Vet Res 1991;52:1170–2.
34. Barbet JL, Snook T, Gay JM, et al. ABCB1-1 Delta (MDR1-1 Delta) genotype is associated with adverse reactions in dogs treated with milbemycin oxime for generalized demodicosis. Vet Dermatol 2009;20:111–4.
35. Kozan E, Sevimli FK, Birdane FM, et al. Efficacy of eprinomectin against Toxacara canis in dogs. Parasitol Res 2008;102:397–400.
36. Doscher ME, Wood IB, Pankavich JA, et al. Efficacy of nemadectin, a new broad-spectrum endectocide, against natural infections of canine gastrointestinal helminths. Vet Parasitol 1989;34:255–9.
37. Yas-Natan E, Shamir M, Kleinbart S, et al. Doramectin toxicity in a collie. Vet Rec 2003;153:718–20.
38. Geyer J, Klintzsch S, Meerkamp K, et al. Detection of the nt230(del4) MDR1 mutation in White Swiss Shepherd dogs: case reports of doramectin toxicosis, breed predisposition, and microsatellite analysis. J Vet Pharmacol Ther 2007;30:482–5.
39. McKellar QA, Benchaoui HA. Avermectins and milbemycins. J Vet Pharmacol Ther 1996;19:331–51.
40. Chittrakarn S, Janchawee B, Ruangrut P, et al. Pharmacokinetics of ivermectin in cats receiving a single subcutaneous dose. Res Vet Sci 2009;86:503–7.
41. Baraka OZ, Mahmoud BM, Marschke CK, et al. Ivermectin distribution in the plasma and tissues of patients infected with Onchocerca volvulus. Eur J Clin Pharmacol 1996;50:407–10.
42. González Canga A, Sahagún Prieto AM, José Diez Liébana M, et al. The pharmacokinetics and metabolism of ivermectin in domestic animal species. Vet J 2009;179:25–37.
43. Gokbulut C, Karademir U, Boyacioglu M, et al. Comparative plasma dispositions of ivermectin and doramectin following subcutaneous and oral administration in dogs. Vet Parasitol 2006;135(3–4):347–54.

44. Al-Azzam SI, Fleckenstein L, Cheng KJ, et al. Comparison of the pharmacokinetics of moxidectin and ivermectin after oral administration to beagle dogs. Biopharm Drug Dispos 2007;28:431–8.
45. Eraslan G, Kanbur M, Liman BC, et al. Comparative pharmacokinetics of some injectable preparations containing ivermectin in dogs. Food Chem Toxicol 2010; 48(8–9):2181–5.
46. Vanapalli SR, Hung YP, Fleckenstein L, et al. Pharmacokinetics and dose proportionality of oral moxidectin in beagle dogs. Biopharm Drug Dispos 2002;23: 263–72.
47. Lallemand E, Lespine A, Alvinerie M, et al. Estimation of absolute oral bioavailability of moxidectin in dogs using a semi-simultaneous method: influence of lipid co-administration. J Vet Pharmacol Ther 2007;30:375–80.
48. Sarasola P, Jernigan AD, Walker DK, et al. Pharmacokinetics of selamectin following intravenous, oral and topical administration in cats and dogs. J Vet Pharmacol Ther 2002;25:265–72.
49. Martinez M, Modric S, Sharkey M, et al. The pharmacogenomics of P-glycoprotein and its role in veterinary medicine. J Vet Pharmacol Ther 2008;31:285–300.
50. Lespine A, Dupuy J, Alvinerie M, et al. Interaction of macrocyclic lactones with the multidrug transporters: the bases of the pharmacokinetics of lipid-like drugs. Curr Drug Metab 2009;10:272–88.
51. Calabrese EJ. P-glycoprotein efflux transporter activity often displays biphasic dose-response relationships. Crit Rev Toxicol 2008;38:473–87.
52. Tranquilli WJ, Paul AJ, Seward RL. Ivermectin plasma concentrations in collies sensitive to ivermectin-induced toxicosis. Am J Vet Res 1989;50:769–70.
53. Coelho JC, Tucker R, Mattoon J, et al. Biliary excretion of technetium-99m-sestamibi in wild-type dogs and in dogs with intrinsic (ABCB1-1Delta mutation) and extrinsic (ketoconazole treated) P-glycoprotein deficiency. J Vet Pharmacol Ther 2009;32: 417–21.
54. Mealey KL, Waiting D, Raunig DL, et al. Oral bioavailability of P-glycoprotein substrate drugs do not differ between ABCB1-1Delta and ABCB1 wild type dogs. J Vet Pharmacol Ther 2010;33:453–60.
55. Mealey KL, Munyard KA, Bentjen SA. Frequency of the mutant MDR1 allele associated with multidrug sensitivity in a sample of herding breed dogs living in Australia. Vet Parasitol 2005;131:193–6.
56. Han JI, Son HW, Park SC, et al. Novel insertion mutation of ABCB1 gene in an ivermectin-sensitive Border Collie. J Vet Sci 2010;11:341–4.
57. Bissonnette S, Paradis M, Daneau I, et al. The ABCB1-1Delta mutation is not responsible for subchronic neurotoxicity seen in dogs of non-collie breeds following macrocyclic lactone treatment for generalized demodicosis. Vet Dermatol 2009;20: 60–6.
58. Hugnet C, Lespine A, Alvinerie M. Multiple oral dosing of ketoconazole increases dog exposure to ivermectin. J Pharm Pharm Sci 2007;10:311–8.
59. Dunn ST, Hedges L, Sampson KE, et al. Pharmacokinetic interaction of the antiparasitic agents ivermectin and spinosad in dogs. Drug Metab Dispos 2011;39:789–95.
60. Sherman JG, Paul AJ, Firkins LD. Evaluation of the safety of spinosad and milbemycin 5-oxime orally administered to Collies with the MDR1 gene mutation. Am J Vet Res 2010;71:115–9.
61. Saunders NR, Habgood MD, Dziegielewska KM. Barrier mechanisms in the brain, II. Immature brain. Clin Exp Pharmacol Physiol 1999;26:85–91.
62. Leuschen MP, Nelson RM Jr. Telencephalic microvessels of premature beagle pups. Anat Rec 1986;215:59–64.

63. Daood M, Tsai C, Ahdab-Barmada M, et al. ABC transporter (P-gp/ABCB1, MRP1/ABCC1, BCRP/ABCG2) expression in the developing human CNS. Neuropediatrics 2008;39:211–8.
64. Tsai CE, Daood MJ, Lane RH, et al. P-glycoprotein expression in mouse brain increases with maturation. Biol Neonate 2002;81:58–64.
65. Pekcec A, Schneider EL, Baumgartner W, et al. Age-dependent decline of blood-brain barrier P-glycoprotein expression in the canine brain. Neurobiol Aging 2011;32:1477–85.
66. Wyse CA, McLellan J, Dickie AM, et al. A review of methods for assessment of the rate of gastric emptying in the dog and cat: 1898-2002. J Vet Intern Med 2003;17:609–21.
67. Cooney DO. Activated charcoal in medical applications. New York: Dekker; 1995. p. 85–8, 310–3, 426–31.
68. Beasley VR, Dorman DC. Management of toxicoses. Vet Clin North Am Small Anim Pract 1990;20:307–37.
69. Lovell RA. Ivermectin and piperazine toxicoses in dogs and cats. Vet Clin North Am Small Anim Pract 1990;20:453–68.
70. Bond GR. The role of activated charcoal and gastric emptying in gastrointestinal decontamination: a state-of-the-art review. Ann Emerg Med 2002;39:273–86.
71. Dorrington CL, Johnson DW, Brant R, et al. The frequency of complications associated with the use of multiple-dose activated charcoal. Ann Emerg Med 2003;41:370–7.
72. Mealey KL. Ivermectin: macrolide antiparasitic agents. In: Peterson ME, Talcott PA, editors. Small animal toxicology. St Louis (MO): Saunders Elsevier; 2006. p. 785–94.
73. D'Hulst C, Atack JR, Kooy RF. The complexity of the GABAA receptor shapes unique pharmacological profiles. Drug Discov Today 2009;14:866–75.
74. Clarke DL, Lee JA, Murphy LA, et al. Use of intravenous lipid emulsion to treat ivermectin toxicosis in a Border Collie. J Am Vet Med Assoc 2011;239:1328–33.
75. Wright HM, Chen AV, Talcott PA, et al. Intravenous fat emulsion (IFE) for treatment of ivermectin toxicosis in 3 dogs ACVIM Forum abstract N-1. J Vet Intern Med 2011;25:725.
76. O'Brien TQ, Clark-Price SC, Evans EE, et al. Infusion of a lipid emulsion to treat lidocaine intoxication in a cat. J Am Vet Med Assoc 2010;237:1455–8.
77. Jamaty C, Bailey B, Larocque A, et al. Lipid emulsions in the treatment of acute poisoning: a systematic review of human and animal studies. Clin Toxicol (Phila) 2010;48:1–27.
78. Rothschild L, Bern S, Oswald S, et al. Intravenous lipid emulsion in clinical toxicology. Scand J Trauma Resusc Emerg Med 2010;18:51.
79. Lucas-Meunier E, Fossier P, Baux G, et al. Cholinergic modulation of the cortical neuronal network. Pflugers Arch 2003;446:17–29.
80. Trailovic SM, Varagic VM. The effect of ivermectin on convulsions in rats produced by lidocaine and strychnine. Vet Res Commun 2007;31:863–72.
81. Gwaltney-Brant SM, Rumbeiha WK. Newer antidotal therapies. Vet Clin North Am Small Anim Pract 2002;32:323–39.
82. Mealey KL. Pharmacogenetics. Vet Clin North Am Small Anim Pract 2006;36:961–73.
83. Mealey KL, Northrup NC, Bentjen SA. Increased toxicity of P-glycoprotein-substrate chemotherapeutic agents in a dog with the MDR1 deletion mutation associated with ivermectin sensitivity. J Am Vet Med Assoc 2003;223:1453–5.
84. Balayssac D, Authier N, Cayre A, et al. Does inhibition of P-glycoprotein lead to drug-drug interactions? Toxicol Lett 2005;156:319–29.

85. Joint WHO/FAO Expert Committee on Food Additives. 696. Ivermectin (WHO Food Additives Series 27). 1991. Available at: http://www.inchem.org/documents/jecfa/jecmono/v27je03.htm. Accessed November 20, 2011.

86. Roberts G; for Joint WHO/FAO Expert Committee on Food Additives. 854. Doramectin (WHO Food Additives Series 36). 1996. Available at: http://www.inchem.org/documents/jecfa/jecmono/v36je02.htm. Accessed November 20, 2011.

87. Heartgard Chewables for Cats package insert. Duluth, GA: Merial Limited; 2011. Available at: http://heartgard.us.merial.com/pdf/HEARTGARD-Chewables-for-Cats.pdf. Accessed November 20, 2011.

88. Novotny MJ, Krautmann MJ, Ehrhart JC, et al. Safety of selamectin in dogs. Vet Parasitol 2000;91:377–91.

89. Paul AJ, Tranquilli WJ, Hutchens DE. Safety of moxidectin in avermectin-sensitive collies. Am J Vet Res 2000;61:482–3.

90. ProHeart 6 package insert. New York: Pfizer; 2010. Available at: https://animalhealth.pfizer.com/sites/pahweb/US/EN/Products/PublishingImages/ProHeart%206%20Prescribing%20Information%20Sept%202010.pdf. Accessed November 20, 2011.

91. Delucchi L, Castro E. Use of doramectin for treatment of notoedric mange in five cats. J Am Vet Med Assoc 2000;216:215–6.

92. Interceptor Flavor Tabs package insert. Greensboro (NC): Novartis Animal Health US; 2009. Available at: http://www.interceptor.novartis.us/resources/INT_product_label_info.pdf. Accessed November 20, 2011.

93. Revolution package insert. New York: Pfizer; 2010. Available at: https://animalhealth.pfizer.com/sites/pahweb/US/EN/Documents/Prescribing%20Info%20or%20Package%20Inserts/US_EN_REVOLUTION_PI.pdf. Accessed November 20, 2011.

94. Advantage Multi for Cats package insert. Shawnee Mission (KS): Bayer HealthCare; 2006. Available at: http://www.bayerdvm.com/Resources/Docs/Advantage-Multi-Cat-Label.pdf. Accessed November 20, 2011.

95. Advantage Multi for Dogs package insert. Shawnee Mission (KS): Bayer HealthCare; 2009. Available at: http://www.bayerdvm.com/Resources/Docs/AdvMulti_Dog_041610.pdf. Accessed November 20, 2011.

96. Woodward K; for Joint WHO/FAO Expert Committee on Food Additives. 855. Moxidectin (WHO Food Additives Series 36). 1996. Available at: http://www.inchem.org/documents/jecfa/jecmono/v36je03.htm. Accessed November 20, 2011.

Toxicology of Newer Insecticides in Small Animals

Tina Wismer, DVM*, Charlotte Means, DVM, MLIS

KEYWORDS

- Insecticides • Toxicity • Insect growth regulators • Spinosads
- Organophosphates/carbamates • Pyrethrins/pyrethroids
- Fipronil • Sulfluramid • Hydramethylnon

In the broadest definition, a pesticide (from fly swatters to chemicals) is a substance used to eliminate a pest. A pest can be insects, mice or other animals, weeds, fungi, or microorganisms like bacteria and viruses. An ideal pesticide would be specific to, safer, and highly efficacious in eliminating the target pest. Humans, domestic animals, wildlife, and the environment would have minimal to no impact. This ideal pesticide would have a short half-life and break down into nontoxic components. It would be inexpensive and easy to apply. The ideal pesticide has not yet been discovered.

However, although not perfect, newer insecticides are significantly safer. These insecticides are able to target physiologic differences between insects and mammals, resulting in greater mammalian safety. This chapter briefly reviews toxicity information of both older insecticides, like organophosphates (OPs), carbamates, pyrethrins, and pyrethroids, as well as some newer insecticides.

ORGANOPHOSPHATES AND CARBAMATES

OPs and carbamates are used to control insect and nematode infestations. They are available as sprays, pour-ons, oral anthelmentics, baits, collars, dips, dusts, granules and foggers.[1] OPs and carbamates competitively inhibit acetylcholinesterase (AChE) by binding to its esteric site.[2] With AChE bound, acetylcholine (ACh) accumulates at nerve junctions in muscles, glands, and the central nervous system (CNS). The excessive ACh causes excessive stimulation of smooth muscle and glandular secretions. At skeletal muscle junctions, the excessive ACh is partly stimulatory (fasciculations) and partly inhibitory (muscle weakness).

After binding, the bonds of some compounds actually strengthen with time, known as aging. This "aging" renders the enzyme unusable (covalent bonding). Inhibition of

The authors have nothing to disclose.
ASPCA Animal Poison Control Center, 1717 South Philo Road, Suite 6, Urbana, IL 61802, USA
* Corresponding author.
E-mail address: tina.wismer@aspca.org

Table 1
Common AChE inhibitors (OPs and carbamates)

Highly toxic	
LD_{50} <50 mg/kg	aldicarb, coumaphos,[a] disulfoton, famphur, methomyl, parathion, phorate, terbufos
Moderately toxic	
LD_{50} 50–1000 mg/kg	acephate, carbaryl, chlorpyrifos,[a] diazinon, phosmet, propoxur, trichlorfon[a]
Low toxicity	
LD_{50} >1000 mg/kg	dichlorvos,[a] dimethoate, malathion, fenthion,[a] temephos, tetrachlorvinphos

[a] Compounds that have caused clinical neuropathy in humans.
Data from Hayes WJ Jr. Pesticides studied in man. Baltimore (MD): Williams & Wilkins; 1982. p. 284–435.

AChE by OPs tends to be irreversible, while inhibition by carbamates is reversible.[3] Recovery of AChE activity after irreversible binding occurs only through the synthesis of new enzymes.[3]

OPs and carbamates are quickly absorbed after dermal, oral, and inhalation exposures.[1] Clinical signs of toxicosis can occur in minutes to hours of exposure, depending on the dose, route, and toxicity of the compound. OPs and carbamates distribute quickly in the body. Most, with the exception of chlorinated OPs (ie, chlorpyrifos), do not accumulate in fat. OPs and carbamates are hydrolyzed in the body. The toxicity and duration of clinical signs depend on treatment, dose, compound, and species of animal (**Table 1**).[4] Cats are considered more susceptible to AChE inhibitors than are dogs in general.[5] Very young, very old, and debilitated animals are also more susceptible.

OPs and carbamates produce muscarinic, nicotinic, and CNS signs. The muscarinic signs include the "SLUDDE" signs (salivation, lacrimation, urination, defecation, dyspnea, emesis) as well as miosis and bradycardia. Dyspnea is due to increased bronchial secretions. Sympathetic stimulation can override the muscarinic signs and result in mydriasis and tachycardia.[4] The nicotinic effects include muscle tremors, fasiculations, weakness, ataxia, and paresis progressing to paralysis.[6] The CNS signs are characterized by hyperactivity, ataxia, seizures, and coma.[6] CNS signs usually occur with high doses or from the highly toxic compounds. Death is due to respiratory failure or cardiac arrest.[6]

OP-induced delayed neuropathy (OPIDN) in animals is characterized by hindlimb ataxia, hypermetria, and proprioceptive deficits. Clinical signs of delayed neuropathy usually begin 2 to 3 weeks after exposure and are thought to be due to phosphorylation of neurotoxic esterase (not from inhibition of AChE).[4] Acute pancreatitis (protracted vomiting, diarrhea that can often be hemorrhagic, increased pancreatic enzymes) can follow OP exposure, due to ACh release from pancreatic nerves and prolonged hyperstimulation of pancreatic acinar cells.[4] The species that are more sensitive to the delayed neurotoxic effects of organophosphorus esters accumulate the esters more rapidly and eliminate them more slowly (chickens > cats > rodents).[7]

If OP/carbamate poisoning is suspected from the clinical signs, a test dose of atropine can be given. Take the baseline heart rate and then administer a preanesthetic dose of atropine sulfate (0.02 mg/kg) IV. If the heart rate increases and the pupils dilate, look elsewhere for the cause of the signs as it takes roughly 10 times the preanesthetic dose (0.2 mg/kg) to resolve clinical signs caused by OP/carbamate insecticides.[4]

AChE activity can be measured in serum, plasma, or whole blood. Whole blood is preferred as in most animal species 80% or more of the total blood AChE activity is in the red blood cells (RBCs). AChE activity varies widely among species of animals, but generally an AChE activity that is less than 50% of normal indicates significant exposure, while an AChE activity less than 25% of normal plus the presence of characteristic clinical signs (SLUDDE, nicotinic signs) indicates toxicosis.[4] After death, AChE activity can be checked in the brain or eye (retina). As AChE activity varies among the regions of the brain, one half of the brain or whole eye (frozen or chilled) should be submitted for testing.[8] Blood and brain AChE does not always correlate well with the severity of clinical signs.[8] Animals that die rapidly may not have depressed (brain or blood) AChE activity. Carbamates are reversible inhibitors of AChE and the results may be normal even when characteristic clinical signs of toxicosis are present. A definitive diagnosis can be reached by finding an anticholinesterase insecticide in the tissue or body fluids (gastrointestinal [GI] tract, liver, skin, blood, etc), presence of clinical signs, and significantly depressed cholinesterase activity (OPs). AChE activity can remain depressed for 6 to 8 weeks with an OP exposure.

If the animal is asymptomatic, decontamination can include emesis (if oral ingestion) and administration of activated charcoal.[4] Due to the quick onset of seizures with the highly toxic AChE inhibitors, do not recommend inducing emesis at home. With dermal exposures to OPs and carbamates, wash the animal with liquid dish detergent and water. Wear gloves and ensure adequate ventilation.

If symptomatic, stabilize the animal and control seizures (diazepam, barbiturates) before proceeding. Oxygen and/or endotracheal intubation may be needed in small animals. A high dose of atropine sulfate (0.2 mg/kg) is given to control the muscarinic signs (SLUDDE). Give one-fourth of the initial dose IV and the rest IM or SQ. Atropine will not reverse nicotinic effects (muscular weakness, etc) or CNS effects (seizures). Atropine blocks the effects of accumulated ACh at the synapse and should be repeated as needed to control bradycardia and increased bronchial secretions.[4] Glycopyrrolate may also be used to control the muscarinic signs (0.01–0.02 mg/kg IV).

Oximes are used to reverse the neuromuscular blockade and nicotinic signs. Oximes should be given as soon as possible because they cannot reverse binding once aging has occurred. Pralidoxime chloride (2-PAM; Protopam) is the most common oxime used to treat OP toxicosis in the United States (20 mg/kg IM or IV bid; continue until nicotinic signs are present. Discontinue after 3 or 4 treatments if no response or if you see aggravation of nicotinic signs). Oximes are not used during carbamate intoxications. Diphenhydramine may also help to combat muscle weakness and tremors, although the usefulness of this treatment has not been established.[5] The prognosis depends on the type of OP/carbamate involved, exposure amount (dose), and treatment measures. Prognosis is considered good unless the animal shows signs of respiratory distress (increased pulmonary secretions, respiratory paralysis)r or seizures.

PYRETHRINS/PYRETHROIDS

Pyrethrins are botanical insecticides obtained from *Chrysanthemum cinerariaefolium*. Pyrethrums are plant-derived (natural) while pyrethroids are synthetic analogs of pyrethrins and have been modified to remain stable in sunlight. Pyrethroids are divided into type I, which do not contain a cyano group, and type II, which contain an alpha cyano group (**Table 2**). Etofenprox is a nonester pyrethroid-like insecticide. Pyrethrins/pyrethroids are often formulated with insect growth regulators

Table 2	
The two types of pyrethroids	
Type I	allethrin, bifenthrin, bioresmethrin, permethrin, phenothrin, resmethrin, sumithrin, tefluthrin, tetramethrin
Type II	cyfluthrin, cyhalothrin, cypermethrin, cyphenothrin, deltamethrin, fenpropathrin, fenvalerate, flucythrinate, flumethrin, fluvalinate, tralomethrin

(methoprene), synergists, solvents (petroleum distillates, acetone), and other carriers (isopropanol). In some situations, the inert ingredients may cause more adverse effects than the insecticide.[9] Pyrethroids cause a rapid "knockdown" of insects, but because pyrethroids are rapidly metabolized, some insects may recover. Synergists such as pipernyl butoxide or MGK-264 are frequently added to the products to increase toxicity to insects.[9,10]

Pyrethroids modulate gating kinetics by slowing the closing of sodium gates. Type II pyrethroids cause a longer duration of the sodium current in the axon than type I pyrethroids and pyrethrins. Thus, type 1 pyrethroids tend to cause tremors and seizures. Type II pyrethroids cause depolarizing conduction blocks with weakness and paralysis. Type II pyrethroids are considered more toxic than type I. Paresthesia is thought to result from direct action on sensory nerve endings. Pyrethrins/pyrethroids can be absorbed dermally, orally, and via inhalation. In animals, dermal absorption is limited due to intradermal metabolism. Pyrethrins/roids are highly lipophilic and distribution to tissues (fat, CNS, peripheral nervous system) is rapid. They are also quickly metabolized and eliminated primarily through the urine. The actual kinetics varies with the specific agent.[9,11] Pyrethroids are generally considered safe when used per label directions. Oral LD_{50} varies with specific agents. Cats are especially sensitive to concentrated pyrethrins/pyrethroids available in monthly spot-ons (permethrin, phenothrin, etc), although individual sensitivity exists. Some cats are sensitive enough that casual contact with a dog treated with a spot-on containing concentrated permethrin (45%–65% permethrin) can cause clinical signs.

Paresthesia is common in all species of animal following dermal application. Paresthesia includes ear twitching, paw and/or tail flicking, hiding, hyperexcitability, and hyperesthesia. Many topical sprays are formulated with isopropyl alcohol and heavy application can result in clinical signs resembling alcohol toxicity (sedation, lethargy, and ataxia). Presence of alcohol in the formulation also frequently causes a taste reaction (drooling, foaming, excessive licking motions, and vomiting).[9,10]

Concentrated pyrethroids (monthly spot-ons) are most likely to cause toxicity, especially in cats. Clinical signs of pyrethrin/pyrethroidstoxicity in cats include paresthesia, generalized tremors, shaking, ataxia, drooling, seizures, and death. Rarely, myoglobinuria will develop (most likely due to shaking/tremors) resulting in acute renal failure. Dogs typically develop signs of paresthesia (shaking of legs, mild muscle fasciculation, rubbing of application site, agitation, nervousness) after dermal application.[9,12] When ingested, granular bifenthrin products designed for lawn use appear to result in vomiting, diarrhea, ataxia, tremors and sometimes seizures in dogs (ASPCA APCC, unpublished data, 2011).

Taste reactions are treated with a taste treat such as milk or tuna. For dermal exposures to spot-ons, bathing multiple times with a liquid dishwashing liquid is important. Paresthesia to spot-ons may be treated by rubbing vitamin E oil on the application area. Corn or olive oil may be used as well. Tremoring or seizing animals should be stabilized before bathing. Methocarbamol (50 mg/kg IV; repeat as needed;

maximum dose 330 mg/kg/d) works well for controlling tremors. Diazepam can be tried in mild cases. For severe tremors or seizures, a constant rate infusion (CRI) of propofol, barbiturates, or gas anesthesia can also be used. Body temperature should be closely monitored. Many cats present hyperthermic due to muscle activity, but after bathing and stabilization, the temperature will drop. IV fluids are recommended. IV lipid emulsion therapy (see article elsewhere in this issue) is has been suggested for resolving severe tremors and seizures from permethrin toxicosis. Some clinicians claim that cats treated with lipid emulsions typically show faster recoveries (ASPCA APCC, unpublished data, 2011).

AVERMECTINS

For details, see article by Merola and Eubig elsewhere in this issue.

IMIDACLOPRID

Imidacloprid was the first neonicotinoid insecticide registered for use. It is approved as a topical spot-on for dogs and numerous products for agricultural and yard use.[13] Imidacloprid mimics the action of ACh in insects; however, imidacloprid is not degraded by AChE. Imidacloprid binds to the postsynaptic nicotinic ACh receptor. This results in persistent activation, preventing impulse transmission and a buildup of ACh. This leads to hyperexcitation, convulsions, paralysis, and insect death. The binding affinity of imidacloprid at the nicotinic receptors in mammals is much less compared to binding affinity in insects. Imidacloprid is most effective against insects with large numbers of nicotinergic ACh receptors. Thus, fleas are susceptible to imidacloprid but ticks are not.[14,15] It has been hypothesized that there are 2 binding sites, based on a rat study, with different affinities for imidacloprid. Based on the study, imidacloprid has both agonistic and antagonistic effects on nicotinic ACh receptor channels.[15]

Imidacloprid is absorbed rapidly and almost completely from the GI tract. It is metabolized in the liver to 6-chloronicotinic acid, an active metabolite. Imidacloprid is widely distributed to tissues but does not accumulate and has poor penetration of the blood-brain barrier, contributing to mammalian safety. Elimination is primarily via urine (70%–80%) and feces (20%–30%). Dermal exposures have practically no systemic absorption. Imidacloprid is spread across the skin via translocation. The product is found in hair follicles and shed with hair and sebum.[13,14]

Dermal hypersensitivity to topical products may occur. Erythema, pruritic, and alopecia may be noted at the application site. Oral ingestions of topical preparations can cause drooling or vomiting. Oral ulcers and gastritis have been seen in cats dosed orally.[14] Large ingestions of agricultural or yard use products, although rare, may result in clinical signs similar to nicotine toxicosis. These signs may include lethargy, drooling, vomiting, diarrhea, ataxia, and muscle weakness.[13]

Imidacloprid has a wide margin of safety. In safety studies, topical applications at 50 mg/kg did not cause adverse effects; the NOEL (no effect level) 1-year feeding study in dogs was 41 mg/kg. Imidacloprid is labeled for use in pregnant animals. Topical products have been labeled for puppies and kittens as young as 7 weeks.[14,16]

Treatment for dermal hypersensitivity includes bathing with a liquid dishwashing detergent or follicle flushing shampoo. In cases with severe pruritis, antihistamines or corticosteroids may be required. Most oral exposures can be treated by diluting with milk or water. Most cases of vomiting will be self-limiting. If massive ingestions occur, treatment for clinical signs is symptomatic and supportive; no specific antidote exists.

NITENPYRAM

Nitenpyram is an insecticide in the neonicotinic class. Nitenpyram is an over-the-counter tablet developed as an oral adult flea insecticide. Nitenpyram is considered safe for pregnant and lactating animals. Nitenpyram works systemically and fleas begin to die within 30 minutes. Off-label use includes treating maggot infestations.[17] The mechanism of action is similar to other neonicotinic insecticides (imidacloprid). Neonicotinic insecticides have little to no binding to vertebrate peripheral ACh receptors.[18]

Nitenpyram is rapidly and almost completely absorbed. The peak plasma level is 1.21 hours for dogs and 0.63 hour for cats. The half-life is 2.8 hours in the dog and 7.7 hours in the cat. Nitenpyram has almost no tissue accumulation. It is primarily eliminated via the urine unchanged (94%).[18]

Nitenpyram has a wide margin of safety. Adult dogs and cats were dosed up to 10 times a therapeutic dose daily for 1 month without adverse effects.[19] Cats receiving 125 mg/kg (125 times therapeutic dose) did exhibit hypersalivation, lethargy, vomiting, and tachypnea. These clinical signs typically developed within 2 hours of treatment and resolved within 24 hours.[17,19]

Reported clinical signs are generally associated with the flea die-off and are not related to the medication. Reported signs include pruritis, hyperesthesia, hyperactivity, panting, agitation, excessive grooming, trembling, and ataxia. Signs are usually self-limiting and resolve without any treatment.[17]

FIPRONIL

Fipronil is a phenylpyrazole insecticide. Fipronil is approved as a spot-on or spray as well as ant and roach baits and seed and soil treatments.[20] Fipronil binds to GABA receptors of insects and blocks chloride passages (GABA antagonist). GABA receptors normally have an inhibitory effect but the net result of fipronil is stimulation of the nervous system and, ultimately, insect death. Fipronil has significantly less binding affinity for mammalian GABA receptors because of differences in receptor configuration.[14, 21]

Fipronil does not readily penetrate the skin, although it is lipid soluble. When applied topically, it is found on the hair shaft and in the stratum corneum and epidermis and accumulates in the sebaceous glands.[14] Orally, fipronil is absorbed slowly. It distributes to a number of tissues, including the GI tract, adrenal glands, and abdominal fat. Fipronil is metabolized by the liver and excreted in the feces and urine.[14]

Fipronil may cause dermal hypersensitivity-type reaction in sensitive animals. Erythema, pruritis, irritation, and alopecia at the application site are the most commonly noted signs from topical exposures. Many of these reactions may be related to the carriers. Typically, dermal hypersensitivity will develop within hours to a couple of days of application and last 24 to 48 hours. Oral ingestions may cause taste reactions (hypersalivation, foaming, gagging), retching, and vomiting. Gastritis has been reported after ingestion of spot-on products and is most likely related to carriers rather than the fipronil. Rarely, in cases of massive ingestions, ataxia, tremors, and seizures are possible. Extralabel use of fipronil on rabbits is known to cause severe and potentially fatal seizures.[14,20]

Fipronil has a wide margin of safety in laboratory animals. There is no reported LD_{50} for dogs and cats. The oral LD_{50} in rats and mice is 97 and 95 mg/kg, respectively. Dogs appear to be more sensitive than cats to fipronil.[20]

Treatment for dermal hypersensitivity includes bathing with a liquid dishwashing detergent by 48 hours after the topical application. Antihistamines and steroids may be used if pruritis is present. After oral exposures, taste reactions are treated by diluting with milk or water. If significant vomiting or gastritis is present, antiemetics and GI protectants may be needed. Fluids and other supportive care should be started, and tremoring or seizing animals should receive methocarbamol, diazepam, or barbiturates as needed.[14]

BORATES

Borate compounds used as insecticides include boric acid, sodium tetraborate pentahydrate, boric acid, disodium octaborate tetrahydrate, and sodium metaborate.[22,23] Borates are generally considered to be cytotoxic to all cells and are irritating to mucous membranes.[24] The mechanisms of the systemic effects of borates are not known.[23]

Borates are rapidly absorbed through mucous membranes, abraded skin, and the GI tract. Borates are not absorbed across intact skin.[22,24] Boric acid is found in all tissues, except the brain, within 30 minutes after oral exposure.[24] Peak CNS concentration occurs within 3 hours.[24] Borates are concentrated in the kidney and excreted without change.[22,24] Preexisting renal disease may slow excretion and increase toxicity. The half-life in dogs is 12 hours.[22]

The most common signs seen in dogs and cats after oral ingestion of borates are vomiting, lethargy, hypersalivation, and anorexia (ASPCA APCC, unpublished data, 2011). Renal failure and seizures are reported in the literature but are rarely seen in small animals due to the small amounts involved. The signs occur within a few hours after exposure and last a couple of hours. No deaths or serious systemic toxic effects were found in dogs given 1.54 to 6.51 g/kg of borax or 1 to 3.09 g/kg of boric acid orally.[24] Young animals are likely more susceptible than adults to the toxic effects.

Treatment is symptomatic and supportive. Activated charcoal poorly binds to boric acid (30 g of charcoal is required to adsorb 380 mg of boric acid).[25] Antiemetics or GI protectants may be given. Fluid diuresis should be started if a large exposure occurs. Animal studies suggested that the use of N-acetylcysteine chelation therapy may increase the excretion of boron and reverse boron-induced oliguria.[22]

HYDRAMETHYLNON

Hydramethylnon is a trifluoromethyl aminohydrazone. It is the only member in this class of insecticide. Hydramethylnon is used to control ants, cockroaches, and termites. It is often used in single bait stations (ant and roach motels) or granular products, especially for fire ants. Hydramethylnon works by inhibiting the electron transport system, thus blocking the production of ATP. This decreases mitochondrial oxygen consumption. The slow disruption in energy metabolism and loss of ATP result in inactivity, paralysis, and insect death. The mechanism of action is similar to that of sulfluramid and rotenone.[14] Hydramethylon is poorly absorbed. More than 95% is excreted unchanged in the feces. Material absorbed is slowly metabolized. In rats, 72% was eliminated in 24 hours and 92% in 9 days.[14]

Hydramethylnon has a wide margin of safety in animals. Orally, it is considered only slightly toxic. Rat oral LD_{50} ranges from 1100 to 1300 mg/kg. The dermal LD_{50} in rabbits is greater than 5000 mg/kg. In 26-week feeding studies in dogs, 3 mg/kg increased liver weights and liver:body weight ratios; 90-day studies in dogs at 6 mg/kg/d caused decreased feed consumption, decreased body weight, and testicular atrophy.[14]

It is rare for any significant clinical signs to develop. Most cases cause only mild gagging or vomiting. In cases where the dose consumed is greater than 90 mg/kg, mild ataxia or tremors may be seen. There is a risk for foreign body obstruction if large pieces of plastic from bait traps are swallowed. Decontamination is required only in large ingestions. Clinical signs are generally self-limiting. Symptomatic and supportive care should be administered as needed.

SPINOSAD

Spinosad is found as granules or sprays for agricultural and lawn use and chewable tablets for dogs to kill fleas.[26] A spot-on containing spinetoram, a related compound, is available for use on cats to kill fleas. Spinosad is a tetracyclic macrolide. It is a combination of spinosyn A and spinosyn D.[26] Spinosyns are produced from the naturally occurring bacterium *Saccharopolyspora spinosa*, an aerobic, nonantibiotic actinomycete. Spinosad activates nicotinic ACh receptors. Treated insects develop involuntary muscle contractions and tremors. Continued hyperexcitation results in prostration, paralysis, and flea death. Spinosad is not known to interact with the binding sites of other nictotinic or GABAergic insecticides (imidacloprid, nitenpyram, fipronil, mibemycin, etc). Spinosad is more selective for insect versus vertebrate nicotinic AChRs.[26]

Spinosad is quickly absorbed after oral ingestion and peak blood concentrations occur within 1 to 6 hours depending on the dose.[27] Spinosad is well distributed throughout the body with the highest concentrations found in fat, liver, kidneys, and lymph nodes.[27] Spinosad is biotransformed with glutathione conjugates and eliminated in the feces (70%–90%) via the bile.[28] Most of the radiolabeled agent is excreted within 24 hours. Elimination from the thyroid is much slower and can result in higher concentrations in the thyroid as compared to other tissues. The half-life of spinosad is 25 to 42 hours.[28]

Canine daily doses of 100 mg/kg for 10 consecutive days (16.7 times the maximum recommended monthly dose) caused vomiting and transient mild elevations in ALT.[26] Phospholipidosis (vacuolation) of the lymphoid tissue was seen in all dogs.[26] Cats dosed at 80 to 120 mg/kg experienced vomiting.[26]

The most common adverse clinical effects seen after ingestion are vomiting and lethargy. These signs usually begin within a few hours of exposure.[26] Ataxia, inactiveness, anorexia, diarrhea, and tremors have also been reported. Concurrent administration of spinosad to animals receiving high doses of ivermectin therapy (eg, demodicosis doses) can result in mild to moderate ivermectin toxicity.[26] It is recommended that dogs receiving extralabel doses of ivermectin not receive concurrent treatment with spinosad.[26] In an overdose situation, induction of emesis and administration of activated charcoal are rarely needed. Most treatment is symptomatic and supportive and includes managing vomiting and diarrhea.

INDOXACARB

Indoxacarb is found in insect baits (ant and roach) for home use and granules and liquids for agricultural use.[29] Recently, a spot-on containing indoxacarb has been introduced for use on dogs and cats. Indoxacarb acts by blocking sodium channels in the nervous system of insects. It is an oxadiazine insecticide despite its name.[30]

Indoxacarb is metabolized in the liver and excreted in both the feces and urine.[31] Most of the dose was excreted within 96 hours. The oral NOEL in dogs is 40 ppm (1.1 mg/kg/d).[32] The most common clinical signs seen in dogs and cats are vomiting, lethargy, diarrhea, and anorexia (ASPCA APCC, unpublished data, 2011). There is one case of a human developing methemoglobinemia after a massive ingestion of indoxacarb (suicide attempt).[33] Treatment is symptomatic and supportive. Due to a low concentration of indoxacarb present in most ant and roach baits, ingestion only requires monitoring for signs of stomach upset.

SULFLURAMID

Sulfluramid (N-ethyl perfluoroctanesulfonamide) is in the chemical class of fluorinated sulfonamides. Sulfluramid is used in ant and roach baits and is impregnated into cardboard to control termites. It is considered a stomach poison.

Sulfluramid is lipid soluble. However, rat studies did not show any tissue accumulation. Cytochrome P450 metabolism produces the deethylated metabolite, perfluorooctane sulfonamide (desethylsulfluramid). The metabolite is a potent oxidative uncoupler and inhibits mitochondrial respiration. Disruption of energy metabolism, and thus the loss of ATP, results in lethargy, paralysis, and death. Based on rat studies, elimination is 56% respiratory, 25% fecal. and 8% urine. The parent compound is about 80% eliminated within 72 hours, while desethylsulfluramid has a half-life of 10.8 days.[34,35]

Sulfluramid has a wide range of safety in vertebrates. The oral LD_{50} in rats varies between 500 and 5000 mg/kg.[26] The most commonly reported clinical sign is mild vomiting. Plastic ingestion in dogs has a risk for foreign body obstruction. High doses in dogs caused transient arrest of spermatogenesis.[36] Treatment is symptomatic and supportive. Manage vomiting with anitiemetics if needed. Most exposures result in self-limiting clinical signs and do not require any treatment.

Environmentally, recent research is looking at long-term exposure to perfluorinated hydrocarbons as suppressants of humoral immunity.[37] The Environmental Protection Agency is phasing out sulfluramid-containing products, primarily due to the long half-life in the environment and potential for reproductive effects. These products are to be phased out by 2016.[38]

ESSENTIAL OILS

Essential oils are produced by plants. The oils are a mixture of terpenes (complex hydrocarbons) and other chemicals. Essential oils give plants their characteristic odors. They vary widely in toxicity. Although the oils have a number of uses, some are used as natural flea and tick treatments on pets (**Table 3** lists the common essential oils used for flea treatments).

Essential oils are rapidly absorbed orally and dermally. Oils are typically metabolized in the liver by glucuronide and glycine conjugates. Cytochrome P-450 enzyme

Table 3	
Common essential oils used for flea treatments	
Common Name and Source of Essential Oil	**Specific Clinical Signs**
Citrus sp (oranges, limes, grapefruit) D-Limonene/linalool	Cats: scrotal dermatitis, profound hypotension (undiluted dips) Rare: immune-mediated dermatopathies (TENS)
Melaleuca alternifolia (tea tree)	Transient hind limb paresis (spot-on), hepatotoxicity
Mentha pulegium Pennyroyal oil, pulegone	Hepatotoxicity
Peppermint, clove, cinnamon, lemongrass, thyme (commercial sprays and spot-ons)	Agitation, tremors, seizures, rarely death

Data from Refs.[40,49–52]

systems in the liver can be induced with repeated exposure to some essential oils. Cats appear to be relatively more sensitive to the effects of essential oil than dogs. Essential oils and their metabolities are primarily eliminated in the urine.[39,40]

The most common clinical signs after dermal exposure include ataxia, muscle weakness, and behavioral abnormalities. Oral ingestions can cause vomiting, diarrhea, and CNS depression. Essential oils can cause aspiration pneumonia if inhaled. Mortality has been reported following the use of melaluca oil in cats (see **Table 3** for clinical signs of specific oils in addition to these common signs).[39,40]

All species of animals may be susceptible to essential oils. Animals with preexisting liver disease have an increased risk of toxicosis. The LD_{50} of essential oils varies widely but typically falls between 2 and 5 g/kg body weight. Mixing oils with organic solvents such as alcohols or the presence of irritated and reddened skin can potentially increase absorption of essential oils resulting in toxicity.[41] The specific mechanism of action is not established.

Dermal exposures require bathing with a liquid dishwashing detergent. Emesis, in most cases, is contraindicated since a risk of aspiration pneumonia exists. Activated charcoal can be given if a large ingestion has occurred. Baseline blood work should be obtained as some oils will cause hepatic damage and acid-base and electrolyte abnormalities. Body temperature should be monitored and corrected as needed. Intravenous fluids can help maintain pressure and hydration status and also aids in renal elimination. Monitor cardiac and respiratory functions as needed. Seizures and tremors usually respond well to diazepam or methocarbamol. Aspiration pneumonia may require oxygen and broad-spectrum antibiotics. Hepatic damage usually responds to good supportive care. The use of SAM-e or milk thistle may be helpful.[40]

LUFENURON

Lufenuron is available as an oral suspension for cats, an injectable for cats, and an oral tablet for dogs. It is approved for use in dogs and cats 6 weeks of age and older for the control of flea populations. It has also been used off label for control of dermatophytosis. Lufenuron, a benzoylphenylurea dieriivative, is a chitin synthesis inhibitor.[42] By stopping polymerization and deposition of chitin, it prevents the eggs from developing into adults.

Only about 40% of an oral dose of lufenuron is absorbed in the small intestine.[42] Absorption is enhanced if administered with a fatty meal. Lufenuron is stored in fat and is slowly redistributed back into the circulation. Lufenuron is not metabolized but excreted unchanged into the bile and eliminated in the feces.

Dogs dosed at 30 times the therapeutic dose for 10 months did not develop and signs of toxicosis.[42] Cats tolerate oral dosages of up to 17 times the therapeutic dose with no adverse effects.[42] Cats do require a substantially higher oral dosage per kilogram than do dogs for equivalent efficacy.

Adverse signs seen after ingestion include vomiting, lethargy, and diarrhea. Injection site pain and swelling can occur in cats. Do not give the injectable product to dogs as they will develop a severe local reaction.[42] Most signs are self-limiting, and treatment, if needed, is symptomatic and supportive.

METHOPRENE

Methoprene is available as suspensions, emulsifiable and soluble concentrates, briquettes, sprays, foggers, baits, and spot-ons. Methoprene is labeled for flea control in dogs and cats, aquatic mosquito control, crop pest control, and home pest control.[43] Methoprene is a juvenile hormone analog. While juvenile hormone concentrations remain high, the insect remains in the same stage and cannot molt.[44] Methoprene is also absorbed by the female flea and affects her ovaries, providing an immediate inhibitory effect.[44]

Methoprene can be absorbed both orally and dermally. It is rapidly excreted, mostly in the urine and feces.[43] Sufficient methoprene is excreted unchanged that the concentration in feces is sufficient to kill some larvae that breed in dung.[45]

Methoprene is considered relatively safe in mammals. The dog oral LD_{50} is greater than 5 g/kg.[43] Younger animals are more susceptible to adverse effects (lethargy, ataxia, rarely tremors) after oral dosing.[43] Oral exposures can cause drooling, vomiting, and lethargy and rarely ataxia or tremors. The ataxia appears within 2 to 8 hours post administration and lasts 6 to 12 hours (ASPCA APCC, unpublished data, 2011). Usually no treatment is necessary if animal has ingested small amount. Local dermal hypersensitivity reactions (redness, itching, rubbing) can be seen in some animals. Most of the symptomatic animals recover without treatment. If the animal is ataxic, prevent further stimulation (provide a quiet and dark environment). Methocarbamol may help with muscle tremors.

PYRIPROXYFEN

Pyriproxyfen is used for insect control on pets, in the home, and on agricultural crops. It is available as a spray, fogger, collar, mousse, shampoo, granule, spot-on, powder, and liquid.[46] Pyriproxyfen is a pyridine-based non-neurotoxic carbamate that does not inhibit cholinesterase. It is an insect juvenile hormone analog. It is both ovicidal and larvicidal.

Pyriproxyfen is quickly absorbed and peak levels are reached in 2 to 8 hours after ingestion.[47] It is metabolized in the liver and excreted mainly in the feces.[44] The oral NOEL in dogs is 100 mg/kg/d for 1 year.[48] Hypersalivation and self-limiting vomiting may be seen with ingestion. Most animals will not need treatment.

SUMMARY

Insecticidal poisoning has become less common in small animal patients as the newer available insecticides are more specific in their mechanisms and target mostly insects, not mammals. This has made many of the newer pesticides safer for use on dogs and cats compared to some of the highly toxic OPs and carbamates available earlier. Serious toxicity problems can still occur, especially with inappropriate use of permethrin-containing spot-ons in cats.

REFERENCES

1. Meerdink GL. Anticholinesterase insecticides. In: Plumlee KH, editor. Clinical veterinary toxicology. St Louis (MO): Mosby; 2004. p. 178–80.
2. Hayes WJ Jr. Pesticides studied in man. Baltimore (MD): Williams & Wilkins; 1982. p 284–435.
3. Osweiler GD. Organophosphorus and carbamate insecticides. In: Toxicology. Philadelphia: Lippincott Williams & Wilkins; 1996. p. 231–6.
4. Fikes JD. Organophosphorus and carbamate insecticides. Vet Clin North Am Small Anim Pract 1990;20:353–67.
5. Nafe LA. Selected neurotoxins. Vet Clin North Am Small Anim Pract 1988;18:593–604.
6. Humphreys DJ. Veterinary toxicology. 3rd edition. Philadelphia: WB Saunders; 1988.
7. Abou-Donia MB, Graham DG, Ashry MA. Delayed neurotoxicity of leptophos and related compounds: differential effects of subchronic oral administration of pure, technical grade, and degradation products on the hen. Toxicol Appl Pharmacol 1980;53:150–63.

8. Plumlee KH. Total cholinesterase activity in discrete brain regions and retina of normal horses. J Vet Diagn Invest 1997;9:109–10.
9. Volmer PA. Pyrethrins and pyrethroids. In: Plumlee KH, editor. Clinical veterinary toxicology. St Louis (MO): Mosby; 2004. p. 188–90.
10. Proudfoot AT. Poisoning due to pyrethrins. Toxicol Rev 2005;24:107–13.
11. Anadón A, Martínez-Larrañaga MR, Martínez MA. Use and abuse of pyrethrins and synthetic pyrethroids in veterinary medicine. Vet J 2009;182:7–20.
12. Malik R, Ward MP, Seavers A, et al. Permethrin spot-on intoxication of cats: literature review and survey of veterinary practitioners in Australia. J Fel Med Surg 2010;12:5–14.
13. Sheets LP. Imidacloprid: a neonicotinoid insecticide. In: Krieger R, editor. Handbook of pesticide toxicology, volume 2, agents. San Diego (CA): Academic Press; 2001. p. 1123–30.
14. Wismer T. Novel insecticides. In: Plumlee KH, editor. Clinical veterinary toxicology. St Louis (MO): Mosby; 2004. p. 183–6.
15. Nagata K, Song JH, Shono T, et al. Modulation of the neuronal nicotinic acetylcholine receptor channel by the nitromethylene heterocycle imidacloprid. J Pharmacol Exp Ther 1998;285:731–8.
16. Griffin L, Hopkins TJ. Imidacloprid: safety of a new insecticidal compound in dogs and cats. Suppl Compend Contin Educ Pract Vet 1997;19:17–20.
17. Hovda LR, Hooser SB. Toxicology of newer pesticides for use in dogs and cats. Vet Clin North Am Small Anim Pract 2002;32:455–67.
18. Vo DT, Hsu WH, Abu-Basha EA, et al. Insect nicotinic acetylcholine receptor agonists as flea adulticides in small animals. J Vet Pharmacol Ther 2010;33:315–22.
19. Witte ST, Luembert LG. Laboratory safety studies of nitenpyram tablets for the rapid removal of fleas on cats and dogs. Suppl Compend Contin Educ Pract Vet 2001;23:7–11.
20. Gupta RC. Fipronil. In: Gupta RC, editor. Veterinary toxicology basic and clinical principles. New York: Academic Press; 2007. p. 502–4.
21. Cole LM, Nicholson RA, Casida JE. Action of phenylpyrazole insecticides at the GABA-gated chloride channel. Pesticide Biochem Physiol 1993;46:47–54.
22. Banner W, Koch M, Capin DM. Experimental chelation therapy in chromium, lead, and boron intoxication with N-acetylcysteine and other compounds. Toxicol Appl Pharmacol 1986;83:142–7.
23. Gosselin RE, Smith RP, Hodge HC. Clinical toxicology of commercial products. 5th edition. Baltimore (MD): Williams & Wilkins; 1984. p. 131–3.
24. Kiesche-Nesselrodt A, Hooser SB. Boric acid. Vet Clin North Am Small An Pract 1990;20:369–73.
25. Oderda GM, Klein-Schwartz W, Insley BM. In vitro study of boric acid and activated charcoal. J Toxicol Clin Toxicol 1987;25:13–9.
26. Comfortis™ (Spinosad) chewable tablets prescribing information package insert. Indianapolis (IN): Eli Lilly and Company; 2007.
27. Robertson-Plouch C, Baker KA, Hozak RR, et al. Clinical field study of the safety and efficacy of spinosad chewable tablets for controlling fleas on dogs. Vet Ther 2008;9:26–36.
28. Bartholomaeus A. Toxicological evaluations: spinosad. IPCS INCHEM: pesticide residues in food 2001. Available at: http://www.inchem.org/documents/jmpr/jmpmono/2001pr12.htm. Accessed July 16, 2011.
29. Crop protection handbook. Willoughby (OH): Meister Publishing; 2004. p. C-280.
30. Narahashi T, Zhao X, Ikeda T, et al. Differential actions of insecticides on target sites: basis for selective toxicity. Hum Exp Toxicol 2007;26:361–6.

31. Tomlin CDS, editor. Indoxacarb (173584-44-6). In: The pesticide manual, a world compendium. Surrey (UK): British Crop Protection Council; 2009.
32. California Environmental Protection Agency/Department of Pesticide Regulation; Toxicology data review summaries: indoxacarb. Available at: http://www.cdpr.ca.gov/docs/toxsums/toxsumlist.htm. Accessed July 16, 2011.
33. Prasanna L, Manimala Rao S, Singh V, et al. Indoxacarb poisoning: an unusual presentation as methemoglobinemia. Indian J Crit Care Med 2008;12:198–200.
34. Grossman MR, Mispagel ME, Bowen JM. Distribution and tissue elimination in rats during and after prolonged dietary exposure to a highly fluorinated sulfonamide pesticide. J Agric Food Chem 1992;40;2505–9.
35. Manning RO, Bruckner JV, Mispagel ME, et al. Metabolism and disposition of sulfluramid, a unique polyfluorinated insecticide, in the rat. Drug Metab Dispos 1991;19:205–11.
36. Hollingsworth RH. Inhibitors and uncouplers of mitochondrial oxidative phosphorylation. In: Krieger R, editor. Handbook of pesticide toxicology, volume 2, agents. San Diego (CA): Academic Press; 2001. p. 1244–6.
37. Peden-Adams MM, EuDaly JG, Dabra S, et al. Suppression of humoral immunity following exposure to the perfluorinated insecticide sulfluramid. J Toxicol Environ Health A 2007;70:1130–41.
38. Fluoride Action Network Pesticide Project. Sulfluramid. Available at: http://www.fluoridealert.org/pesticides/sulfluramid-page.htm. Accessed June, 20, 2011.
39. Means C. Selected herbal hazards. Vet Clin North Am Small Anim Pract 2002;32:367–82.
40. Means C. Essential oils. In: Plumlee KH, editor. Clinical veterinary toxicology. St Louis (MO): Mosby; 2004. p. 149–50.
41. Wolfe A. Essential oil poisoning. Clin Toxicol 1999;37:721–7.
42. Stansfield DG. A review of safety and efficacy of lufenuron in dogs and cats. Canine Pract 1997;22:34–48.
43. Environmental Protection Agency. R.E.D. facts: methoprene. Washington, DC: Office of Pesticides and Toxic Substances; 1991.
44. Palma KG, Meola SM, Meola RW. Mode of action of pyriproxyfen and methoprene on eggs of Ctenocephalides felis felis (Siphonaptera: pulicidae). J Med Entomol 1995;30:421–6.
45. McEwen FL, Stephenson GR. The use and significance of pesticides in the environment. New York: John Wiley and Sons; 1979.
46. U.S. Environmental Protection Agency/Office of Pesticide Program's Chemical Ingredients Database on Pyriproxyfen (95737-68-1). Available at: http://ppis.ceris.purdue.edu/htbin/epachem.com. Accessed May 15, 2011.
47. Matsunaga H, Yoshino H, Isobe N, et al. Metabolism of pyriproxyfen in rats. 1. Absorption, disposition, excretion, and biotransformation studies with phenoxypheny[l-14C]pyriproxyfen. J Agric Food Chem 1995;43:235–40.
48. Federal Register. Available at: http://www.epa.gov/EPA-PEST/1999/October/Day-21/p27398.htm. Accessed June 30, 2011:56681.
49. Frank AA, Ross JL, Sawwell BK. Toxic epidermal necrolysis associated with flea dips. Vet Hum Toxicol 1992;34:57–61.
50. Rosenbaum MR, Kerlin RL. Erythema multiforme major and disseminated intravascular coagulation in a dog following application of a d-limonene-based insecticidal dip. J Am Vet Med Assoc 1995;207:1315–9.
51. Lee JA, Budgin JB, Mauldin EA. Acute necrotizing dermatitis and septicemia after application of a d-limonene-based insecticidal shampoo in a cat. J Am Vet Med Assoc 2002;221:258–62.
52. Sudekum M, Poppenga RH, Raju N. Pennyroyal oil toxicosis in a dog. J Am Vet Med Assoc 1992;200:817–8.

Common Rodenticide Toxicoses in Small Animals

Camille DeClementi, VMD[a,b,]*, Brandy R. Sobczak, DVM[a]

KEYWORDS

- Rodenticide • Anticoagulant • Bromethalin • Cholecalciferol

This article focuses on the 3 most commonly used rodenticide types: anticoagulants, bromethalin, and cholecalciferol. Since there are multiple types of rodenticides available on the market and the color of the bait is not coded to a specific type of rodenticide, it is important to verify the active ingredient in any rodenticide exposure. Additionally, many animal owners may use the term "D-con" to refer to any rodenticide regardless of the actual brand name or type of rodenticide. Rodenticide baits are most typically formulated as bars. Loose bait such as pellets are no longer produced for consumer sale according to new Environmental Protection Agency (EPA) risk mitigation rules; however, this form (loose bait) may be seen for quite some time while older products are used up. The EPA released their final ruling on rodenticide risk mitigation measures in 2008 and all the products on the market had to be compliant by June 2011. The purpose of the measures is to reduce exposures to children and nontarget species including wildlife. After June 2011, consumer products may not contain the second-generation anticoagulants brodifacoum, difethialone, difenacoum, and bromadiolone and instead must contain either first-generation anticoagulants or nonanticoagulants including bromethalin and cholecalciferol.[1] These regulations are likely to cause an increase in the number of bromethalin and cholecalciferol cases seen in veterinary clinics.

ANTICOAGULANT RODENTICIDES

The discovery of the causative agent of sweet-clover poisoning in cattle, dicoumarol, led to the development of the anticoagulant rodenticides. Cattle suffering from this type of poisoning developed internal bleeding; therefore, dicoumarol was tested as a rodenticide. Warfarin, named after the Wisconsin Alumni Research Foundation (WARF), was the first compound marketed as an anticoagulant rodenticide. The

The authors have nothing to disclose.

[a] ASPCA Animal Poison Control Center, 1717 South Philo Road, Suite 36, Urbana, IL 61802, USA

[b] Department of Veterinary Biosciences, College of Veterinary Medicine, University of Illinois, Urbana, IL, USA

* Corresponding author. ASPCA Animal Poison Control Center, 1717 South Philo Road, Suite 36, Urbana, IL 61802.

E-mail address: camille.declementi@aspca.org

first-generation anticoagulants were created during the 1940s and 1950s. They required continuous exposure to achieve rodent control. The second-generation anticoagulant rodenticides (SGARs), including brodifacoum, difethialone, difenacoum, and bromadiolone, were developed in the subsequent decades as rodents developed resistance to the first-generation anticoagulants. SGARs were formulated to be more palatable to rodents, more effective, faster, and longer acting.[2] Although chlorophacinone and diphacinone were developed after warfarin like the SGARs listed above, they differ structurally and the EPA has not placed the same restrictions on their use.[1,2]

Warfarin and pindone are short-acting anticoagulants with shorter half-lives (<24 hours) compared to the long acting products whose half-lives are up to 6 days.[3] The long-acting anticoagulants include diphacinone, difethialone, chlorophacinone, brodifacoum, and bromadiolone. Veterinarians are well-trained to use their knowledge and judgement to make treatment decisions for their patients according to each unique case. As a general guideline, the ASPCA Animal Poison Control Center (APCC) recommends decontamination if and as needed and monitoring (prothrombin PT] time or activated partial thromboplastin time [APTT]) or treatment with vitamin K_1 (if and as needed) when the ingested dose of warfarin is greater than 0.5 mg/kg and other anticoagulants is greater than 0.02 mg/kg.

Exposure in domestic pets occurs through ingestion of the product from the bait container or from the environment to which the rodents have carried the bait. Now that the EPA is requiring consumer products be contained in a tamper-resistant bait stations and has prohibited the sale of pelleted formulations to consumers, hopefully pets will be protected from finding a rodent's hoard of product. For anticoagulants, toxicosis from a pet ingesting rodents poisoned by the bait (also called relay toxicosis) is of limited concern since the amount of rodenticide in the rodent is small. However, if the pet is very small and ingests a large number of the poisoned rodents, relay toxicosis is possible. For example, a barn cat that preys on rodents as its main source of nutrition could become intoxicated if those rodents were poisoned by an anticoagulant rodenticide.[3]

Pathophysiology and Clinical Signs

The anticoagulant rodenticides cause their effects by interfering with the production of the clotting factors II, VII, IX, and X by the liver. In the normal production of these factors, vitamin K_1 is converted to vitamin K_1 epoxide. The enzyme vitamin K_1 epoxide reductase then converts vitamin K_1 epoxide back to the active form of vitamin K_1. This cycle repeats over and over to create active clotting factors. The anticoagulants inhibit vitamin K_1 epoxide reductase, thereby leading to depletion of active vitamin K_1 and the halt of the production of active clotting factors.[3,4]

During the first 36 to 72 hours following ingestion of the anticoagulant, the patient is usually clinically normal as the clotting factors are slowly depleted. Usually within 3 to 5 days, enough clotting factors are depleted for hemorrhage to develop. It is possible in some patients with underlying illnesses (such as preexisting bleeding disorders or hepatic disease), depletion of coagulation factors may occur sooner, resulting in hemorrhage as early as 24 to 48 hours following exposure.

Many poisoned animals are not presented to the veterinarian until clinical signs develop. It is important to remember that hemorrhage can occur anywhere in the body; however, the most common clinical signs are dyspnea, coughing, lethargy, and hemoptysis.[3] Bleeding into body cavities such as the chest, abdomen, and joints is also common. Many patients present with vague clinical signs of lethargy, weakness, and anemia without any overt external hemorrhage, although some animals may present with frank external hemorrhage from surgical or traumatic sites, the gastro-intestinal (GI) tract, or orifices. Abdominal distention, exophthalmia, lameness, bruising, hematomas, or muffled heart sounds are also possible. Bleeding into the brain or spinal cord may result in severe central nervous system (CNS) disturbances, seizing, paresis, paralysis, or acute death.[3] Tracheal constriction due to thymic, peritracheal, or laryngeal bleeding may result in severe dyspnea.[2]

Diagnosis

Because it has the shortest half-life, factor VII is the first one affected. Depletion of factor VII leads to an elevation of the PT. PIVKA, the collective term for the precursors of the vitamin K–dependent clotting factors, also becomes increased. The PT may be elevated within 36 to 72 hours. Beyond 72 hours, as other factors become depleted, elevations in APTT and activated clotting time (ACT) will develop. Clinical pathologic abnormalities can include anemia, thrombocytopenia, hypoproteinemia, and de-creases in CO_2 and Po_2.[2]

Diagnosis is based on history of exposure, compatible clinical signs, and laboratory results indicative of coagulopathy. Differential diagnoses should include congenital and acquired coagulopathies, and other causes of anemia (eg, trauma, etc). Coagu-lation panels may aid in the differentiation of anticoagulant rodenticide from other coagulopathies. Serum chemistry profiles to detect hepatic or other systemic disease that might affect blood clotting may be indicated.[4] Anticoagulant toxicosis may be worsened in cases of significant hepatic disease due to impaired ability to synthesize coagulation factors and decreased metabolism of ingested rodenticide.

Treatment

For patients that have recently ingested an anticoagulant rodenticide, decontamina-tion by emesis (with 3% hydrogen peroxide or apomorphine) is indicated as long as the patient does not have any underlying conditions that would make inducing emesis contraindicated (including seizure disorder and significant cardiovascular disease). The bar forms of bait may remain in the stomach for a period of time, allowing for effective emesis as long as 4 to 8 hours after ingestion. If emesis is unsuccessful or contraindi-cated, the clinician may give one dose of activated charcoal with a cathartic.[3]

In asymptomatic patients, the clinician may choose to either begin prophylactic vitamin K_1 therapy or monitor PT and only place the patient on vitamin K_1 if the PT becomes elevated. If PT is monitored, a baseline should be run and then repeated at 48 and 72 hours after exposure. The baseline PT is important to determine if any previous exposures may have occurred of which the owner was not aware. No treatment with vitamin K_1 is necessary if the PT remains normal after 72 hours. However, any elevation in the PT warrants full treatment with vitamin K_1. The clinician should remember that vitamin K_1 administration could result in falsely normal PT values because new clotting factor synthesis only requires 6 to 12 hours. Therefore, if PT is being monitored, no vitamin K_1 should be given. The dosage of vitamin K_1 is 3 to 5 mg/kg divided bid and given orally with a fatty meal to enhance absorption. For the short-acting anticoagulant rodenticides (warfarin and pindone), the duration of treatment with vitamin K_1 is 14 days; for bromadiolone, 21 days; and for the other SGARs, 4 weeks.[2] Sometimes, if the ingested dose of anticoagulant is very high, more than 4 weeks of treatment with vitamin K_1 may be necessary (see later).

For symptomatic patients, stabilization is critically important. Oxygen may be needed for dyspnea. Transfusions with whole blood or fresh or fresh frozen plasma may be necessary to replace blood and clotting factors. Once the patient is bleeding, decontamination is not indicated since the exposure would have occurred multiple days prior. Once stabilized, the patient should be started on oral vitamin K_1. Vitamin K_1 should not be given by injection due to risk of hematoma formation or risk of bleeding at the venipuncture and possible risk of anaphylactic reaction. Oral administration is ideal, because vitamin K_1 will be delivered directly to the liver where the clotting factors are activated through the portal circulation. The patient should be hospitalized until the PT is normal and can then be sent home to continue oral vitamin K_1 therapy for the durations recommended earlier. If the active ingredient of the anticoagulant product is unknown, continue vitamin K_1 therapy for at least 4 weeks.

For all patients, it is advisable to check a PT at 48 to 72 hours following the last dose of vitamin K_1. Vitamin K_1 should be continued for 1 additional week or longer if the PT is still increased. This may happen when the pet ingests large amounts of bait. If possible, avoid the use of other highly protein-bound drugs (corticosteroids; NSAIDs, etc) during the treatment, and instruct the owner to restrict exercise during this time. The prognosis is excellent in patients treated before clinical signs develop. If the patient presents after bleeding has started, the prognosis will depend on the severity and the location of the bleeding. For example, a patient that bled into the brain and presented seizing will have a much more guarded prognosis will than a patient that bled into a joint and presented with lameness.[3]

BROMETHALIN

Bromethalin is a neurotoxin, which inhibits mitochondrial energy function (adenosine triphosphate [ATP]) production within the brain.[5] It is available in pelleted forms such as place packs, blocks or bars of bait, and baited worms. The pellets and bait bars are 0.01% bromethalin. Usually the place packs are 0.75 oz of bait, and the bars are 0.5 oz, which is equivalent to 2.13 mg/pack and 1.42 mg/bar of bromethalin, respectively. The baited worms are 0.025% bromethalin and weigh 5 g, which would be 1.25 mg of bromethalin per worm.

Pathophysiology and Clinical Signs

Bromethalin is readily absorbed from the gastrointestinal tract and can peak in the plasma within several hours after ingestion (4 hours within the rat). It is metabolized in the liver via mixed-function oxygenases. The N-demethylated metabolite desmethyl bromethalin is much more toxic than the parent compound. Both bromethalin and desmethyl bromethalin have a wide distribution within the body. The highest levels are found within the fat and brain due to the highly lipophilic nature of bromethalin. Excretion is very slow and occurs through the bile, with evidence of some enterohepatic recirculation. The plasma half-life in rats is approximately 5 to 6 days.[5,6]

Bromethalin and desmethyl bromethalin uncouple oxidative phosphorylation, which is critical for brain and cellular function. As a result, cellular and tissue ATP is decreased and sodium–potassium ion channel pumps are affected. This leads to electrolyte imbalances and a fluid shift into myelinated areas of the brain and spinal cord.[6] Cerebral lipid peroxidation may also occur, which then damages organelles and cellular membranes. A chain reaction of progressive and irreversible cellular damage and necrosis can then develop.[7]

Clinical signs of bromethalin toxicosis are often dose-dependent and can manifest as 2 different syndromes. High doses of bromethalin can cause a "convulsant syndrome," which usually is seen at doses greater than or equal to the LD_{50} for a species. In both dogs and cats, clinical signs may include hyperesthesia, hyperexcitability, tremors, seizures, circling, vocalization, mild to severe CNS depression, hyperthermia, and death. Signs may occur within 4 to 18 hours of ingestion.

Lower doses of bromethalin (less than the LD_{50}) lead to a "paralytic syndrome." With these exposures, the onset of clinical signs is slower and sometimes delayed. Signs may take 1 to 7 days to develop, initially manifesting as ataxia, CNS depression, paresis of the hindlimbs, then progressing to paralysis several days later. Clinical effects may continue to worsen over the next 1 to 2 weeks.[5,8] Additional findings may include upper motor neuron signs: proprioceptive deficits, loss of deep pain, exaggerated pelvic limb reflexes, and increased bladder tone. Animals with a dull mentation may progress to a comatose or semicomatose state.[6] Cats may occasionally exhibit abdominal distention and ileus. Other clinical signs in dogs and cats may include anorexia, vomiting, extensor rigidity, positional nystagmus, anisocoria, dysphonia, fine muscle tremors, recumbency, tachypnea, dysuria, absent menace response, abnormal papillary light reflex, and opisthotonus. A decerebrate posture and seizures may occur in the terminal stages, and death may be from respiratory depression.[5,8,9]

Cats are much more sensitive to bromethalin, and the guinea pig is the most resistant, since this species has much lower N-demethylase activity. The LD_{50} in guinea pigs is greater than 1000 mg/kg orally, and 13 mg/kg in rabbits. For dogs, the oral LD_{50} is 3.65 mg/kg, with a minimum lethal dose (MLD) of 2.5 mg/kg. The LD_{50} in cats is much lower, 0.54 mg/kg, with an MLD of 0.45 mg/kg.[6]

Animals may develop clinical signs of toxicosis at even lower doses though, as some individuals may be more sensitive than others.[5] Based on clinical cases reported to the ASPCA APCC, clinical signs and death have been reported in dogs exposed to bromethalin at doses as low as 0.46 mg/kg (ASPCA APCC Database, unpublished data, 2001–2011). Cats have developed clinical signs after doses as low as 0.24 mg/kg (ASPCA APCC Database, unpublished data, 1998–2000).[10] The risk for relay toxicosis after ingesting an animal that died from bromethalin is low. However, it is theoretically possible in cats that feed mainly on rodents that have died of bromethalin poisoning, as cats are much more sensitive than other species.

Diagnosis

An antemortem diagnosis is most often made based on the history of bait ingestion and the development of clinical signs. Frequently, owners may not know the bait was consumed until they notice that the stool is discolored (often green). Performing a rectal exam may aid in determining how recent the ingestion was or if there are multiple animals involved. Clinical lab tests are often unremarkable and nondiagnostic. An increase in cerebrospinal fluid (CSF) pressure may or may not be present in symptomatic animals. If it is increased, it is usually not as high as that in animals with head trauma. The reason for this may be from the edema being confined within the myelin sheaths. Analysis of the CSF is often normal, without any evidence of inflammation.[5]

Postmortem diagnosis is often based on histologic changes in the CNS and possible detection of residues. Grossly in dogs, cerebral edema is usually mild. In fatal ingestions, histologic lesions include spongy degeneration of the white matter in the optic nerve, cerebrum, cerebellum, brain stem, and spinal cord. Myelin and cellular edema and vacuolization are also seen.[5,8] Although the white matter is primarily affected, vacuolization can occasionally be seen in the cerebral cortical gray matter. No peripheral nerve lesions occur.[9] Detection of bromethalin in the stomach contents, ascites, fat, liver, kidney, and brain may also be performed at select veterinary laboratories.[6,8]

Table 1
The ASPCA APCC's decontamination recommendations for bromethalin ingestion

Time Since Exposure	Dose Ingested[a]	Action
Dogs		
<4 hours	0.1–0.49 mg/kg	Emesis or 1 dose of activated charcoal
>4 hours	0.1–0.49 mg/kg	One dose of activated charcoal
<4 hours	0.5–0.75 mg/kg	Emesis and 3 doses of activated charcoal over 24 hours
>4 hours	0.5–0.75 mg/kg	Three doses of activated charcoal over 24 hours
<4 hours	>0.75 mg/kg	Emesis and 3 doses of activated charcoal a day for 48 hours
>4 hours	>0.75 mg/kg	Three doses of activated charcoal a day for 48 hours
Cats		
<4 hours	0.05–0.1 mg/kg	Emesis[b] or 1 dose of activated charcoal
>4 hours	0.05–0.1 mg/kg	One dose of activated charcoal
<4 hours	0.1–0.3 mg/kg	Emesis and 3 doses of activated charcoal over 24 hours
>4 hours	0.1–0.3 mg/kg	Three doses of activated charcoal over 24 hours
<4 hours	>0.3 mg/kg	Emesis and 3 doses of activated charcoal a day for 48 hours
>4 hours	>0.3 mg/kg	Three doses of activated charcoal a day for 48 hours

[a] *Note:* 1 oz of 0.01% bromethalin bait contains 2.84 mg of bromethalin.
[b] *Note:* emesis in cats can be induced with xylazine 0.4–0.5 mg/kg IM or IV and reversed with yohimbine (0.1 mg/kg IV); emesis success with xylazine in cats is approximately 43% in cats (ASPCA APCC, unpublished data, 2009).

Treatment

In the asymptomatic animal, decontaminate by inducing emesis if the exposure was within the past 4 hours. If the ingestion was more than 4 hours earlier, single or repeated doses of activated charcoal may be indicated, depending on the amount consumed (**Table 1**). Cats may need longer treatment and multiple charcoal doses due to their greater sensitivity to bromethalin.[5]

For animals that are given activated charcoal, especially those given repeated doses, obtaining baseline serum sodium is recommended prior to administration due to potential of development of hypernatremia. Intravenous fluid administration and monitoring in the clinic for 4 hours may also be warranted with administration of a single dose of charcoal. Serum sodium should be closely monitored for patients receiving repeated charcoal doses. Some animals can have an osmotic fluid shift after charcoal administration, and the chances of hypernatremia may increase after multiple doses. Development of hypernatremia can cause CNS signs within the first 4 hours of dosing activated charcoal (ataxia, tremors, depression), which could be mistaken for bromethalin toxicosis. If these signs develop, repeat a serum sodium level and compare it to the baseline. It is also recommended to reduce the subsequent doses of charcoal by half after giving the initial dose. (For example, if a 10-lb dog is given 30 mL of activated charcoal, the rest of the doses should be decreased to 15 mL.) The first dose can be given with a cathartic such as sorbitol, and the subsequent doses without a cathartic, to reduce the risk of electrolyte derangements. The charcoal can be repeated at 8-hour intervals. If it is not being passed in the stools prior to the next dose, give the animal a warm water enema to move the charcoal out of the GI tract. This can also provide electrolyte-free water to the body, if the sodium is starting to become elevated.

Symptomatic bromethalin patients are difficult to treat successfully, especially if the patient is showing serious CNS effects. If signs are less severe, such as ataxia or depression, some animals may recover with supportive care over a period of 2 to 4 weeks. However, some animals may have permanent neurologic dysfunction. In patients with tremors, seizures, coma, or paralysis, the prognosis is poor to grave.

Cerebral edema can be treated with mannitol and corticosteroids, but often signs return once therapy is discontinued. Side effects of mannitol are dehydration, hypernatremia, hyperkalemia, hypotension, pulmonary edema, and renal failure. Rehydrating these animals may worsen the CNS signs. Furosemide may be an alternative to mannitol to reduce these risks and may be combined with dexamethasone. Tremors and seizures can be treated with methocarbamol, diazepam, or barbiturates. Recumbent animals may need nutritional support and good nursing care to prevent decubital ulcers and pneumonia.[5,6]

CHOLECALCIFEROL

The chemical name of vitamin D_3 is cholecalciferol. Vitamin D_3 is required by the body and is acquired in mammals as part of the diet or by dermal exposure to ultraviolet light.[11,12] An understanding of the metabolic pathway of cholecalciferol is important to a discussion of intoxication by cholecalciferol rodenticides. In the liver, cholecalciferol is metabolized to calcifediol (25-hydroxycholecalciferol). This conversion has limited negative feedback; therefore, a large ingestion of cholecalciferol will lead to a significant increase in calcifediol.[13] Calcifediol is then metabolized by the kidney to calcitriol (1,25-dihydroxycholecalciferol), which is the most active metabolite. As calcitriol concentrations increase, a negative feedback mechanism halts the production of calcitriol; however, calcifediol continues to be produced in high enough amounts to lead to clinical effects.[13] Since calcifediol has a very long half-life,[12] poisoned patients may require treatment for an extended period of time.

Pathophysiology and Clinical Signs

The metabolites of cholecalciferol cause their effects by increasing serum calcium and phosphorus.[13] They act to increase intestinal absorption of calcium, stimulate calcium and phosphorus transfer from bones into the plasma, and enhance renal tubular reabsorption of calcium. Within 48 hours of exposure, patients may develop vomiting, lethargy, and muscle weakness as a result of the increased plasma concentration on the cells in the body.[13] Prolonged elevation of serum calcium and phosphorus can lead to tissue mineralization. Tissue mineralization in the kidneys can lead to acute renal failure. Decreased functioning of the GI tract, skeletal and cardiac muscle, blood vessels, and ligaments can result from mineralization in these areas.[13]

The literature suggests that clinical signs can be seen at cholecalciferol dosages of 0.5 mg/kg.[11] This dosage corresponds to a 50-lb dog ingesting only 0.5 oz of a typical 0.075% cholecalciferol bait; therefore, even small ingestions may warrant treatment. The ASPCA APCC recommends decontamination when the ingested dose is greater than 0.1 mg/kg.

Clinical signs typically occur within 12 to 36 hours of ingestion of the rodenticide. The common clinical signs seen with cholecalciferol toxicosis include vomiting, anorexia, depression, polyuria, and polydipsia. Acute renal failure can develop within

24 to 72 hours. If the patient survives the initial clinical signs, they may have long-term effects relating to mineralization of their tissues and organs.[13]

Diagnosis

Often the diagnosis is made based on the history of ingestion and the development of clinical signs. Some owners may also notice bait in the stool. A rectal exam may help confirm ingestion and rule in or rule out other pets in the household that may have also been exposed. Clinical laboratory tests to perform include serum phosphorus levels, calcium (total and ionized), blood urea nitrogen (BUN), and serum creatinine. A urinalysis may show isosthenuria.[12] Be certain that the blood sample is not hemolyzed or lipemic, as this can lead to a falsely elevated total calcium. Young animals will also have elevated calcium levels from bone growth. Ionized calcium (iCa) is affected by the pH of blood or serum. An acidic pH will dissociate calcium from protein and will increase iCa. An alkaline pH occurs when samples are exposed to air. With loss of carbon dioxide, calcium will bind to protein and decrease iCa, so samples should be collected and handled anaerobically.[14] A reference lab is ideal for testing iCa, since some in-house analyzers may not be accurate.[15]

After acute exposures, the serum phosphorus is often the first laboratory elevation that is seen ($>7-8$ mg/dL). This is then followed by an increase in serum calcium (13–20 mg/dL), and these changes can occur within 24 to 72 hours after ingestion. Radiography or ultrasonography may help in diagnosing soft tissue mineralization in symptomatic animals.[11,14]

Specific antemortem testing includes 25(OH)D$_3$ (calcifediol or 25-hydroxycholecalciferol), which is the primary circulating metabolite of cholecalciferol. Ionized calcium and serum intact parathyroid hormone (PTH) levels may also be of value. In animals that have ingested cholecalciferol, the 25-hydroxycholecalciferol levels will be increased at least 15 times above normal. In some patients, levels may remain elevated for weeks to months. The iCa is also elevated, and the PTH is low.[12,14] Testing for 1,25-dihydroxycholecalciferol (calcitriol) and other vitamin D$_3$ analogs such as calcipotriene is not readily available.[11] Calcitriol has a short half-life and often peaks within the serum on the fourth day after ingestion, then rapidly declines. The homeostatic negative control mechanism for calcium is not triggered until 4 days after exposure.[16]

Postmortem diagnosis is more difficult. The kidney is the best organ to use for detecting 25-hydroxycholecalciferol levels. Plasma and serum samples can be used as well. On gross necropsy, the stomach may be empty from vomiting and anorexia, and animals are often dehydrated. Gastric ulceration with hemorrhage may also be present, and the gastric mucosa may be hyperemic and swollen. The kidneys may be normal in appearance or look mottled. The lungs may look hemorrhagic, edematous, or normal.[12] Additionally, there is soft tissue mineralization within the heart, kidneys, GI tract, skeletal muscles, ligaments, and tendons. Azotemic ulcers may be evident in the oral cavity.[11] Histopathologic findings may include soft tissue mineralization of the great vessels, stomach, kidneys, and lungs but are not pathognomonic. Within the heart and arteries, the atria and aorta have the most evidence of mineralization. Within the vessels, it is often within the smooth muscles. Myocardial degeneration may be present within the heart, including mineralized and necrotic myocytes. The stomach may have mineralization within the smooth muscles and the lamina propria. The stomach wall is often congested, with the mucosal epithelium showing erosion, necrosis, sloughing, and hemorrhage. These lesions are often located near bands of mineralization. The kidneys often have evidence of mineralization within the glomerulus, convoluted tubules, and the blood vessels, resulting in epithelial cell necrosis and cellular debris. Protein cast formation may also be observed. Within the lungs, the alveolar septae are often thickened, with hemorrhage and mineralization.[11,12]

Treatment

In the asymptomatic animal, decontaminate by inducing emesis if the exposure was within the past 4 hours. If the ingestion was more than 4 hours earlier, administer activated charcoal if the animal has not been vomiting prior to presentation. There is evidence of enterohepatic recirculation of cholecalciferol, so repeated doses of activated charcoal may be needed[11] (see treatment recommendations for bromethalin for charcoal administration suggestions). The use of cholestyramine resin has shown some benefit in reducing vitamin D_3 levels in humans. Cholestyramine can be tried as an adjunct treatment in dogs at 0.3 to 1 g/kg PO 3 times a day for 4 days. This can be given between activated charcoal doses (eg, activated charcoal, then give cholestyramine in 4 hours, repeat charcoal in 8 hours, then give cholestyramine in 4 hours, etc). Baseline serum chemistries of total calcium, ionized calcium, phosphorus, BUN, and creatinine should be obtained and monitored every 24 hours for 4 days. If these remain normal, no additional treatment is needed.

In symptomatic animals, treatment is aimed at correcting the hypercalcemia. Often animals have been vomiting and are anorexic; therefore, rehydration and diuresis should be instituted first with 0.9% sodium chloride (NaCl) at 2 to 3 times maintenance fluid rate. After the animal is rehydrated, then loop diuretics and glucocorticoids can be instituted.[14,17,18] Sodium ions enhance calcium excretion by reducing tubular calcium reabsorption and enhancing calciuresis. Furosemide enhances calcium renal excretion by decreasing sodium and chloride reabsorption across the loop of Henle, which diminishes the positive potential across the tubule. Thiazide diuretics should be avoided, as these can decrease calciuresis. Monitoring hydration status is critical with diuretic use. Prednisone aids in suppression of bone resorption. It also reduces the absorption of calcium by the intestines and increases the urinary excretion of calcium by reducing absorption by the distal tubules. If the patient is acidotic, sodium bicarbonate may decrease iCa as calcium ions bind to plasma proteins and bicarbonate. The dose is 1 to 4 mEq/kg slowly IV, and effects may last up to 3 hours. If the serum phosphorus is elevated, phosphate binders such as aluminum hydroxide given orally are beneficial. A diet low in phosphorus and calcium should be fed for at least 4 weeks.[11,12,14] (See **Box 1** for medication doses.)

Patients that are severely affected or whose calcium levels continue to rise despite therapy will need more aggressive treatment. The preferred drug to use is pamidronate disodium, which is a bisphosphonate that inhibits bone resorption. It is administered slowly intravenously within 0.9% sodium chloride. The drug can inhibit bone resorption for a long duration, but some animals do need a second infusion. Elevations in BUN and creatinine can occur after administration, so animals should be maintained on IV fluids during this time, and until calcium levels normalize. The pamidronate treatment may need to be repeated in 5 to 7 days of the initial dose. The cost of pamidronate may be high, but it often lowers the calcium within 24 to 48 hours after dosing. Monitoring renal values are important when using this drug, and caution should be used in animals with azotemia.[11,12,19] In humans, side effects of pamidronate include hypocalcemia, hypophosphatemia, hypokalemia, and hypomagnesemia.[17] Monitoring these parameters in veterinary patients is recommended.

If pamidronate is unavailable, another option is calcitonin salmon but it is less effective. It also has a very short half-life (2 to 4 hours), and must be given intramuscularly multiple times a day for several weeks. It works by reducing the activity and formation of osteoclasts, and the decrease in calcium is rapid. Vomiting

Box 1

ASPCA APCC recommended management of hypercalcemia associated with cholecalciferol and vitamin D analogs (revised November 2011)

Stabilize animal as needed (fluids, antiemetics, antiseizure medications, etc)

Decontamination

- Less than 4 hours post ingestion-emesis (3% *hydrogen peroxide*, 2.2 mL/kg PO maximum 3 tablespoons (may repeat once); or use *apomorphine 0.03 mg/kg IV; Activated charcoal* (6–12 mL/kg PO, repeat ½ of the initial dose q8–12h for 2–3 doses). Monitor for hypernatremia in patients receiving activated charcoal.

- Greater than 4 hours post ingestion—*activated charcoal*—use caution to avoid aspiration; contraindicated in vomiting animals; Monitor serum calcium and phosphorous for 4 days (see below).

- Cholestyramine has been shown to be effective in lab animals and humans to enhance excretion of vitamin D by binding to bile acids. Dose: 0.3-1 g/kg PO TID for 4 days.

Laboratory monitoring

- Baseline calcium, phosphorus, BUN, creatinine; complete serum biochemistry is recommended especially in older animals or animals with previously existing health problems.

- If Ca, P, BUN, Cr are normal on presentation—monitor Ca, P, BUN, Cr q12h for at least 4 days. Phosphorus tends to elevate before calcium. Treatment may be discontinued if 96-hour values are normal.

- If Ca, P, BUN, and/or Cr are abnormal on presentation—go to Hypercalcemia Management protocol below:

- Monitor Ca × P product—if > 60, then chances of soft tissue mineralization increases. To compute, take Ca level (in mg/dL) and multiply by P level (in mg/dL); eg, if Ca = 14 and P = 5, then Ca × P = 70 and there is risk of soft tissue mineralization; some labs may report values in units other than mg/dL—be sure to convert to mg/dL before calculating the product. Young dogs may have higher baseline serum calcium and phosphrous levels. In these dogs, Ca × P product between 60-95 may be normal. Do not just look at this value only; other trends (elevation in serum calcium and phosphorous and comparison with baseline values) should also be considered when interpreting the results. Most dogs with persistent significant hypercalcemia show signs of anorexia, and lethargy and some GI signs. Some increase in Ca × P product in the absence of clinical signs or other electrolyte changes may not be significant.

Hypercalcemia management protocol I (preferred)—Pamidronate is a bisphosphonate used in humans to treat hypercalemia of malignancy.

- *IV Normal saline (0.9% NaCl)*; twice maintenance; forced diuresis; maintain diuresis until calcium levels have dropped

- *Furosemide*—2.5–4.5 mg/kg PO tid to qid or 0.5 mg/kg/h via continuous IV infusion; avoid thiazide diuretics as they reduce renal excretion of calcium

- *Dexamethasone*—l mg/kg SQ divided qid or *prednisone*—2–3 mg/kg PO bid

- *Pamidronate* (Aredia®)—1.3–2 mg/kg; dilute in normal saline and administer IV over a 2-hour period

Hypercalcemia management protocol II—The authors believe that this protocol is less desirable, as calcitonin is not consistent in its ability to lower serum calcium, and some dogs become refractory to calcitonin. Additionally, in experimental dogs, concurrent use of pamidronate and calcitonin resulted in greater soft tissue mineralization than when either drug was used alone.

- *IV Normal saline*; twice maintenance; forced diuresis; maintain diuresis until calcium levels have dropped

- *Furosemide*—2.5–4.5 mg/kg PO tid to qid or 0.5 mg/kg/h via continuous IV infusion; avoid thiazide diuretics as they reduce renal excretion of calcium
- *Dexamethasone*—I mg/kg IV or SQ divided qid or *prednisone*—2–3 mg/kg PO bid
- *Salmon calcitonin* (Calcimar®) 4–6 U/kg SQ bid–tid

Once Ca levels have stabilized

- Wean off fluids and monitor Ca, P, BUN, and Cr at least every 24 hours. If BUN and Cr are elevated, treat for acute renal failure (ie, maintain fluid diuresis). If calcium level starts to rise, re-institute fluid therapy and consider another dose of pamidronate (generally expect this to occur within 5–7 days after first dose). In our experience, most dogs given pamidronate have required only one dose, although some have needed repeated doses.
- Switch to an oral corticosteroid and furosemide; if lab values remain normal 5–7 days after discontinuing IV fluids, gradually wean off of these medications over 1–2 weeks
- Aluminum hydroxide–30–90 mg/kg/day PO in divided doses as needed if phosphorus level remains elevated.
- Closely monitor appetite—development of anorexia may be an indication that the calcium level has risen. Monitor Ca, P for a minimum of 5–7 days after those values have returned to normal. Then 2–3 times a week for 2 weeks, and then weekly for 2 weeks. Feed a low Ca diet during this time period.
- Monitor for hypocalcemia

and anorexia are often side effects, and animals often become refractory to treatment within a few days. Combining pamidronate and calcitonin is used in human medicine but is not recommended in veterinary patients since studies do not show any benefit when used together in dogs, and it potentially may worsen the outcome.[14,20]

Saline diuresis should be continued until the serum calcium levels return to normal. Fluid therapy in symptomatic patients may be needed for 1 week or longer because the half-life of cholecalciferol is very long (29 days). Furosemide and prednisone may need to be continued for 1 to 2 weeks after the animal is off of fluids and then gradually tapered. After fluid therapy has stopped, the calcium levels should be monitored every 24 hours for 96 hours, then twice a week for 2 weeks, then once a week for 2 weeks, to make sure there is not a relapse.[11,14,20]

SUMMARY

This article covers the pathophysiology, clinical signs, diagnosis and treatment for the three most commonly encountered rodenticides: anticoagulants, bromethalin and cholecalciferol. Anticoagulants cause coagulation abnormalities and bleeding, bromethalin is a neurotoxin and cholecalciferol leads to increased serum calcium and phosphorus which causes renal failure. Risk mitigation policies implemented by the EPA beginning in June 2011 are likely to cause an increase in the number of bromethalin and cholecalciferol cases seen in veterinary clinics.

REFERENCES

1. US Environmental Protection Agency. Final risk mitigation decision for ten rodenticides. Available at: http://www.epa.gov/opp00001/reregistration/rodenticides/finalriskdecision.htm. Accessed May 11, 2011.
2. Murphy MJ. Anticoagulant rodenticides. In: Gupta RC, editor. Veterinary toxicology basic and clinical principles. New York: Elsevier; 2007. p. 525–47.

3. Merola V. Anticoagulant rodenticides: deadly for pests, dangerous for pets. Vet Med 2002;97:716–22.

4. Sheafor SE, Couto CG. Clinical approach to a dog with anticoagulant rodenticide poisoning. Vet Med 1994;94:466–71.

5. Dorman DC. Bromethalin. In: Peterson ME, Talcott PA, editors. Small animal toxicology. 2nd edition. St Louis (MO): Elsevier Saunders; 2006. p. 609–18.

6. Dorman D. Bromethalin. In: Plumlee KH, editor. Clinical veterinary toxicology. St Louis (MO): Mosby; 2004. p. 446–8.

7. Osweiler GD. The action of poisons. In: Toxicology. Baltimore (MD): Williams and Wilkins; 1996. p. 17–22.

8. Dorman DC, Simon J, Harlin KA, et al. Diagnosis of bromethalin toxicosis in the dog. J Vet Diagn Invest 1990;2:123–8.

9. Dorman DC, Zachary JF, Buck WB. Neuropathologic findings of bromethalin toxicosis in the cat. Vet Pathol 1992;29:139–44.

10. Dunayer E. Bromethalin: the other rodenticide. Vet Med 2003;98:732–6.

11. Morrow CK, Volmer PA. Cholecalciferol. In: Plumlee KH, editor. Clinical veterinary toxicology. St Louis (MO): Mosby; 2004. p. 448–51.

12. Rumbeiha WK. Cholecalciferol. In: Peterson ME, Talcott PA, editors. Small animal toxicology. 2nd edition. St Louis (MO): Elsevier Saunders; 2006. p. 629–42.

13. Morrow C. Cholecalciferol poisoning. Vet Med 2001;96:905–11.

14. Rosol TJ, Chew DJ, Nagode LA, et al. Disorders of calcium: hypercalcemia and hypocalcemia. In: DiBartola SP, editor. Fluid therapy in small animal practice. 2nd edition. Philadelphia: WB Saunders; 2000. p. 108–62.

15. Tappin S, Rizzo F, Dodkin S, et al. Measurement of ionized calcium in canine blood samples collected in prefilled and self-filled heparinized syringes using the i-STAT point-of-care analyzer. Vet Clin Pathol 2008;37(1):66–72.

16. Rumbeiha WK, Braselton WE, Nachreiner RF, et al. The postmortem diagnosis of cholecalciferol toxicosis: a novel approach and differentiation from ethylene glycol toxicosis. J Vet Diagn Invest 2000;12:426–32.

17. Kadar E, Rush JE, Wetmore L, et al. Electrolyte disturbances and cardiac arrhythmias in a dog following pamidronate, calcitonin, and furosemide administration for hypercalcemia of malignancy. J Am Anim Hosp Assoc 2004;40:75–81.

18. Jensterle M, Pfeifer M, Sever M, et al. Dihydrotachysterol intoxication treated with pamidronate: a case report. Cases J 2010;3:78–93.

19. Gwaltney-Brant SM, Rumbeiha WK. Newer antidotal therapies. Vet Clin Small Anim 2002;32:323–39.

20. Rumbeiha WK, Kruger JM, Fitzgerald SF, et al. Use of pamidronate to reverse vitamin D_3-induced toxicosis in dogs. Am J Vet Res 1999;60:1092–7.

Toxicology of Explosives and Fireworks in Small Animals

Patti Gahagan, DVM[a], Tina Wismer, DVM[b],*

KEYWORDS

- Explosives • Nitrates • Explosive detection dogs/working dogs
- Fireworks • Barium • Chlorates

Exposure to explosives and fireworks in dogs can result in variable severity of clinical signs depending on presence of different chemicals and the amount. The risk can be lessened by proper education of dog handlers and owners about the seriousness of the intoxications.

EXPLOSIVES

An explosive is any material that can undergo rapid and self-propagating decomposition, resulting in the liberation of heat and the production of energy, most commonly through the expansion of gases. The released energy has a number of potential uses. These include commercial applications such as blasting in mines and quarries, demolition in the construction industry, military applications, and firearms applications.

There are over 300 materials classified by the Bureau of Alcohol, Tobacco, Firearms, and Explosives (ATF) as explosive materials.[1] It is beyond the scope of this article to deal with each of these materials from a toxicity standpoint. However, explosive materials can be grouped according to similarity of chemical structure, which makes evaluation of the toxicity potential much easier to understand.

Explosives are classified based on the rapidity of the decomposition and resultant energy wave as either low-order explosives or high explosives. Examples of low-order explosives include pipe bombs, gunpowder, and petroleum-based bombs. High explosives propagate a supersonic shockwave when the explosive material decomposes into hot, rapidly expanding gases. Examples of high explosives include trinitrotoluene (TNT), cyclonite (RDX), and pentaerythritol tetranitrate (PETN) (**Table 1** provides a glossary of abbreviations).

The authors have nothing to disclose.
[a] Novartis Animal Health US, Inc, 3200 Northline Avenue, Suite 300, Greensboro, NC 27408, USA
[b] ASPCA Animal Poison Control Center, 1717 South Philo Road, Suite 36, Urbana, IL 61802, USA
* Corresponding author.
E-mail address: tina.wismer@aspca.org

Table 1	
Glossary of abbreviations	
Abbreviation	**Definition**
ANFO	Ammonium nitrate/fuel oil
Blackpowder	Potassium nitrate + carbon + sulfur
C4	RDX + plasticizer
EGDN	Ethylene glycol dinitrate
NC	Nitrocelluose
NG	Nitroglycerine
PETN	Pentaerythritol tetranitrate
RDX	Research Department Explosive; cyclotrimethylenetrinitramine, also known as cyclonite, hexogen, and T-4
Semtex	RDX + PETN
Smokeless powder	Nitrocellulose based propellant (gunpowder)
TNT	Trinitrotoluene

Explosives can also be classified as primary, secondary, or tertiary based on how easily the decomposition process can be initiated. Primary explosives are used to ignite secondary explosives. Examples of primary explosives include lead azide (LA), lead styphnate (LS), and nitroglycerin (NG). Blasting caps contain primary explosives and are used to ignite secondary explosives to initiate the decomposition process. Secondary explosives are much more stable than primary explosives and detonate only under specific circumstances. Examples of secondary explosives include TNT and RDX. Tertiary explosives are quite insensitive to shock and cannot be reliably detonated by primary explosives. Typically, a small amount of a secondary explosive (ignited by a small amount of a primary explosive) is used to detonate tertiary explosives. Ammonium nitrate and fuel oil (ANFO) is an example of a tertiary explosive.[1]

Most explosives are tightly regulated, with access limited by various agencies, most notably the ATF. Exposure of small animals to explosive materials is limited primarily to dogs and will most commonly result from improper or negligent storage of materials, stolen materials no longer being handled appropriately, and training aids used to train explosives detection dogs.

Explosives detection dogs working in actual field conditions (not in training scenarios) are unlikely to suffer from toxic ingestions as they are trained extensively not to touch or otherwise interfere with explosives. A working dog that violates this training in actual field conditions is more likely to be seriously injured or killed by an explosion than to suffer any toxicity. Therefore, it is dogs in training that are most likely to consume explosive agents. Careful training techniques that limit the novice dog's ability to come in contact with and consume training aids make oral exposures uncommon.

While the specific odors that explosives detection dogs are trained to detect may vary based on specific needs, these dogs are commonly trained to alert on 6 specific odors: black powder or smokeless powder; commercial dynamite containing ethylene glycol dinitrate (EGDN) or NG; RDX; PETN; TNT (military dynamite); and slurries/water gel explosives.[2] Therefore, these are the explosives most likely to be encountered by a training dog in a clinical setting.

Many low explosives are also tightly regulated and not likely to be ingested by dogs. However, some agents used in explosives are readily available without restriction and pose toxic concerns to companion animals. These agents include the petroleum distillates and nitrates, including fertilizers. Though most commonly thought of in its use as an explosive, NG is also available as a medicine (vasodilator) and could potentially be ingested in households as well.

Nitroaromatics

Trinitrotoluene (TNT) is a nitroaromatic compound most commonly used by the military as a booster for other high explosives. It is also used in commercial mining operations. TNT and other nitroaromatic compounds easily penetrate the skin. Dermal exposure can cause methemoglobinemia, anemia, local dermal irritation, and hepatic injury. Urinary bladder tumors have been associated with chronic dermal TNT exposure in humans.[3] Dermal exposures are rare in dogs. If dermal exposure does occur, decontamination by bathing with a liquid dishwashing detergent should be instituted. Gloves should be worn to protect the bather. Any dermal lesions should be treated symptomatically and supportively.

An acute inhalation exposure in dogs can cause mild and transient respiratory irritation. Removal to fresh air is usually the only treatment needed. If significant respiratory signs do occur, institute symptomatic and supportive care.

Dogs are more likely to be exposed via ingestion of negligently handled or stored materials. Acute oral single-dose LD_{50} values have not been established for TNT in dogs, but short-term (90-day) oral LD_{50} values were 1320 and 794 mg/kg in male and female rats, respectively, and 660 mg/kg in male and female mice. The animals developed tremors followed by mild seizures 1 to 2 hours after dosing. Doses of 20 mg/kg/d for 13 weeks caused anemia with reduced erythrocytes, hemoglobin, and hematocrit in dogs. Other effects included splenomegaly with hemosiderosis, hepatomegaly, elevated serum cholesterol levels, and depressed serum glutamic pyruvic transaminase activity in dogs. The "no observable effect" level for dogs was 0.2 mg/kg/d.[4] A 6-month oral toxicity study of TNT in dogs demonstrated the major toxic effects to be hemolytic anemia, methemoglobinemia, hepatic injury, splenomegaly, and death at doses ranging from 0.5 to 32 mg/kg/d. Because all doses caused effects, a "no observable effect" level was not established although only the highest dose (32 mg/kg) was lethal.[5]

Dogs known to have ingested TNT that present to a clinic should undergo decontamination since the amounts needed to cause significant signs in an acute oral exposure are not known. If the ingestion is within 4 hours of exposure and the dog is asymptomatic, emesis induction with apomorphine is a reasonable option. Depending on the amount recovered, N-acetylcysteine (Mucomyst; 140 mg/kg PO or IV then 70 mg/kg PO q8h for 5 to 7 treatments), which helps maintain or restore glutathione levels, may be prudent to help prevent/treat methemoglobinemia. It has been shown to reduce chemically induced methemoglobinemia in vitro.[6] However, there is some question as to whether it will be effective in treating methemoglobinemia formation resulting from nitrite toxicity.[7] In human medicine, methylene blue is the preferred agent for treating methemoglobinemia secondary to nitrate toxicity.[8] In dogs, methylene blue is not commonly used because it is not readily available to veterinarians. It can be administered IV as a 1% solution at 1.5 mg/kg. Repeat in 30 minutes once if needed. Monitoring liver values for animals showing significant clinical signs is also recommended.

Nitramines

The most prominent nitramine explosive in use today is cyclonite, also known as RDX or hexahydro-1,3,5-trinitro-1,3,5-triazine. It exhibits a high degree of stability so it poses little risk for spontaneous detonation. It is commonly combined with plasticizers to make C-4. It is also commonly combined with PETN to form Semtex. PETN is a nitrate ester (discussed later) in the next section.

While inhalation of cyclonite can cause numerous signs, including seizures, this is not likely clinically relevant in dogs as they are more commonly exposed to the plasticized form rather than the crystalline form found in manufacturing plants.[9] Similarly, there is little concern for significant dermal absorption in dogs exposed to the plasticized form.[10]

Following ingestion of cyclonite, absorption is slow.[11] The peak plasma level in humans is 24 hours.[12] In rats, a plateau was reached within several hours but remained stable for 24 hours.[13] The elimination half-life in humans is 15 hours.

There is conflicting information regarding the LD_{50} of cyclonite, probably because of the wide variability of granulation. The LD_{50} of coarse granular cyclonite is 3 times higher than that of fine powder.[14] One study lists the LD_{50} for dogs as 6 mg/kg, while another lists the "no observable effect level" at 10 mg/kg/d for 3 months.[15] In a study of 7 female dogs fed a diet of cyclonite at 50 mg/kg/d for 6 days per week for 6 weeks, one dog died at the end of the fifth week from excessive congestion of the walls of the small intestines.[14]

Despite being an organic nitrate–based explosive, cyclonite does not seem to cause nitrate-like toxicity. It is a corrosive irritant of the eyes, skin, mucus membranes, and respiratory tract but mainly acts as a neurotoxicant. There is some evidence that limbic structures in the central nervous system (CNS) may be involved in cyclonite-induced seizure susceptibility.[16] In dogs ingesting cyclonite, seizures are the most common clinical sign and may occur minutes to hours after ingestion. In published case reports, 100% of exposed dogs outside of a research setting experienced seizures. In the ASPCA Animal Poison Control Center (APCC)'s database, 6 of 11 symptomatic dogs experienced seizures. Metabolic acidosis is a possible sequelae. Vomiting is also a commonly reported clinical sign in dogs. Development of minor methemoglobinemia in humans has been suggested, but this has not been reported in dogs ingesting cyclonite. There has been one documented case of elevated hepatic enzymes in dogs and one reported case of elevated renal values.[12]

Decontamination via emesis (with apomorphine or 3% hydrogen peroxide) induction is reasonable in asymptomatic dogs ingesting cyclonite. Some explosives detection dog handlers are taught to immediately induce vomiting in the field with any ingestion that occurs during training scenarios (P. Gahagan, personal communication, 2009). Although there may be some concern for inducing vomiting with an agent known to possess some corrosive potential, the corrosive potential of cyclonite is relatively mild compared to the risk of seizure activity. If cyclonite is mixed with more corrosive materials, the risk of significant corrosive injury should be considered in determining whether to induce vomiting. Activated charcoal may be helpful in reducing absorption. Because of slow and delayed absorption of cyclonite, activated charcoal may be beneficial when there is a delay between ingestion and seeking medical assistance. The addition of a cathartic such as sorbital or magnesium sulfate to activated charcoal may decrease gastrointestinal (GI) transit time and lessen the absorption of cyclonite.

Clinically affected dogs should be treated supportively. Seizures are typically well controlled with diazepam (0.5–2 mg/kg IV). In one case, diazepam was used CRI to control seizures.[11] Other antiseizure medication such as phenobarbital or propofol can also be tried if diazepam does not seem to control seizures well. Intravenous fluids for general support are indicated for seizing dogs. Cessation of seizures generally corrects resultant metabolic acidosis, but acid-base status should also be monitored. GI protectants such as famotidine or other H2 blockers along with sucralfate should be given to protect the GI mucosa. Antiemetics such as maropitant (1 mg/kg subcutaneously once a day) or metoclopramide can be used to control vomiting.

Most dogs recover with good supportive care. Depending on the dose, duration of signs can range between 24 and 72 hours. Outside of a research setting, there are no reported deaths from ingestion of cyclonite.

Nitrate Esters

There are 4 nitrate esters commonly used in explosives applications: nitrocellulose (NC), NG, PETN, and ethylene glycol dinitrate (EGDN). Both NG and PETN are also used pharmacologically as potent vasodilators.

NC is a highly flammable compound used as a propellant or low-order explosive. By itself it is considered nontoxic. The toxic concern when nitrocellulose is ingested is more related to compounds with which it may be combined rather than the nitrocellulose itself. If ingested as a sole agent, the only expected signs would be mild, self-limiting GI upset secondary to dietary indiscretion.

NG is used in the manufacture of dynamite, gunpowder, and rocket propellants. In addition to its uses in the fields of weapons and explosives, it is also used in human medicine to alleviate the pain associated with angina pectoris and in veterinary medicine as a vasodilator.

With ingestion of NG, the most common sign is hypotension. As with most agents with toxic potential, the dose determines the severity of hypotension. When considering NG as an explosive agent, it would be rare for a dog to ingest just NG. It would be much more common for there to be a co-ingestion of other agents. The other agent would likely be responsible for the main clinical signs, but with NG as a component, blood pressure monitoring would be important. For most symptomatic dogs that have ingested explosive materials containing NG, the use of intravenous fluids may be adequate to treat the risk for hypotension in such ingestions.

Because of its nitrate contents, NG has the potential for causing methemoglobinemia. However, this rarely occurs in dogs as monogastrics compared to ruminants are less likely to convert nitrate to nitrite, which is responsible for oxidizing hemoglobin to methemoglobin. There are some human case reports involving methemoglobinemia, but these involved chronic use of NG and often resulted only in clinically insignificant methemoglobinemia. In dogs, mild methemoglobinemia was induced with a daily dose of 25 mg/kg for 12 months.[17] Significant methemoglobinemia is not expected with acute ingestions of NG in dogs. Dogs ingesting explosive materials containing NG should be treated symptomatically. Most signs in affected dogs will likely be from the non-NG components of the material ingested.

PETN is another nitrate ester commonly used in explosives applications. It is a major component of detonating cord and is also used in blasting caps and other types of detonators. It is also mixed with cyclonite to form the explosive Semtex. Structurally, PETN resembles NG. As such, it also has pharmacological uses for the treatment of angina pectoris and for its vasodilatory effects in humans. The pharmacologic formulation includes a lactose stabilizer. Removing this stabilizer creates its explosive potential.

In one study, dogs were given 5 mg/kg of PETN via orogastric tube. A gradual fall in blood pressure occurred, but it spontaneously resolved.[18] PETN is also absorbed via the respiratory tract in dogs with similar changes in blood pressure.[18] These studies were conducted with pharmacologic preparations of PETN. Ingestion and inhalation of the less stable explosive formulations may yield different results. As with

NG, there is a potential for hypotension following ingestion of PETN containing explosive materials, but the bulk of the clinical signs will likely be more related to the other components. For example, ingestion of Semtex will cause primarily signs related to the cyclonite component although monitoring of blood pressure as part of the treatment is prudent.

EGDN is the fourth nitrate ester used in explosives applications. The only commercial use is in the production of dynamite, most commonly as an EGDN/NG mixture. Ingestion of dynamite will most likely cause GI upset. With sufficient ingestions, there may be a potential for hypotension, depression, bradycardia and respiratory depression due to the combined effects of EGDN and NG.

Dogs ingesting dynamite may spontaneously decontaminate themselves by vomiting. For those who do not vomit spontaneously, induction of emesis is prudent. With larger ingestions, activated charcoal following emesis induction is reasonable, followed by monitoring of heart rate and blood pressure. Fluids will both help support the blood pressure, lessening the risk for hypotension.

Ammonium Nitrate and Fuel Oil (ANFO)

ANFO has largely replaced dynamite in many commercial mining operations. It also has many military applications. Many explosive slurries and gels are ANFO based. Technically ANFO is a blasting agent—a combination of an inorganic nitrate and a carbonaceous fuel. Adding an explosive ingredient such as TNT changes the classification to an explosive.

Ammonium nitrate when ingested will cause primarily GI signs. Vomiting and diarrhea are both common. Even with large ingestions, GI signs tend to predominate. Methemoglobinemia is rare with nitrate ingestion in dogs compared to the more sensitive ruminants.

Fuel oils used in ANFO are hydrocarbon-based petroleum distillates. Ingestion of petroleum distillates most commonly causes GI signs. When vomiting occurs, there is also the risk of aspiration. The risk for aspiration is related to the volatility of the particular petroleum distillate. The upright stance of humans puts them at higher risk for aspiration following ingestion of petroleum distillates compared to quadrupeds like dogs. While possible, ingestion of less volatile petroleum distillates by dogs does not commonly cause aspiration. Ingestion of petroleum distillates may also cause CNS signs including depression, ataxia, seizure, or coma. The mechanisms involved are not fully understood, but theories include hydrocarbons having direct CNS toxic effects.

Because of the explosive potential for ANFO, the individual components are not stored together. Therefore, dogs are more likely to ingest the individual components than ingesting the mixed ANFO products. Ingesting a mixture rather than single petroleum distillate will lower the risk for aspiration as solids are less likely to be aspirated than volatile liquids. Treatment is symptomatic and supportive. In most cases it is best to avoid inducing vomiting. However, if other, more toxic substances were ingested concurrently with ANFO, inducing vomiting should be considered.

Lead-Based Explosives

The lead-based explosives are primary explosives and include LA and LS. Neither of these is currently produced in the US because of toxic and environmental concerns. There are, however, still stockpiles of LA and LS left over from the Vietnam era and used by the military to make primers.[19] Though highly toxic due to their lead content, because LA and LS are both primary explosives, an animal attempting to ingest them is more likely to suffer extensive trauma from detonation than to safely ingest enough to cause lead toxicosis.

The toxic potential of lead is well known in small animal medicine. When ingested, lead affects the CNS and stability of the red blood cell membrane and causes neuronal damage, cerebral edema, demyelination, and decreased nerve conduction. Several veterinary toxicology books have excellent discussions on lead poisoning and its treatment. The readers are encouraged to seek advice from these articles if they suspect lead poisoning from ingestion of lead-based explosive.

FIREWORKS

Fireworks are low explosive pyrotechnic devices.[20] Fireworks are divided into 2 main classes: consumer and professional. Consumer fireworks can be purchased by the general public and include firecrackers, rockets, and smoke bombs. Professional (display) fireworks are restricted use and are paper or pasteboard tubing filled with combustible materials.[20] Fireworks contain multiple ingredients that produce either noise, light, smoke, or floating materials. These include fuel (usually black powder), oxidizers (nitrates, chlorates, or perchlorates), color-producing compounds, binders, and reducing agents (sulfur, charcoal).[20] Colors in fireworks are produced by a combination of different metals. The toxicity will vary depending on the compounds contained in the firework. Spent (used) fireworks can have a different composition from unused and the kinetics and toxicity can vary (increased or decreased).[21]

Laboratory testing is available for most components of fireworks. However, due to the time needed to get results, most lab tests are not clinically useful. Emesis may be induced if the animal is asymptomatic and only if noncorrosive agents were ingested. Milk or water can be used to dilute corrosive agents. A gastric lavage can be performed if a large amount of noncorrosive agents were ingested. If corrosive compounds have been ingested, gastroprotectants should be started (sucralfate, H2 blockers like famotidine, etc). The animal may need an esophagostomy or gastrostomy tube if severe oral or esophageal burns are evident. Silver sulfadiazine can be used topically for dermal burns. Activated charcoal does not bind to chlorates or heavy metals and should also not be used if corrosive agents were ingested.

The exact composition of the firework is often unknown, so treatment is tailored toward supportive care. Monitoring of renal and liver enzymes may be needed in affected animals for up to 72 hours post ingestion. Oxygen should be administered if the animal appears cyanotic. Intravenous fluids should be used to maintain normal blood pressure and urine production. Ingestion of wood, plastic, metal, or paper components can lead to foreign body obstruction or perforation of the digestive tract.

Aluminum

Aluminum salts are commonly used in sparklers because they produce silver and white flames and sparks.[20] Aluminum is poorly absorbed from the GI tract. Acute aluminum toxicity is unlikely in a healthy patient.[22]

Antimony

Antimony (antimony sulfide) is used to produce glitter effects. Antimony compounds are poorly absorbed from the GI tract, but they are locally corrosive.[23] Antimony toxicosis is very rare. Ingestion can cause oral ulcers, vomiting, and bloody diarrhea. GI protectants such as famotidine or sucralfate may help reduce GI irritation.

Barium

Barium salts (barium chloride, barium nitrate) are added to fireworks to produce green colors and to help stabilize other volatile elements.[20] The oral absorption of barium is dependent on the solubility of the particular barium salt but is generally rapid. Barium can cause severe hypokalemia by blocking the exit of potassium from skeletal muscle.[24] Barium stimulates skeletal, smooth, and cardiac muscle, causing vomiting, diarrhea, salivation, hypertension, and arrhythmias within hours after exposure.[24] Peak serum concentrations are reached usually within 2 hours.[25] Signs can progress to tremors, seizures, paralysis, mydriasis, tachypnea, respiratory failure, and cardiac shock.[24] If no signs develop within 6 to 8 hours of exposure, none will be expected. Barium is radiopaque, and magnesium sulfate can be used to precipitate barium in the GI tract and prevent further absorption.[24] Potassium chloride can be used to correct hypokalemia and related cardiac arrhythmias.[24] Monitor changes in other electrolytes and correct as needed.

Beryllium

Beryllium produces white sparks when used in fireworks. It is very poorly absorbed from the GI tract, but inhalation can be problematic.[26] Inhaled beryllium is cytotoxic to alveolar macrophages, causing cell death and interstitial fibrosis.[23] Pneumonitis, dyspnea, and pulmonary edema can develop, but exposure to beryllium through inhalation in dogs is very unlikely. Beryllium is also known to be carcinogenic. Oral exposure in dogs may result in self-limiting vomiting.

Calcium

The addition of calcium to fireworks can produce orange colors or can be added to deepen other colors.[20] Calcium salts are poorly absorbed from the GI tract. Most acute oral ingestions of calcium salts produce mild vomiting and diarrhea. Calcium chloride is corrosive and can cause GI hemorrhage. Hypercalcemia is not likely. Sodium chloride diuresis along with furosemide can be used to enhance calcium excretion.[27]

Cesium

Cesium (cesium nitrate) produces indigo colors in fireworks. The toxicity of cesium salts is rarely of importance.[28] The metal can cause dermal burns due to its reactivity with water and oxygen.

Chlorates

Chlorates are found in fireworks as a component of many oxidizers and are used to strengthen the color of the flame. Chlorates are locally irritating and can cause vomiting and diarrhea.[29,30] Orally, chlorates are well absorbed with slow excretion through the kidney (unchanged). Chlorates can cause damage to the proximal renal and renal vasoconstriction.[30] Chlorates are also potent oxidizing agents. The oxidation of red blood cells causes hemolysis and methemoglobinemia. Development of methemoglobinemia can be delayed for 1 to 10 hours post exposure. The oral LD_{50} in the dog is 1 g/kg.[29] Elevations in renal enzymes and hyperkalemia can also be seen.[21]

Gastric lavage with mineral oil has been suggested to prevent absorption of chlorates.[29] The mineral oil can be mixed with 1% sodium thiosulfate for increased efficacy. Methylene blue (1% injectable solution at 1 to 1.5 mg/kg IV, repeat once in 30 minutes if needed) can be used to convert chlorate-induced methemoglobin back to hemoglobin, although methylene blue is not readily available in most veterinary clinics.[29] If no methylene blue is available, *N*-acetylcysteine (140 mg/kg IV or PO then 70 mg/kg PO q8h for 5 to 7 treatments) and ascorbic acid can be tried (20 to 30 mg/kg IM q8h) in treating methemoglobinemia. Do not use ascorbic acid if aluminum has been ingested as it can enhance aluminum absorption and brain aluminum accumulation. Sodium thiosulfate can also be used to inactivate chlorate ions. On necropsy, chocolate-colored blood and tissues (methemoglobinemia), dark kidneys, and renal tubular necrosis are indicative of chlorate intoxication.[29]

Copper

Copper salts (copper chloride, copper halides) are used to produce blue colors in fireworks.[31] Copper salts are locally corrosive but have minimal absorption.[31] Absorbed copper can cause hemolysis. Metallic copper has little to no toxicity.

Iron

Iron provides gold sparks in fireworks.[20] Iron absorption is a regulated process and excess iron has a corrosive effect on the GI tract.[32] Vomiting, diarrhea, and severe GI irritation/ulcers can result. Excess absorbed iron causes free radical formation and lipid peroxidation. The liver is the most affected organ. Peak serum iron concentrations occur in 2 to 6 hours after ingestion. Large iron ingestion can cause CNS depression, acidosis, liver failure, and shock prior to death. Magnesium hydroxide will combine with iron to form FeOH, which is poorly absorbed. Deferoxamine is an iron chelator (ascorbic acid increases effectiveness), but it can potentially cause blindness and ototoxicity.[33] Care should be taken if giving deferoxamine to working or service dogs.

Lithium

Lithium carbonate can be used to add red coloration to the fireworks.[20] Soluble lithium salts are quickly absorbed from the GI tract. Lithium affects neuronal metabolism in the CNS, nerve excitation, and synaptic transmission.[34] Peak plasma levels are reached within 2 to 5 hours. Vomiting is common, and higher doses can cause tremors, ataxia, and seizures. Diuresis with 0.9% NaCl will increase excretion of lithium.

Magnesium

Adding magnesium to fireworks gives white sparks and improved brilliance. Magnesium absorption occurs in the small intestine. Magnesium salts stimulates GI motility and fluid secretions, leading to diarrhea. Large amounts of absorbed magnesium can cause neuromuscular blockade by inhibiting the release of acetylcholine, resulting in flaccid paralysis, hypotension, respiratory depression, and electrocardiographic changes (bradycardia, prolonged PR and QRS interval).[35] Elevations in renal enzymes can also be seen (rare). Intravenous calcium gluconate can reverse respiratory depression induced by hypermagnesemia.[36] Animals with ileus are more at risk for developing magnesium toxicosis.

Nitrates

Nitrates are oxidizing compounds found in fireworks.[20] Sodium nitrate can be added to make gold or yellow colors. Nitrates are converted in vivo to nitrites. Nitrites cause methemoglobinemia. Monogastric animals have limited ability to perform this action, so they usually do not develop methemoglobinemia with acute ingestions.[37]

Phosphorus

Phosphorus can be found in the fuel part of the firework or can be added for glow-in-the-dark effects. Phosphorus can be absorbed orally, dermally, or by inhalation. The white phosphorus found in fireworks can cause severe hemorrhagic gastroenteritis, abdominal pain, muscular weakness, and possible cardiovascular collapse.[38] When serum phosphorus levels rise, it binds with calcium (calcium phosphate), leading to hypocalcemia, which can be treated with intravenous calcium gluconate. Hepatic and renal injury can also be seen. N-Acetylcysteine can be used to protect against phosphorus-induced liver injury.[39] Phosphorus can also cause electrocardiographic changes (QRS or QT interval changes, ventricular arrhythmias). Decontamination with a copper sulfate (20 to 100 mL of 0.2% to 0.4% copper sulfate) or potassium permanganate (2 to 4 mL/kg, 1:10,000 solution) gastric lavage has been suggested to decrease absorption of phosphorus. Phosphorus absorption is enhanced when given with alcohols or fats, so do not dilute with milk. Treatment may include use of GI protectants (famotidine and carafate), intravenous fluids, and monitoring of hepatic and renal functions.

Potassium

Potassium (potassium nitrate, potassium perchlorate) plays many roles in fireworks. It provides a violet color and is part of the black powder explosive and oxidative mixture. Potassium is quickly absorbed from the proximal GI tract. Excess potassium causes depolarization of cardiac muscle and increases cardiac muscle excitability, leading to hypotension or hypertension, cardiac dysrhythmias (peaked T waves, small P waves, QRS widening becoming progressively prolonged), heart block, and cardiac arrest.[40] However, animals with normal renal function usually have minimal toxicity consisting of GI signs only. If the animal becomes symptomatic and shows evidence of hyperkalemia, the use of intravenous sodium bicarbonate will help the patient's hyperkalemia by shifting potassium intracellularly. Other measures to treat hyperkalemia can be used as needed (0.9% saline; 5% dextrose; insulin-dextrose combination etc).

Rubidium

Rubidium (rubidium nitrate) is used in fireworks for its violet color and as an oxidizer.[41] Rubidium is considered to be of low toxicity.

Strontium

Strontium (strontium carbonate) is added to fireworks for its brilliant red color and ability to stabilize firework mixtures.[42] It is commonly used because it is inexpensive. Acute ingestions are not expected to cause serious health problems. Signs of mild stomach upset can be seen in dogs.

Sulfur

Sulfur (sulfur dioxide) is found in black powder and reducing agents.[20] Vomiting and diarrhea are common following ingestion.[43] Sulfur can be converted to hydrogen sulfide in the colon by bacteria. Hydrogen sulfide can cause ataxia, arrhythmias, collapse, unconsciousness, pulmonary edema, and death, but these signs from sulfur ingestion are not expected.

Titanium

Titanium is added to fireworks to produce silver sparks. Titanium is biologically inert and practically nontoxic.[44] There is poor GI absorption and the unchanged metal is excreted in the feces.

Zinc

Zinc produces smoke effects in fireworks. Zinc salts are corrosive and produce vomiting, diarrhea, and GI ulcers.[45] Absorption of soluble zinc salts is highly variable. Zinc metal can be ionized in the stomach and absorbed. Once absorbed, zinc causes hemolytic anemia and secondary renal failure. Zinc may be chelated with calcium disodium EDTA, BAL, or D-penicillamine once it is no longer in the GI tract.[45] Most cases of zinc toxicosis do not require treatment with a chelating agent. Zinc toxicosis in dogs usually requires administration of intravenous fluids and monitoring for hemoglobinuria and renal functions.

SUMMARY

Exposure to explosives and fireworks in dogs can result in variable severity of clinical signs depending on presence of different chemicals and the amount. The risk can be lessened by proper education of dog handlers and owners about the seriousness of the intoxications. Most animals will recover within 24 to 72 hours with supportive care. Cyclonite, barium, and chlorate ingestion carries a risk of more severe clinical signs.

REFERENCES

1. Commerce in explosives; list of explosive materials. Fed Reg 2010;75:70291–3.
2. International Police Work Dog Association Explosives Detection Certification Rules, revised September 2010. Available at: www.ipwda.org/explosives.php. Accessed June 30, 2011.
3. Explosives: Nitroaromatics. GlobalSecurity.org Web site. www.globalsecurity.org/military/systems/munitions/explosives-nitroaromatics.htm. Accessed June 30, 2011.
4. Dilley JV, Tyson CA, Spanggord RJ, et al. Short-term oral toxicity of 2,4,6-trinitrotoluene in mice, rats, and dogs. J Toxicol Environ Health 1982;9:565–85.
5. Levine BS, Rust JH. Six month oral toxicity study of trinitrotoluene in beagle dogs. Toxicology 1990;63:233–44.
6. Wright RO, Magnani B, Shannon MW, et al. N-Acetylcysteine reduces methemoglobin in vitro. Ann Emerg Med 1996;28:499–503.
7. Tanen DA, LoVecchio F, Curry SC. Failure of intravenous N-acetylcysteine to reduce methemoglobin produced by sodium nitrite in human volunteers: a randomized controlled trial. Ann Emerg Med 2000;35:369–73.
8. Herman MI, Chyka PA, Butlse AY. Methylene blue by intraosseous infusion for methemoglobinemia. Ann Emerg Med 1999;33:111–3.
9. Explosives: Nitramines. GlobalSecurity.org Web site. Available at: www.globalsecurity.org/military/systems/munitions/explosives-nitramines.htm. Accessed June 30, 2011.
10. US Dept of Health and Human Services. Occupational Safety and Health Guideline for Cyclonite, 1995. Available at: www.cdc.gov/niosh/docs/81-123/pdfs/0169.pdf. Accessed June 30, 2011.
11. Bruchim Y, Saragusty J, Weisman A, et al. Cyclonite (RDX) intoxication in a police working dog. Vet Rec 2005;157:354–6.
12. Fishkin RA, Stanley SW, Langston CE. Toxic effects of cyclonite (C-4) plastic explosive ingestion in a dog. J Vet Emerg Crit Care 2008;18:537–40.

13. Faust RA. Toxicity summary for hexahydro-1,3,5-trinitro-1,3,5-triazine (RDX). Oak Ridge (TN): Oak Ridge National Laboratory; 1994.

14. Bingham E, Cohrssen B, Powell CH. Patty's toxicology, vols. 1–9. 5th edition. New York: John Wiley & Sons; 2001. p. 616.

15. De Cramer KG, Short RP. Plastic explosive poisoning in dogs. J S Afr Vet Assoc 1992;63:30–1.

16. Burdette LJ, Cook LL, Dyer RS. Convulsant properties of cyclotrimethylenetrinitramine (RDX): spontaneous audiogenic and amygdaloid kindled seizure activity. Toxicol Appl Pharmacol 1988;93:436–44.

17. Ellis HV 3rd, Hong CB, Lee CC, et al. Subacute and chronic toxicity studies of trinitroglycerin in dogs, rats, and mice. Fundam Appl Toxicol 1984;4(Pt 1):248–60.

18. von Oettingen WF, Donahue DD. Acute toxic manifestations of PETN. US Public Health Bull 1944;282:23–30.

19. Oyler KD, Cheng G, Mehta N, et al. Green explosives: potential replacements for lead azide and other toxic detonator and primer constituents, 27th Army Science Conference proceedings. Available at: www.armyscienceconference.com. Accessed June 30, 2011.

20. Gondhia R. The chemistry of fireworks. Available at: www.ch.ic.ac.uk/local/projects/gondhia/composition.html. Accessed June 30, 2011.

21. Wismer TA. Matches and fireworks. In: Osweiler GD, Hovda LR, Brutlag AG, et al, editors. Blackwell's Five-minute veterinary consult clinical companion small animal toxicology. Ames (IA): Wiley-Blackwell; 2011. p. 568–73.

22. Henry DA, Goodman WG, Nudelman RK. Parenteral aluminum administration in the dog: I. Plasma kinetics, tissue levels, calcium metabolism, and parathyroid hormone. Kidney Int 1984;25:362–9.

23. Gwaltney-Brant SM. Heavy metals. In: Haschek WM, Rousseaux CG, Wallig MA, editors. Handbook of toxicologic pathology. 2nd edition. San Diego (CA): Academic Press; 2002. p. 701–33.

24. Roza O, Berman LB. The pathophysiology of barium: hypokalemic and cardiovascular effects. J Pharmacol Exp Ther 1971;177:433–9.

25. Johnson CH, VanTassell VJ. Acute barium poisoning with respiratory failure and rhabdomyolysis. Ann Emerg Med 1991;20:1138–42.

26. Hathaway GJ, Proctor NH, Hughes JP. Proctor and Hughes' Chemical hazards of the workplace. 4th edition. New York: Van Nostrand Reinhold Company; 1996. p. 77–8.

27. Suki WN, Yium JJ, Von Minden M. Acute treatment of hypercalcemia with furosemide. N Engl J Med 1970;283:836–40.

28. ATSDR (Agency for Toxic Substances & Disease Registry). Cesium. Available at: www.atsdr.cdc.gov/ToxProfiles/TP.asp?id=578&tid=107. Accessed June 30, 2011.

29. Sheahan BJ, Pugh DM, Winstanley EW. Experimental sodium chlorate poisoning in dogs. Res Vet Sci 1971;12:387–9.

30. Lee DBN, Brown DL, Baker LRI. Haematological complications of chlorate poisoning. Br Med J 1970;2:31–2.

31. Thompson LJ. Copper. In: Gupta RC, editor. Veterinary toxicology. New York: Elsevier; 2007. p. 427–9.

32. Hooser SB. Iron. In: Gupta RC, editor. Veterinary toxicology. New York: Elsevier; 2007. p. 433–7.

33. Chen SH, Liang DC, Lin HC, et al. Auditory and visual toxicity during deferoxamine therapy in transfusion-dependent patients. J Pediatr Hematol Oncol 2005;27:651–3.

34. Brent J, Klein LJ. Lithium. In: Brent J, Wallace KL, Burkhart KK, et al, editors. Critical care toxicology: diagnosis and management of the critically poisoned patient. Philadelphia: Elsevier Mosby; 2005. p. 523–32.

35. Cumpston KL, Erickson TB, Leikin JB. Poisoning in pregnancy. In: Brent J, Wallace KL, Burkhart KK, et al, editors. Critical care toxicology: diagnosis and management of the critically poisoned patient. Philadelphia: Elsevier Mosby; 2005. p. 134.

36. Brühwiler H, Häfliger M, Lüscher KP. Severe accidental magnesium poisoning in a twins pregnancy in the 32nd week of pregnancy. Geburtshilfe Frauenheilkd 1994;54: 184–6.

37. Casteel SW, Evans TJ. Nitrate. In: Plumlee KH, editor. Clinical veterinary toxicology. St Louis (MO): Mosby; 2004. p. 127–30.

38. Thompson LJ. Phosphorus. In: Gupta RC, editor. Veterinary toxicology. New York: Elsevier; 2007. p. 473–4.

39. Panganiban LR. Value of N-acetylcysteine in the management of "Watusi"-induced hepatotoxicity [abstract 127]. Vet Hum Toxicol 1993;35:348.

40. Mattu A, Brady WJ, Robinson DA. Electrocardiographic manifestations of hyperkalemia. Am J Emerg Med 2000;18:721–9.

41. Lenk W, Prinz H, Steinmetz A. Rubidium and rubidium compounds. In: Ullmann's Encyclopedia of industrial chemistry. Weinheim: Wiley-VCH Verlag GmbH & Co; 2010. Available at: http://onlinelibrary.wiley.com/doi/10.1002/14356007.a23_473. pub2/full. Accessed June 30, 2011.

42. Patnaik P. Handbook of inorganic chemicals. New York: McGraw-Hill; 2002. p. 884.

43. Hall JO. Sulfur. In: Gupta RC, editor. Veterinary toxicology. New York: Elsevier; 2007. p. 465–9.

44. Goyer RA, Clarkson TW. Toxic effects of metals. In: Klaassen CD, editor. Casarett & Doull's toxicology: the basic science of poisons. 6th edition. New York: McGraw-Hill; 2001. p. 857.

45. Garland T. Zinc. In: Gupta RC, editor. Veterinary toxicology. New York: Elsevier; 2007. p. 470–2.

Mushroom Poisoning Cases in Dogs and Cats: Diagnosis and Treatment of Hepatotoxic, Neurotoxic, Gastroenterotoxic, Nephrotoxic, and Muscarinic Mushrooms

Birgit Puschner, DVM, PhD[a],*, Colette Wegenast, DVM[b]

KEYWORDS

- Amanita • Amanitins • Hepatotoxic mushrooms
- Gastrointestinal irritation • Liver failure • Neurotoxicosis
- Toxicosis

There is no simple test that distinguishes poisonous from nonpoisonous mushrooms, and accurate mushroom identification will require consultation with an experienced mycologist. Although it is estimated that only a few species are lethal, it is not clear how many of the mushrooms worldwide contain potentially toxic compounds. New species are being discovered continuously, and for many species, toxicity data are unavailable. In the United States, mushroom poisonings of humans and animals continue to be a medical emergency and demand extensive efforts from clinicians and toxicologists. It is challenging to establish a confirmed diagnosis of mushroom poisoning in animals because of limited diagnostic assays for toxin detection. Currently, only the detection of amanitins, psilocin, and psilocybin is available at select veterinary toxicology laboratories. Thus, only limited data on confirmed mushroom poisonings in animals exist. Because the risk of animals to ingest toxic mushrooms, particularly in dogs due to their indiscriminant eating habits, is much

---

The authors have nothing to disclose.
[a] Department of Molecular Biosciences, School of Veterinary Medicine, University of California, 1120 Haring Hall, Davis, CA 95616, USA
[b] Animal Poison Control Center, American Society for the Prevention of Cruelty to Animals (ASPCA), ASPCA Midwest Office, 1717 South Philo Road, Suite 36, Urbana, IL 61802, USA
* Corresponding author.
E-mail address: bpuschner@ucdavis.edu

Vet Clin Small Anim 42 (2012) 375–387
doi:10.1016/j.cvsm.2011.12.002
0195-5616/12/$ – see front matter © 2012 Elsevier Inc. All rights reserved.

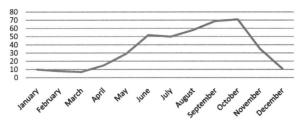

Fig. 1. ASPCA APCC average number of reported mushroom exposure cases by month (January 1, 2006–January 1, 2011).

greater than the risk for humans, mushroom poisoning in animals is likely underreported.

Human and animal mushroom poisoning cases can be reported to the North American Mycological Association's Mushroom Poisoning Case Registry. Reports may be submitted online at www.sph.umich.edu/~kwcee/mpcr. In addition, the website provides a list of volunteers willing to assist in the identification of mushrooms. The volunteers are listed by region. Alternatively, many universities have lists of mycologists available for assistance.

INCIDENCES

The ASPCA Animal Poison Control Center (APCC) received 2090 incident reports of potential mushroom exposures in animals between January 1, 2006, and December 31, 2010. A majority of these exposures were reported in dogs. These cases on average involved 433 canine and 6 feline exposures per year (some incidents involved multiple animals). During this period, there were also reports of mushroom exposure in 7 caprine, 2 mustelid, 1 avian, 1 lagomorph, and 1 marsupial case. The fall months (September and October) had the highest number of cases reported to the APCC (**Fig. 1**). Regionally, in the continental United States, the Northeast region had the largest annual average number of reported potential exposures (**Fig. 2**). In the majority (94.6%) of the reported exposures, the type of mushroom ingested was unknown at the time of the original call to the APCC; thus, the agent was classified as "unknown mushroom." These data reflect overall trends, but due to reporting and identification constraints, they are not representative of confirmed exposures/diagnoses of mushroom poisonings. Improved identifications and reporting in small animals may increase the accuracy of incidence data in the future.

HEPATOTOXIC MUSHROOMS

The majority of confirmed mushroom poisoning cases reported in animals are caused by hepatotoxic mushrooms that contain cyclopeptides. While a number of mushroom genera (*Amanita, Galerina, Lepiota, Cortinarius, Conocybe* spp) contain the hepatotoxic cyclopeptides,[1] *Amanita phalloides* is considered most toxic worldwide. *A phalloides*, also known as Death Cap (**Fig. 3**), is found throughout North America with 2 distinct ranges: one on the West Coast from California to British Columbia and one on the East Coast from Maryland to Maine.[2] The mushroom grows commonly in association with oaks, birch, and pine and is the species most frequently resulting in fatalities in humans[3] and probably also in dogs. *A phalloides* is particularly common in the San Francisco Bay area and is most abundant in warm, wet years. The large fruiting bodies appear in the late summer and fall and have a smooth, yellowish-green

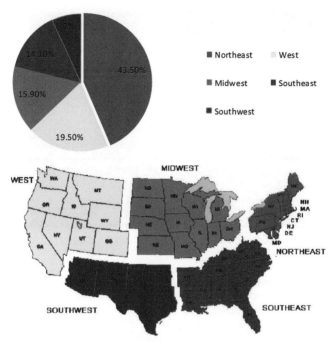

Fig. 2. ASPCA APCC average annual number of reported mushroom exposures by region (January 1, 2006–January 1, 2011).

to yellowish-brown cap, white gills, a white ring around the upper part of the stem (veil), and a white cup-like structure around the base of the stem (volva). *A ocreata*, also referred to as the Western North American destroying angel (**Fig. 4**), grows exclusively along the Pacific Coast from Baja California to Washington and is commonly found in sandy soils under oak or pine. *A ocreata* occurs commonly in

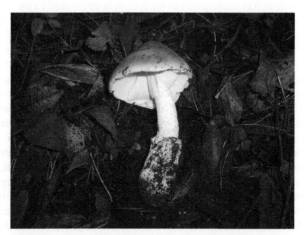

Fig. 3. *Amanita phalloides.* (*Courtesy of* Dr R. Michael Davis, UC Davis.)

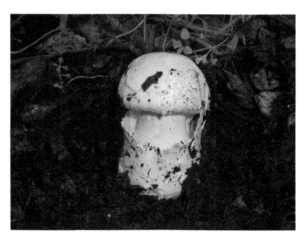

Fig. 4. *Amanita ocreata.* (*Courtesy of* Dr R. Michael Davis, UC Davis.)

California. The fruiting bodies are usually found in later winter and spring and have a white or cream-colored cap, white, short gills, a white stem with a white, thin, broken, partial veil, and a white, thin volva.

These toxic species contain a number of different toxins, most notably the amatoxins, which include the hepatotoxic amanitins responsible for most poisonings and fatalities. In humans, the estimated oral LD_{50} of α-amanitin is 0.1 mg/kg body weight, which is similar to an oral LD_{50} for methyl-γ-amanitin in dogs of 0.5 mg/kg body weight.[4] On average, species of *A phalloides* and *A ocreata* contain 1.5 to 2.3 mg amanitins per gram of mushroom dry weight.[5] Therefore, one mushroom cap can contain a lethal dose for an animal or a human.

Amanitins inhibit RNA polymerase II, which shuts down transcription and leads to decreased protein synthesis.[6] Cells with a high metabolic rate, including hepatocytes, crypt cells, and proximal convoluted tubules of the kidneys, are most prone to the toxic effects. Apoptosis of hepatocytes[7] and amanitin-induced insulin release[8] are additional effects that contribute to the pathogenesis.

Differences in bioavailability account for differences in species sensitivities. The rate of gastrointestinal (GI) absorption of amanitins is estimated to be much greater in dogs than in mice and rabbits; rats appear relatively resistant to the toxic effects of amanitins. Once absorbed, α-amanitin is taken up by hepatocytes via OATP1B3, an organic anion-transporting polypeptide.[9] Amanitins do not undergo metabolism and are primarily excreted unchanged in urine with a small amount (up to 7%) eliminated in bile. Amanitins are detectable in serum and urine well before any clinical sign of poisoning, whereas routine laboratory tests such as complete blood count and serum chemistry profiles are unremarkable until liver or kidney damage has occurred. In humans with *A phalloides* exposure, α- and β-amanitins are present in plasma for up to 36 hours and in urine for up to 72 hours post exposure.[10] The plasma half-life of amanitins in dogs is short ranging from 25 to 50 minutes. Plasma and urine amanitin concentrations do not seem to correlate with the clinical severity or outcome.

Amanitin poisoning is clinically divided into 4 phases, although not all cases present with those 4 consecutive stages. The initial phase is a latency period of approximately 6 to 12 hours, during which no clinical signs of illness occur after the ingestion. During the second phase, poisoned animals develop GI signs (vomiting, diarrhea, evidence of abdominal pain, lethargy, anorexia) between 6 and 24 hours after ingestion. After a period of "false recovery" of 12 to 24 hours, which signifies the third phase of poisoning, fulminant liver failure develops. During this third phase, close monitoring of liver and kidney function is essential in order to prevent misdiagnosis. After the GI phase, severe hypoglycemia as a result of breakdown of liver glycogen can occur.[11] Fifty percent of dogs given lethal doses of amanitins or pieces of A phalloides died from hypoglycemia 1 to 2 days after exposure.[4] The fourth and final phase begins 36 to 48 hours after exposure and is characterized by fulminant hepatic failure with subsequent coagulation disorders, encephalopathy, and renal failure. Significant elevations in serum of aspartate aminotransferase (AST), alanine aminotransferase (ALT), alkaline phosphatase, and bilirubin are commonly observed.[12] Puppies, or dogs that ingest large amounts of amanitins, can die of amanitin poisoning rapidly, within 24 hours.[13]

A tentative diagnosis of hepatotoxic mushroom toxicity can be made based on history of exposure (witness or suspected exposure), a latency period of 6 to 12 hours before clinical signs are seen and the types of clinical signs present. Confirmatory diagnosis is made by detection of α-amanitin in serum, urine, gastric contents, suspect mushroom, liver, or kidney.[14] This testing is provided by select veterinary toxicology laboratories. The well-known Meixner test (also known as the newspaper test of Wieland) should not be relied on alone for amanitin identification.[15] Rapid confirmation of amanitins in suspect exposures assists in the early recognition of exposure and timely therapeutic intervention, while a negative result can prevent unnecessary hospitalization. Serum and urine samples should be collected and frozen at various time points beginning as early after exposure as possible. Amanitin has been detected in livers and kidneys of dogs dying from amanitin poisoning. In humans, amanitin concentrations have been detected in liver and kidney up to 22 days post ingestion and at later time points. Kidneys appear to contain higher concentrations than liver. At necropsy, the liver is often swollen, without any other significant gross abnormalities. Histopathologically, the liver shows massive hepatocellular necrosis with collapse of hepatic cords[11] and acute tubular necrosis in dogs that developed renal failure.

There is no specific antidote to treat amanitin intoxication. Despite the evaluation of numerous treatment options, no specific therapy has proved to be effective and the mortality rate in dogs is high. The key elements of treatment are close monitoring, fluid replacement, and supportive care. Activated charcoal at 1 to 2 g/kg PO with or without a cathartic like sorbitol (do not use a cathartic if diarrhea is present) followed by 2 or 3 half-doses within 24 hours of exposure is recommended. In the past, multidose activated charcoal was recommended. However, recent data indicate that interruption of the enterohepatic circulation of amanitin is unlikely to be effective after 24 hours.[16] Dextrose, vitamin K_1, blood products, and intravenous fluids must be considered as beneficial therapeutic agents for case management. In Europe, a silibinin-containing product (Legalon-Sil; Madaus Inc, Cologne, Germany) is a well-established and approved treatment for amanitin poisonings in humans.[17] Silibinin, or silybin, the main component of silymarin, which is extracted from the common milk thistle, Silybum marianum, reduces the uptake of amanitins into hepatocytes.[18] In dogs, 50 mg/kg of silibinin IV given at 5 and 24 hours after exposure to A phalloides was shown to be effective.[19] Other options may include use of nonspecific hepatoprotective agents like N-acetylcysteine (Mucomyst; Bristol-Myers Squibb Company, New York, NY, USA) or S-adenosylmethionine (SAMe), although their efficacy remains undetermined. Penicillin G at 1000 mg/kg IV given at 5 hours after dogs were exposed to A phalloides was also effective in reducing amanitin uptake into the hepatocytes. However, the efficacy of penicillin G in humans with amanitin poisoning is questionable. Manage vomiting as needed with metoclopramide (0.2 to 0.4 mg/kg subcutaneously or intramuscularly every 6 hours or maropitant 1 mg/kg subcutaneously once a day).

NEUROTOXIC MUSHROOMS
Hydrazines

Hydrazines are toxins in false morels, *Gyromitra* spp, which are found throughout the North America, especially under conifers and aspens. Gyromitrin, the toxin, is estimated to be present at 0.12% to 0.16% in fresh *G esculenta*. While the estimated lethal dose of gyromitrin in humans is 20 to 50 mg/kg for adults and 10 to 30 mg/kg for children,[20] such data are unavailable for dogs or cats. But gyromitrin poisoning is rarely reported in veterinary medicine; only one case report, in a 10-week-old dog, exists.[21] The dog vomited 2 to 3 hours after chewing on a mushroom later identified as *G esculenta,* became lethargic and comatose 6 hours post-ingestion, and died 30 minutes later. Gyromitrin is a direct irritant resulting in vomiting and diarrhea within 6 to 12 hours after exposure. The toxin is hydrolyzed in the stomach to monomethyl-hydrazine, which depletes pyridoxal 5-phosphate, ultimately resulting in decreased γ-aminobutyric acid (GABA) concentrations and increased glutamic acid concentrations.[22] Clinically, seizures can develop. Additional metabolites of gyromitrin can also result in hemolysis and liver and kidney failure. Diagnosis of gyromitrin poisoning is primarily based on the identification of the mushroom as detection of gyromitrin is not routinely available. Treatment of gyromitrin poisoning is mainly supportive, including correction of fluid and electrolyte imbalances. Pyridoxine can be given intravenously to dogs at 75 to 150 mg/kg body weight during acute phases of seizure activity.[23] Diazepam can also be considered for seizure control at 0.5 to 1.0 mg/kg IV to effect.

Isoxazoles

Ibotenic acid and muscimol are chemically classified as isoxazoles, which are most commonly associated with exposures to *Amanita pantherina* (panther cap, panther agaric) and *Amanita muscaria* (fly agaric). These mushrooms are found throughout the United States but are most abundant in the Pacific Northwest in the summer and fall, where they are often found in coniferous and deciduous forests. Clinical signs of poisoning in humans are seen with exposures greater than 6 mg of muscimol or 30 to 60 mg of ibotenic acid.[24] The concentration of ibotenic acid in *A muscaria* is estimated to be at 100 mg/kg fresh, while the concentration of muscimol is less than 3 mg/kg fresh weight. Therefore, an average-size, 60- to 70-g fruiting body of *A muscaria* can contain a toxic concentration of isoxazoles. While the toxicity of isoxazoles is not well documented in dogs, postmortem examination of puppies indicated that the ingestion of a single *A pantherina* can be lethal.[25] Although both muscimol and ibotenic acid are present in the mushrooms, muscimol is further derived from ibotenic acid by spontaneous decarboxylation, which can occur during drying of the mushroom, during digestion in the stomach, or after absorption in a variety of tissues. Therefore, muscimol is considered the major toxin responsible for causing clinical signs of toxicosis. Muscimol increases the membrane permeability for anions resulting in a slight, short-lasting hyperpolarization and associated decreased excitability of the receptive neuron. Muscimol also acts on GABA$_A$ receptors and has a depressant action.[26] Neurologic signs in animals include disorientation, opisthoto-nus, paresis, seizures, paddling, chewing movements, miosis, vestibular signs (ataxia, head tilt, nystagmus, circling, etc), respiratory depression, and, in severe cases, coma. In humans, muscimol intoxication is referred to as the "pantherine-muscaria" syndrome, which is characterized by mydriasis, dryness of the mouth, ataxia, confusion, euphoria, dizziness, and tiredness within ½ to 2 hours of ingestion, followed by full recovery within 1 to 2 days. Similar clinical signs have been described in cats,[27] while favorable[28] and lethal outcomes have been described in dogs with isoxazole exposure.[25,29] Diagnosis of isoxazole poisoning is primarily based on the history of exposure to a mushroom, quick onset of clinical signs (within hours of exposure), the type of clinical signs (hallucinations and other central nervous system [CNS] effects), and identification of the mushroom. While muscimol and ibotenic acid are excreted in urine shortly after exposure, routine diagnostic tests are not available. Treatment of isoxazole poisoning is mainly supportive, with special focus on seizure control. Early decontamination (induction of emesis and administration of activated charcoal) can be tried in asymptomatic animals. Because of the GABAergic effects of muscimol and ibotenic acid, medications with GABA agonist effects such as diazepam or phenobarbital should be used with caution. The use of these medications in a poisoned animal to control seizuresmay further aggravates CNS and respiratory depression. Thus, if such drugs are used, the animal's respiration should be carefully monitored for need of mechanical ventilation.

Psilocin and Psilocybin

Mushrooms in the genera *Psilocybe*, *Panaeolus*, *Conocybe*, and *Gymnopilus* contain primarily psilocybin, with some also containing psilocin. These mushrooms grow predominantly in fields and animal pastures in the Northwestern and Southeastern United States. The toxin concentrations in these mushrooms are affected by location, growing conditions, storage conditions, and species. Species common to the Pacific Northwest contain between 1.2 and 16.8 mg/kg psilocybin on a dry weight basis.[30] Oral doses of 10 to 20 mg of psilocybin result in hallucinations in people. Toxicity data for domestic animals do not exist. Psilocin is pharmacologically the most active metabolite of psilocybin after dephosphorylation in plasma, liver, and kidney.[31] Psilocin is structurally similar to serotonin and activates some serotonin receptors in the CNS,[32] leading to lysergic acid diethylamine (LSD)-like clinical effects. In the United States, United Kingdom, and Germany, psilocybin and psilocin are classified as controlled substances, and mushrooms containing those substances are called magic or hallucinogenic mushrooms. People consuming those mushrooms generally have hallucinations for approximately 1 hour, and have full recovery within 12 hours. In dogs, exposure to psilocybin containing mushrooms can result in aggression, ataxia, vocalization, nystagmus, seizures, and increased body temperature.[33] Exposure can be confirmed by detection of psilocin and psilocybin in urine by select veterinary diagnostic laboratories. Because of the short-lasting effects, mild cases may resolve themselves without treatment. Symptomatic and supportive treatment may be necessary when severe clinical signs are present. Seizures can be controlled with diazepam or phenobarbital.

MUSCARINE-CONTAINING MUSHROOMS

The most common muscarine-containing mushrooms include *Inocybe* spp and *Clitocybe* spp. The largest numbers of mushroom species that contain significant amounts of muscarine belong in these 2 genera.[34] These mushrooms are often described as nondescript little brown mushrooms, although some may be other colors such as white or cream.[34] They can be found in forests, lawns, and parks. These mushrooms most commonly fruit in summer and fall, although some fruit year round.[34] Several other genera such as *Mycena*, *Boletus*, *Entoloma*, and *Omphalotus* are suspected to contain significant muscarine levels.[34–36] Muscarine is also present in low concentrations in other mushrooms such as *Amanita muscaria*.[34]

Muscarine is a thermostable muscarinic receptor agonist that binds to acetylcholine receptors in the peripheral nervous system.[34] Stimulation of postganglionic neurons results in parasympathomimetic effects. Unlike acetylcholine, it is not degraded by acetylcholinesterase and toxicity results from unregulated stimulation at the receptors.[34,37] Organophosphates and carbamates can produce similar muscarinic signs; however, they act by binding acetylcholinesterase, which increases the amount of acetylcholine at the receptors. There may also be muscarinic compounds that produce a histaminic effect resulting in flushing, hypotension, and wheezing.[36]

Clinical signs can occur rapidly (often within 5 to 30 minutes) and mostly within 2 hours of ingestion.[34,36,37] Signs may include **s**alivation, **l**acrimation, **u**rination, **d**iarrhea, **d**yspnea, and **e**mesis (often described by the acronym SLUDDE). Dyspnea may develop in response to increased bronchial secretions and bronchoconstriction. Bradycardia, miosis, hypotension, and abdominal pain are also possible. In the author's experience, dogs suspected of ingesting muscarinic mushrooms often present with a history of acute onset of vomiting, severe diarrhea, and ptyalism. The saliva may be described as thick and ropey. Differential diagnoses include exposure to pesticides such as organophosphates, and carbamates and mycotoxins like slaframine. Exposure to cholinesterase-inhibiting pesticides such as organophosphates and carbamates may also result in nicotinic signs such as tremors, muscle weakness, and seizures. Unlike these pesticides, muscarine does not stimulate nicotinic receptors or cross the blood-brain barrier.[34,36,37] Consequently, nicotinic and direct CNS effects are not expected. Depression may develop as a result of hypotension or hypoxia.[34]

Diagnosis is based on rapid onset of clinical signs, the type of clinical signs (SLUDDE), and response to treatment. Muscarine has been detected in urine and analysis could be considered for confirmation of exposure.[36] Identification of the mushrooms from the environment and/or vomitus may also be used to support the diagnosis.

Decontamination includes induction of emesis and administration of activated charcoal in asymptomatic animals following ingestion of mushrooms. The rapid onset of signs (which may include vomiting) following muscarinic mushroom ingestion often makes decontamination unfeasible. Atropine competes with muscarine at the receptors and is the recommended treatment. In dogs and cats, the beginning dosage is 0.04 mg/kg with one fourth of the dose given intravenously and the remainder given subcutaneously or intramuscularly (American Society for the Prevention of Cruelty to Animals, Animal Poison Control Center, Antox™, unpublished data, 2011). The dosage can be titrated up and repeated if needed to control severe signs. Overatropinization should be avoided and can result in anticholinergic signs, including tachycardia, hyperthermia, behavior changes, and GI stasis. Signs typically respond well to atropine and resolve within 30 minutes of administration. Without treatment, signs may persist for several hours. Supportive care (intravenous fluids) should be provided as needed. The prognosis, in most cases, is good and long-term effects are not expected.

MUSHROOMS RESULTING IN GASTROINTESTINAL IRRITATION

Mushrooms that result in primarily GI signs are grouped under this category. Specific genera include *Agaricus*, *Boletus*, *Chlorophyllum*, *Entoloma*, *Gomphus*, *Hebeloma*, *Lactarius*, *Naematoloma*, *Omphalotus*, *Ramaria*, *Rhodophyllus*, *Russula*, *Scleroderma*,

Tricholoma, and others. These mushrooms have a wide distribution and variation in appearance and substrate.

The toxins in most species have not been identified. Illuden S is thought to be a toxic component in some *Omphalotus* and *Lampteromyces* species.[38] Illudens can be cytotoxic and have produced hemorrhagic lesions in animal studies.[36,38] *Omphalotus illudens* also produces a muscarine-like effect although muscarine has not been isolated from this mushroom.[39] Suspected toxins in other species include Monoterpenes, norcaperatic acid, hebeleomic acid A, cucurbitane trierpene glycosides, lectins, marasmane/lactarane sesquiterpenes, and phenolethylamines. Proposed mechanisms include hypersensitivity, idiosyncratic reactions, some enzyme deficiencies, and local GI irritation.[40] Some of the mushrooms in this category are considered edible, although even the edible species can result in GI signs in sensitive individuals. Some of the toxins may be inactivated by cooking.

The onset of clinical signs is fairly fast and signs are expected within 15 minutes to several hours after ingestion. Vomiting, diarrhea, and abdominal discomfort are common signs. Other signs may include lethargy, hypersalivation, hematemesis, and hematochezia. Secondary electrolyte abnormalities and hypovolemia may develop. A 1-year-old cat ingested one-half of an *Agaricus* spp cap and developed foaming, vomiting, diarrhea, and disorientation. Hematemesis developed in another cat that ingested an unknown species of *Russula*. The mushroom was described as having a shellfish odor, which may have attracted the cat.[40] There is also a report of a 7-month-old pot bellied pig that developed vomiting, weakness, hypothermia, abdominal pain, tachycardia, and tachypnea within 1 hour of ingestion of *Scleroderma citrinum*. The pig died within 5 hours despite treatment with fluids and dexamethasone.[40] Differential diagnoses for GI irritant mushrooms include many other causes of acute gastroenteritis such as dietary indiscretion, garbage poisoning, foreign body ingestion, pancreatitis, bacterial or viral gastroenteritis, ingestion of corrosive or irritating agents, and ingestion of GI irritant plants.

Diagnosis is supported by the history, clinical signs, and evidence of mushrooms in the vomitus. The mushrooms should be saved for identification. It is important to note that GI upset is also an initial sign following ingestion of more dangerous hepatotoxic and nephrotoxic mushrooms, although the onset is typically more delayed. A complete blood count, chemistry panel, and radiographs may be performed to assess the clinical picture and help rule out other causes for the signs. In severe cases, electrolyte and acid-base status should be monitored and corrected as needed.

Decontamination includes emesis and activated charcoal in asymptomatic animals following ingestion of mushrooms. The potential rapid onset of vomiting may make decontamination following ingestion of GI irritant mushrooms less feasible. Treatment is symptomatic and supportive and depends on the extent of signs. Intravenous fluids are recommended to maintain hydration. Sucralfate, H2 blockers (famotidine), and/or proton pump inhibitors (omeprazole) may be used to reduce mucosal irritation. Vomiting should be controlled with antiemetics such as maropitant and metoclopramide. Many cases are self-limiting and resolve without treatment. The severity of signs depends on the type of mushroom, amount ingested, and individual sensitivity. In most cases, the prognosis is good and full recovery is expected within a few hours to days.

NEPHROTOXIC MUSHROOMS

Some species of mushrooms in the genus *Cortinarius* are nephrotoxic. These mushrooms were first noted to be toxic in Poland in the 1950s.[34,36,41] Although they are found throughout Europe and North America, reports of toxicity have been rare in North America. There is a report of a woman who developed renal failure after ingesting *Cortinarius orellanosus* mushrooms from under an oak tree in Michigan.[42] To the author's knowledge, there have been no confirmed cases of accidental animal poisoning resulting from nephrotoxic mushrooms in North America.

The mushrooms are often a rusty or reddish brown color.[36] Webcap is a common name used for some of these nephrotoxic mushrooms due to the presence of a cortina or spider-web like veil that connects the edge of the cap to the stem in the immature stages. The cortina is not recognizable in adult mushrooms.[35,36] *Cortinarius* sp grows in forests and mountains and is rare in urban areas.[34] These mushrooms most commonly fruit between August and October.[43]

The bipyridyl toxin orellanine is thought to be the main toxin in *Cortinarius* sp mushrooms. Orelline and orellinine are 2 thermal and photo degradation products that have been identified. These toxins are thought to inhibit protein synthesis in renal tubular epithelium. Another theory is that the toxins reduce cellular NADPH, which results in free radical damage, lipid peroxidation, and membrane destruction.[34] There is a lag time between ingestion and development of signs, which suggests metabolism to an active form of the toxin.[34] Another toxin, a cyclopeptide named cortinarin has been isolated from some species. Cortinarins A, B, and C have been described. In the liver, cortinarin A is thought to be metabolized to cortinarin B, which is then converted to its sulfoxide form via cytochrome P450 enzymes. Cortinarins A and B sulfoxide are nephrotoxic. Females seem to be more resistant to the toxin than males. This may be due to differing binding capacities in the cytochrome P450 system.[34] There is still some controversy over the toxins present in *Cortinarius* sp and their relationship to each other and the nephrotoxicity associated with these mushrooms. Toxicity is not affected by cooking, canning, or drying of the mushrooms.[34] Interestingly, experimentation in rats has shown significant individual variation in susceptibility. In one study, 20% to 30% of rats were resistant to toxicity even at high dosages.[44]

There is a latent phase between ingestion and onset of signs. GI signs may occur within 72 hours. Within 3 to 20 days, signs of renal failure may develop. In humans, increased thirst, flank pain, chills, and night sweats have been described. Oliguria followed by diuresis and recovery or chronic renal failure may occur.[36] *Cortinarius orellanus* resulted in signs similar to those noted in humans when given orally to the cat, guinea pig, and mouse experimentally. The main damage was to the renal tubular epithelium.[40] In animals, vomiting, diarrhea, polyuria, polydipsia, abdominal pain, and depression may be noted. Differential diagnoses include other causes for GI upset and acute renal failure such as grape or raisin ingestion, NSAIDs, ethylene glycol, lily ingestion (cats), and leptospirosis.

Diagnostic tests to monitor renal values and a complete clinical assessment include a complete blood count and serum chemistry. In addition, urinalysis may reveal isosthenuria, glucosuria, pyuria, proteinuria, cylinduria, and hematuria. Acid-base status and electrolytes should also be monitored. Liver enzymes are expected to remain normal.[36] Orellanine can be detected in the urine within 24 hours of the exposure. Unfortunately, due to the lag time between ingestion and onset of signs, this may not be clinically useful.[34] The clinical signs and laboratory findings are not specific for *Cortinarius* sp ingestion. Due to the rarity of animal poisoning in North America, diagnosis should be made based on the history, mushroom identification if possible, and ruling out more likely causes of renal failure/damage. Renal biopsy may also be useful. In humans, renal biopsies have revealed interstitial edema, interstitial nephritis, and acute tubular necrosis.[42] Thin-layer chromatography has detected orellanine in renal biopsy samples up to 6 months post ingestion. Orellanine has also been measured in human plasma.[36]

Decontamination includes emesis and activated charcoal in asymptomatic animals following ingestion of mushrooms. However, due to the long latent period, patients may not be presented until days after the exposure and the opportunity for decontamination is missed. Treatment consists of supportive care for renal failure and GI signs. Intravenous fluids, GI protectants (sucralfate, famotidine, rhinitidine, or omeprazole), and antiemetics (maropitant, metoclopramide) may be used. In humans, chronic hemodialysis is often necessary and, in some cases, renal transplant is performed. In humans, forced diuresis is not recommended due to increased renal damage.[41] Furosemide increased toxicity, in rats, when injected prior to C orellanoides ingestion.[44] In animals, peritoneal or hemodialysis could be considered. Experimental treatments, in humans, include use of corticosteroids, N-acetylcysteine, and selenium. The results have not been conclusive.[36]

The prognosis, following ingestion of nephrotoxic Crotinarius sp, varies. There appears to be a dosage-dependent aspect as well as individual variation. In humans, renal failure has been reported to occur in 30% to 40% percent of cases. This may be followed by a slow return to normal function or development into chronic renal failure, which requires hemodialysis and/or transplantation. A shorter latent period usually indicates a worse prognosis.[36]

SUMMARY

There are numerous types of mushrooms that may be ingested by small animals, mostly by dogs. Although many mushrooms are not toxic, there are some types that can result in hepatotoxic, neurologic, cardiovascular, hemolytic, muscarinic, GI, and/or nephrotoxic effects. Gross identification by nonmycologists is often not effective, so it is safest to assume that any mushroom ingested may potentially be toxic until or unless identification is accomplished. It should also be assumed that more than one kind of mushroom could be ingested in a single exposure.

Following ingestion of an unknown mushroom in small animals, decontamination should consist of induction of emesis (3% hydrogen peroxide or apomorphine in dogs and xylazine in cats) followed by administration of activated charcoal (1 to 2 g/kg) orally in asymptomatic animals. The vomitus should be examined for the presence of mushrooms. Mushroom specimens from the vomitus and/or other similar mushrooms from the animal's environment should be saved for identification. Do not save mushrroms in plastic bags. Instead, place them in a paper bag, towel, or a newspaper. Refrigerate the specimen until shipped out for identification. Specimen should be labeled and dated properly. Information regarding a brief history of exposure, chronology of onset time and types of clinical signs, blood and chemistry changes, treatment used, and response to treatment should be sent to the veterinary diagnostic laboratory when needed.

Baseline complete blood count and chemistry panels should be obtained and repeated as needed. The animal should be monitored at the clinic for several hours for the onset of CNS, cardiovascular, muscarinic, and GI signs. Also, during this time, the animal can be monitored for hypernatremia that may occur following administration of activated charcoal. If signs develop, or are present at the time of presentation, the animal should be treated accordingly. If no signs develop, the animal can be monitored on an outpatient basis for the development of delayed (often beyond 6 to 8 hours) GI signs that often precede more severe effects associated with the hepatotoxic, hemolytic, and nephrotoxic mushrooms. Typically signs are expected within 4 hours following ingestion of isoxazoles, GI irritants, muscarine, and psilocybins. If the onset of vomiting, diarrhea, and abdominal pain are delayed beyond 6 to 8 hours, it increases the suspicion that the more serious amatoxin, gyrometrin, or orellanine (rare) toxins have been ingested. In asymptomatic animals, serum chemistries could be monitored daily for up to 4 days post ingestion. SAMe could be initiated as a potential liver protectant in case amatoxin was ingested.

REFERENCES

1. Lincoff G, Mitchel DH. Cyclopeptide poisoning. In: Toxic and hallucinogenic mushroom poisoning. A handbook for physicians and mushroom hunters. New York: Van Nostrand Reinhold Company; 1977. p. 25–48.
2. Wolfe BE, Richard F, Cross HB, et al. Distribution and abundance of the introduced ectomycorrhizal fungus Amanita phalloides in North America. New Phytol 2010;185: 803–16.
3. Mitchel DH. Amanita mushroom poisoning. Annu Rev Med 1980;31:51–7.
4. Faulstich H, Fauser U. The course of Amanita intoxication in beagle dogs. In: Faulstich H, Kommerell B, Wieland T, editors. Amanita toxins and poisoning. Baden-Baden (Germany): Verlag Gerhard Witzstrock; 1980. p. 115–23.
5. Duffy TJ. Toxic fungi of Western North America. March 2008. Available at: http://www.mykoweb.com. Accessed December 6, 2011.
6. Lindell TJ, Weinberg F, Morris PW, et al. Specific inhibition of nuclear RNA polymerase II by alpha-amanitin. Science 1970;170:447–9.
7. Magdalan J, Ostrowska A, Piotrowska A, et al. α-Amanitin induced apoptosis in primary cultured dog hepatocytes. Folia Histochem Cytobiol 2010;48:58–62.
8. De Carlo E, Milanesi A, Martini C, et al. Effects of Amanita phalloides toxins on insulin release: in vivo and in vitro studies. Arch Toxicol 2003;77:441–5.
9. Letschert K, Faulstich H, Keller D, et al. Molecular characterization and inhibition of amanitin uptake into human hepatocytes. Toxicol Sci 2006;91:140–9.
10. Jaeger A, Jehl F, Flesch F, et al. Kinetics of amatoxins in human poisoning: therapeutic implications. J Toxicol Clin Toxicol 1993;31:63–80.
11. Puschner B, Rose HH, Filigenzi MS. Diagnosis of Amanita toxicosis in a dog with acute hepatic necrosis. J Vet Diagn Invest 2007;19:312–7.
12. Kallet A, Sousa C, Spangler W. Mushroom (Amanita phalloides) toxicity in dogs. Calif Vet 1988;42:1, 9–11, 22, 47.
13. Cole FM. A puppy death and Amanita phalloides. Aust Vet Assoc 1993;70:271–2.
14. Filigenzi MS, Poppenga RH, Tiwary AK, et al. Determination of alpha-amanitin in serum and liver by multistage linear ion trap mass spectrometry. J Agric Food Chem 2007;55:784–90.
15. Beuhler M, Lee DC, Gerkin R. The Meixner test in the detection of α-amanitin and false positive reactions caused by psilocin and 5-substituted tryptamines. Ann Emerg Med 2004;44:114–20.
16. Thiel C, Thiel K, Klingert W, et al. The enterohepatic circulation of amanitin: kinetics and therapeutical implications. Toxicol Lett 2011;203:142–6.
17. Karlson-Stiber C, Persson H. Cytotoxic fungi: an overview. Toxicon 2003;42:339–49.
18. Abenavoli L, Capasso R, Milic N, et al. Milk thistle in liver diseases: past, present, future. Phytother Res 2010;24:1423–32.
19. Vogel G, Tuchweber B, Trost W, et al. Protection by silibinin against Amanita phalloides intoxication in beagles. Toxicol Appl Pharm 1984;73:355–62.
20. Schmidlin-Meszaros J. Gyromitrin in Trockenlorcheln [Gyromitra esculenta sicc]. Mitt Geb Lebensm Hyg 1974;65:453–65.
21. Bernard MA. Mushroom poisoning in a dog. Can Vet J 1979;20:82–3.

22. Lheureux P, Penaloza A, Gris M. Pyridoxine in clinical toxicology: a review. Eur J Emerg Med 2005;12:78–85.
23. Villar D, Knight MK, Holding J, et al. Treatment of acute isoniazid overdose in dogs. Vet Hum Toxicol 1995;37:473–7.
24. Halpern JH. Hallucinogens and dissociative agents naturally growing in the United States. Pharmacol Ther 2004;102:131–8.
25. Hunt RS, Funk A. Mushrooms fatal to dogs. Mycologia 1977;69:432–3.
26. Chebib M, Johnston GA. The 'ABC' of GABA receptors: a brief review. Clin Exp Pharmacol Physiol 199;26:937–40.
27. Ridgway RL. Mushroom (Amanita pantherina) poisoning. J Vet Med Assoc 1978;172:681–2.
28. Martin JG. Mycetism (mushroom poisoning) in a dog: case report. Vet Med 1956;51:227–8.
29. Naude TW, Berry WL. Suspected poisoning of puppies by the mushroom Amanita pantherina. J S Afr Vet Assoc 1997;68:154–8.
30. Smolinske SC. Psilocybin-containing mushrooms. In: Spoerke DG, Rumack BH, editors. Handbook of mushroom poisoning—diagnosis and treatment. Boca Raton (FL): CRC Press; 1994. p. 309–24.
31. Grieshaber AF, Moore KA, Levine B. The detection of psilocin in human urine. J Forens Sci 2001;46:627–30.
32. Halberstadt AL, Koedood L, Powell SB, et al. Differential contributions of serotonin receptors to the behavioral effects of indoleamine hallucinogens in mice. J Psychopharmacol 2010. DOI:10.1177/0269881110388326.
33. Kirwan AP. 'Magic mushroom' poisoning in a dog. Vet Rec 1990;126:149.
34. Benjamin DR. Mushrooms: poisons and panaceas. New York: WH Freeman & Co; 1995.
35. Turner NJ, Szczawinski AF. Common poisonous plants and mushrooms of North America. Portland (OR): Timber Press; 1991.
36. POISINDEX® System (intranet database). Version 5.1. Greenwood Village (CO): Thomson Reuters (Healthcare) Inc.
37. Goldfrank LR. Mushrooms. In: Nelson SL, Lewin AN, Howland MA, et al, editors. Goldfrank's Toxicological emergencies. 9th edition. China: McGraw-Hill Companies; 2011. p. 1522–34.
38. Bresinsky A, Besl H. Gastrointestinal syndrome. In: A colour atlas of poisonous fungi. London: Wolfe Publishing; 1990. p. 130.
39. Spoerke D, Rumack BH. Handbook of mushroom poisoning, Boca Raton (FL): CRC Press; 1994.
40. Spoerke D. Mushroom exposure. In: Peterson ME, Talcott PA, editors. Small animal toxicology. Philadelphia: WB Saunders; 2001. p. 571–92.
41. Michelot D, Tebbett I. Poisoning by members of the genus Cortinarius: a review. Mycol Res 1990;94:289–98.
42. Judge BS, Ammirati JF, Lincoff GH, et al. Ingestion of a newly described North American mushroom species from Michigan resulting in chronic renal failure: Cortinarius orellanosus. Clin Toxicol (Phila) 2010;48:545–9.
43. Berger KJ, Guss DA. Mycotoxins revisited: part II. J Emerg Med 2005;28:175–83.
44. Nieminen L, Pyy K. Individual variation in mushroom poisoning induced in the male rat by Cortinarius speciosissimus. Med Biol 1976;54:156–8.

Differential Diagnosis of Common Acute Toxicologic Versus Nontoxicologic Illness

Safdar A. Khan, DVM, MS, PhD

KEYWORDS

- Differential diagnosis • Small animal poisoning
- Toxicologic illness • Nontoxicologic illness

Major Clinical Abnormality	Common Toxicologic Rule Outs	Nontoxicologic Rule Outs
Central nervous system (CNS) abnormalities (excitation and seizures)	**Strychnine** (rapid onset, rigidity, hyperesthesia, wooden horse–like stance) **Metaldehyde** (hyperthermia, tremors, shaking) **Amphetamines, or cocaine** (ingestion in dogs: sympathomimetic effects and hyperthermia) **Tremorgenic mycotoxins** (Penitrem A, roquefortine) from eating moldy foods (gastrointestinal [GI] signs, hyperthermia, and tremors) **Cold medications: pseudoephedrine, ephedrine, some antihistamines** (sympathomimetic effects, hyperthermia) **Organophosphate (OP) or carbamate** pesticides (cholinergic crisis; salivation, lacrimation, urination, diarrhea (SLUD) signs) **Pyrethrins/pyrethroids** type pesticides (especially permethrin in cats: tremors, shaking, ataxia, seizures, GI signs)	**Trauma/head trauma** (outdoor animal, external or internal wounds/injuries) **Meningitis** (fever, hyperesthesia, neck stiffness, and pain) **Hydrocephalus** (large rounded head; ventrolateral deviation of eyes; seizures **Intracranial neoplasia** (primary or secondary brain tumor: older animals)

The author has nothing to disclose.

This article was adapted and modified with permission from Khan SA. Intoxication versus acute, nontoxicologic illness: differentiating the two. In: Ettinger SJ, Feldman EC, editors. Ettinger and Feldman's textbook of veterinary internal medicine. 7th edition. St Louis (MO): Saunders Elsevier; 2010. Chapter 144, p. 549–54; and Khan SA. Investigating fatal suspected poisonings. In: Poppenga RH, Gwlatney-Brant SM, editors. Small animal toxicology essentials. Sussex (UK): John Wiley and Sons; 2010. p. 71–6.

ASPCA Animal Poison Control Center, 1717 South Philo Road, Suite 36, Urbana, IL 61802, USA

E-mail address: safdar.khan@aspca.org

Vet Clin Small Anim 42 (2012) 389–402

doi:10.1016/j.cvsm.2012.01.001

vetsmall.theclinics.com

0195-5616/12/$ – see front matter © 2012 Elsevier Inc. All rights reserved.

Major Clinical Abnormality	Common Toxicologic Rule Outs	Nontoxicologic Rule Outs
	Organochlorine pesticides (tremors, shaking, ataxia, seizures)	Congenital portosystemic shunts (more common in certain breeds, <6 months of age, small liver)
	Chocolate: caffeine, theobromine, methylxanthines (polydipsia, polyuria, excitation, pacing, GI and CV effects)	
	Zinc phosphide: mole or gopher baits (GI signs, shaking, pulmonary edema)	Rabies (acute behavior changes, excitation, paralysis)
	Bromethalin toxicosis: rat or mouse bait (paresis, weakness, ataxia, twitching)	
	Lead (GI signs, nucleated red blood cells [RBCs], basophilic stipling, anemia)	Canine distemper (young dogs: fever, respiratory, GI and CNS signs)
	Metronidazole (toxicosis in dogs with repeated use: nystagmus, ataxia, weakness, paresis, seizures)	Hypocalcemia or hypercalcemia (hypocalcemic tetany, cardiovascular [CV] effects, CNS, renal effects from hypercalcemia)
	Nicotine: tobacco or cigarettes (ingestion in dogs: spontaneous vomiting, shaking, CV effects)	
	Tricyclic antidepressants toxicosis: amitriptyline, clomipramine, imipramine, nortriptyline (agitation, nervousness, ataxia, CV effects; sedation/lethargy at low doses)	Hypoglycemia (disorientation, ataxia, seizures, serum glucose <60 mg/dL)
	Brunfelsia plant ingestion (all parts toxic particularly seeds; strychnine poisoning–like signs; vomiting, tremors, stiffness, seizures	Idiopathic epilepsy (dogs 1–5 years of age: bloodwork normal)
		Polycythemia vera (primary or secondary, PCV 65%–81%, brick-red mucous membrane)
		Uremia (secondary to acute or chronic renal failure [ARF or CRF])
		Endotoxemia/septic shock (hemorrhagic GI signs, progressive weakness, abdominal pain)

Major Clinical Abnormality	Common Toxicologic Rule Outs	Nontoxicologic Rule Outs
CNS abnormalities (CNS depression and seizures)	**Ivermectin, moxidectin, and other avermectin** toxicosis (ataxia, weakness, depression, tremors, seizures, blindness) **Marijuana ingestion** (ataxia, hypothermia, urinary incontinence) **Benzodiazepine ingestion**: alprazolam, clonazepam, diazepam, lorazepam (hyporeflexia, ataxia, CNS excitation: paradoxical reaction) **Barbiturate overdose**: short acting or long acting (coma, hypothermia, weakness, ataxia) **Ethylene glycol**: *see Acute renal failure* (ataxia, drunkenness, disorientation, GI signs) **Methanol or ethanol ingestion** (GI, signs, ataxia, weakness, depression) **Propylene glycol**: antifreeze (depression, ataxia, GI signs) **Baclofen** or other centrally acting muscle relaxant (ingestion in dogs: vocalization, ataxia, disorientation, coma, hypothermia) **Amitraz insecticide** (depression, ataxia, CV effects, paralytic ileus) **SSRI (selective serotonin reuptake inhibitor) and other similar antidepressant** toxicosis (SSRI types like fluoxetine, sertraline, paroxetine; CNS sedation or excitation, ataxia, tremors, seizures, mydriasis, tachycardia)	**Thiamine deficiency in cats** (cats fed mainly fish diet) **Coonhound paralysis** (ascending flaccid paralysis; raccoon exposure within 2 weeks) **Feline infectious peritonitis**: dry form (iritis; fever, weight loss, ataxia, seizures) **Feline leukemia** (lymphadenopathy, nonregenerative anemia) **Feline panleukopenia** (fever, GI signs, ataxia, neutropenia)
Muscle weakness, paresis, paralysis	**Black widow spider bite** (cats: swelling, pain) **2,4-D and other phenoxy herbicides** (in dogs: ataxia, weakness, GI signs) **Metronidazole** *see Seizures* (in dogs: nystagmus, ataxia, weakness, seizures) **Bromethalin** rodenticide (see under *Seizures*; paresis, CNS depression/excitation, twitching, seizures) **Coral snake** envenomation (cats: local swelling, pain, puncture wound) **Macadamia nuts** (ingestion in dogs: weakness, ataxia) **Concentrated tea tree oil** exposure: Melaleuca oil (both cats and dogs: weakness, ataxia, CNS depression)	**Coonhound paralysis** (muscle pain, ascending flaccid paralysis; raccoon exposure within 2 weeks) **Botulism** (ascending paresis and paralysis) **Tick paralysis** (flaccid ascending paralysis) **Aortic thromboembolism** (cold extremities, weakness)

Major Clinical Abnormality	Common Toxicologic Rule Outs	Nontoxicologic Rule Outs
	Albuterol inhalor ingestion/toxicosis (muscle weakness accompanied by severe hypokalemia; tachycardia, agitation)	**Profound anemia** (measure PCV) **Severe hypokalemia** **Hyponatremia** **Tetanus** (hyperesthesia, rigidity, muscle spasm, third eyelid visible) **Severe hypovolemia** **Marked hypothermia or hyperthermia** **Degenerative spinal cord diseases**
Acute blindness	**Lead**, see *Seizures* (GI signs, behavior changes, nucleated RBCs, basophilic stipling) **Ivermectin, moxidectin**, and other avemectin toxicosis, see *Seizures* (ataxia, weakness, seizures, blindness reversible) **Salt poisoning** (in dogs: excessive sodium chloride ingestion, polydipsia, GI signs, tremors, ataxia, seizures, serum sodium >160 mEq/L)	**Retinal detachment or hemorrhage** **Glaucoma** **Trauma** (penetrating injury of head, face) **Acute cataract** **Optic neuritis** **Optic nerve disorders** (optic chiasm, optic radiation, occipital cortex) **Sudden acquired retinal degeneration**
Acute renal failure (ARF)	**Ethylene glycol toxicosis** (ataxia, drunkenness, GI signs, acidosis, azotemia) **Easter lily (*Lilium longiflorum*), Tiger lilies (*Lilium tigrinum, Lilium lancifolium*), Rubrum or Japanese show lilies (*Lilium speciosumf*), Day lilies (*Hemerocallis* sp)** (reported in cats, initially GI signs, azotemia in generally 24–72 hours after ingestion) **Cholecalciferol rodenticide** and other vitamin D₃ analogue: calcipotriene, calcitriol; *see under Hypercalcemia* (initial GI signs, hypercalcemia, hyperphosphatemia, CV, and CNS effects, azotemia)	**Renal infiltration** (with lymphoma) **Renal thromboembolism** **Infectious** (pyelonepheritis, leptospirosis, Rocky Mountain spotted fever, borreliosis, feline infectious peritonitis: cats) **Urinary tract obstruction** **Renal lymphomas** (more in cats than in dogs)

Major Clinical Abnormality	Common Toxicologic Rule Outs	Nontoxicologic Rule Outs
	Grapes and raisins (ingestion in dogs: initial GI signs, then azotemia in >24 hours, possible pancreatitis) **NSAIDs:** ibuprofen, naproxen, nabumetone, piroxicam, carprofen, diclofenac, ketoprofen, indomethacin, ketorolac, oxaprozin, etodolac, flurbiprofen, sulindac (initially GI signs, azotemia in 24–74 hours after ingestion in acute cases) **Zinc toxicosis** see *hemolysis* (GI signs, pancreatitis, hemoglobinuria, anemia, renal failure) **Melamine and cyanuric acid contamination** (outbreak in the United States in 2007 from contaminated dog and cat food: crystaluria, azotemia, GI signs)	**Chronic renal failure** (end stage) **Ischemic renal failure** (hypotension, trauma, shock, congestive heart failure, anaphylaxis) **Neoplasia** (adenocarcinoma in dogs; lymphosarcoma in cats) **Amyloidosis** (immune-mediated) **Hypercalcemia** (due to any cause) **Transfusion reactions** **Myoglobinuria/ hemoglobinuria** (due to any cause)
Acute hepatic damage	**Carprofen** and other NSAID-induced hepatopathies in dogs (within a few days after initiating therapy, GI signs, increased alanine transaminase) **Corticosteroids** (steroid hepatopathy, long-term use) **Phenobarbital** (chronic use) **Mushrooms:** amanita type (delayed onset, 12 hours, GI signs, acute hepatic damage in 1–3 days) **Blue-green algae:** *Microcystis* sp (acute onset, GI signs, shock) **Iron:** multivitamin ingestion (GI signs, shock, acute liver damage in 1–2 days) **Copper** (copper storage disease; certain breeds can accumulate copper over a period of times) **Sago palm or cycad palm:** *Cycas* sp (ingestion: GI signs, liver damage in 1–3 days, seizures) **Acetaminophen toxicosis** (methemoglobinemia within a few hours, GI signs, increased liver enzymes in 1–3 days) **Aflatoxicosis** (dogs: mostly from contaminated dog food, several outbreaks reported in the United States)	**Hepatic lipidosis** (cats: period of stress, anorexia, obese animals) **Hepatic neoplasia** (primary or metastatic, acute or gradual) **Infectious hepatitis** (leptospiros, infectious canine hepatitis, canine herpes virus, cholangiohepatitis, liver abscess, histoplasmosis, cocidiomycosis, babesiosis, toxoplasmosis, some rickettsial diseases, feline infectious peritonitis) **Acute pancreatitis** (systemic) **Septicemia/ endotoxemia** (vomiting, diarrhea, hypothermia, collapse)

Major Clinical Abnormality	Common Toxicologic Rule Outs	Nontoxicologic Rule Outs
	Xylitol *see Hypoglycemia* (ingestion in dogs: hypoglycemia within 12 hours, seizures, acute hepatic damage and coagulopathy in 1–3 days)	**Heat stroke** (high ambient temperature) **Shock** (weak pulse, poor capillary refill time, progressive weakness) **Chronic passive congestion** (secondary to cardiac problems)
Presence of acute oral lesions/ulcers	**Acid ingestion** (corrosive lesions on lips, gums, tongue, salivation, vomiting, fever) **Alkali ingestion** (same as with acid, esophageal perforation more likely) **Cationic detergents**: present in several disinfectants (oral burns, salivation, vomiting, fever) **Alkaline battery** (ingestion: oral burns, salivation, vomiting) **Potpourri ingestion** (oral burns, salivation, vomiting, tongue protrusion, fever) **Bleaches:** sodium or calcium hypochlorite (bleach-like smell, salivation, vomiting, wheezing, gagging) **Ingestion of phenolic compounds** (especially in cats: oral ulcers/lesion may be present, Heinz body anemia and hemolysis may be seen)	**Uremic stomatitis** (azotemia, GI signs) **Periodontal disease** (associated with dental calculus; gingival lesions) **Trauma** (presence of foreign body, grass, stick, bone, porcupine quills) **Electrical cord chewing** (systemic signs such as dyspnea, pulmonary edema) **Systemic lupus erythematosus** and other autoimmune diseases (oral lesions and other systemic and cutaneous signs present) **Infectious** (feline calcivirus infection, feline leukemia virus, feline immunodeficiency virus, feline herpesvirus, nocardiasis, ulcerative necrotizing stomatitis, fusobacterium)

Major Clinical Abnormality	Common Toxicologic Rule Outs	Nontoxicologic Rule Outs
Acute methemoglobinemia, Heinz body anemia, hemolysis or blood loss (anemia)	**Acetaminophen** (chocolate-brown colored mucous membrane within hours, dyspnea) **Local anesthetic** toxicosis: lidocaine, benzocaine, tetracaine and dibucaine (methemoglobinemia, CV and CNS effects) **Phenazopyridine** and other azo dyes toxicosis (methemoglobinemia, hemoglobinuria) **Naphthalene mothball** ingestion (moth ball-like odor in the breath, hemolysis) **Onions and garlic** toxicosis (hemolysis in 2–3 days, anemia, coffee-color urine) **Zinc toxicosis** (metallic object in the GI tract, gastritis, pancreatitis, hemolysis, hemoglobinuria) **Iron** (mostly see GI signs, hepatic damage, or shock) **Anticoagulants rodenticides**: brodifacoum, bromadiolone, chlorophacinone, difethialone, diphacinone, pindone, warfarin (hemorrhaging, increased prothrombin time [PT] or activated partial thromboplastin time [aPTT], dyspnea, weakness) **Copper** (certain breeds of dogs can accumulate copper in the liver) **Rattlesnake** envenomation (swelling, pain, hemoglobinuria) **DL-Methionine toxicosis:** GI signs, ataxia, weakness, possible Heinz body anemia hemolysis in cats with large overdose, less likely in dogs	**Trauma** (overt blood loss) **Immune-mediated hemolytic anemia** **Thrombocytopenia** (drug-induced, infectious or immune mediated) **CRF** (smaller kidneys, azotemia) **Infectious** (ehrlichiosis, feline leukemia, hookworms, *Mycoplasma hemofelis*, babesiosis) **Severe liver diseases** (deficiency of clotting factor can result in bleeding disorders) **Disseminated intravascular coagulation** (secondary to underlying cause such as shock, neoplasia, septicemia, viral infections, pancreatitis) **Inherited bleeding disorders** (von Willebrand disease, factor X deficiency, factor XI deficiency) **Epistaxis** (primary or secondary, trauma, infectious, nasal polyps, malignant neoplasm)

Major Clinical Abnormality	Common Toxicologic Rule Outs	Nontoxicologic Rule Outs
Cardiac abnormalities	**Foxglove**: *Digitalis* sp (plant ingestion: GI signs and cardiac arrhythmias) **Lily of the valley**: *Convallaria majalis* (plant ingestion GI signs and cardiac arrhythmias) **Oleander**: *Nerium oleander* (GI signs and cardiac arrhythmias) **Bufo toads**: *Bufo* sp (GI signs collapse, seizures, and cardiac arrhythmias) **Azalea and other Rhododendron** plant: (GI signs and possible cardiac arrhythmias) **Antidepressant toxicosis**: (CNS signs, anticholinergic effects) **Calcium channel blockers** toxicosis: amlodipine, felodipine, verapamil, diltiazem (hypotension, bradycardia or tachycardia, atrioventricular block, pulmonary edema) **Beta-adrenergic blocking agents** toxicosis: atenolol, metoprolol, propranolol, esmolol (hypotension, tachycardia, bradycardia, weakness **Albuterol inhalor** ingestion/toxicosis: (tachycardia, agitation, premature ventricular contractions [PVCs], hypokalemia) **Alpha-adrenergic receptor agonists** overdose/toxicosis: (amitraz, clonidine; hypotension, weakness, collapse, bradycardia, hypothermia)	**Automobile trauma** (evidence of other injuries) **Gastric dilation and volvulus** (abdominal distention, dyspnea, shock) **Severe anemia** (due to any cause of anemia) **Severe hypokalemia** (due to any cause) **Acidosis** (due to any cause) **Hypoxia** (due to any cause of hypoxia) **Primary heart disease** (cardiomyopathy, valvular heart disease, congenital heart problems, heartworm infestation: heart murmur, cardiomegaly, or evidence of congestive heart failure)
Pulmonary edema	**Paraquat herbicide** (rare; progressive dyspnea, panting, delayed onset after exposure) **Petroleum distillates**: kerosene, gasoline, and other hydrocarbons (hydrocarbon smell in the breath, salivation, vomiting, CNS depression, diarrhea, aspiration) **Zinc phosphide** (GI and CNS signs, pulmonary edema) **Smoke inhalation** (dyspnea, collapse, panting, shock) **Organophosphate or carbamate** pesticides (cholinergic crisis, SLUD signs)	**Cardiogenic** (multiple causes of left ventricular failure) **Noncardiogenic** (seizures, head trauma, electrical shock) **Hepatic disease** (secondary to any cause of hepatic disease) **Renal disease** (any cause of renal disease) **Drowning and near drowning** **Shock** (immune mediated, anaphylactic, trauma, transfusion reactions)

Major Clinical Abnormality	Common Toxicologic Rule Outs	Nontoxicologic Rule Outs
	Some organic arsenicals (mainly injectable, melarsamine)	Neoplasia (primary or secondary)
	Calcium channel blockers toxicosis, see *Cardiac abnormalities* (noncardiogenic pulmonary edema along with cardiac signs)	
GI signs (vomiting, diarrhea, abdominal pain, drooling)	Arsenical herbicides (initial stages: vomiting, abdominal pain, watery diarrhea)	Infectious (feline panleukopenia, canine distemper, canine parvovirus, canine coronavirus, infectious canine hepatitis, leptospirosis, salmonellosis)
	Iron toxicosis (multivitamin ingestion in dogs: initial GI signs within hours)	
	Castor beans: *Ricinus communis* (initial GI signs within several hours)	
	Garbage poisoning (vomiting, diarrhea, dehydration, abdominal pain)	
	Chocolate toxicosis (initial stages: polydipsia, polyuria, vomiting, hyperactivity, tachycardia)	Internal parasites (hookworms)
	Fertilizer ingestion (nitrogen, phosphorous, potash [NPK]: vomiting, diarrhea, polydipsia)	Dietary discretion (recent change in diet)
	Insoluble calcium oxalate containing plants: elephant's ear *Caladium* sp, dumb cane *Dieffenbachia* sp, philodendron *Philodendron* sp, peace lily *Spathiphyllum* sp (vomiting, diarrhea, oral swelling, salivation)	Foreign body (plastic, wood, metal, bones, partial or complete obstruction)
	Endotoxins and enterotoxins: staphylococcal, clostridial, *E coli*, salmonella (severe GI signs, progressive lethargy, dehydration, hypothermia)	Gastric dilation, volvulus, intussusceptions (abdominal distention, pain, dyspnea, shock)
	Zinc oxide (diaper rash ointment ingestion in dogs; mild to severe gastritis)	Liver diseases (secondary to liver disease)
	Zinc phosphide (GI and CNS signs, pulmonary edema; liver and kidney damage possible)	Kidney diseases (secondary to renal disease, postrenal obstruction, uremia)
	NSAID toxicosis (initial stages: GI signs with or without blood)	Metabolic disorders (diabetic ketoacidosis, hypoadrenocorticism)
		Sudden change in the environment (traveling, weather change, boarding, moving)
		Inflammatory bowel disease (generally immune mediated)

Major Clinical Abnormality	Common Toxicologic Rule Outs	Nontoxicologic Rule Outs
Hypernatremia (measured serum sodium >160 in dogs and >165 in cats)	**Paint ball ingestion** (dogs: history of paintball ingestion, polydipsia, vomiting, diarrhea, ataxia) **Salt toxicosis** (history of inducing emesis with sodium chloride, ingestion of excessive amounts of salt-containing objects [eg, Play-Doh] and foods) **Activated charcoal administration** (can occur sporadically in some dogs with both single or multiple doses possibly due to fluid shift in the gut) **Seawater ingestion** (history of visit to a beach, lack of access to fresh water, swimming)	**Due to pure water loss** (nephrogenic diabetes inspidus, heat stroke, fever, burns, no access to water) **Due to hypotonic water loss** (severe diarrhea, vomiting, diabetes mellitus, renal failure, hypoadrenocorticism)
Hypoglycemia	**Ingestion of xylitol-containing products** (ingestion of sugar-free gum, bakery products, hypoglycemia within 12 hours) **Ingestion of oral diabetic/hypoglycemic agents** (sulfonylureas)	**Insulinoma** **Acute hepatic disease** **Functional hypoglycemia** (idiopathic in neonates, severe exercise) **Internal parasitism** **Adrenocortical insufficiency** **Endotoxemia**
Sudden, acute, unattended, or unexplained death (death within 24 hours of being reported healthy or minimal clinical effects)	**4-Aminopyridine**; an avicide, trembling, shaking, CV effects, seizures, death **5-Flurouracil ingestion**; (topical anticancer; available 2%–5% solution/cream; seizures, vomiting, cardiac arrhythmias; acute death possible with large ingestion **5-Hydroxytryptophan (5-HTP) ingestion**; used as over-the-counter sleep aid, antidepressant; accidental ingestion; seizures, hyperthermia; acute death with large ingestions possible **Acetaminophen (cats)**; death likely from methemoglobinemia within hours with large ingestion; cats more sensitive **Albuterol inhaler ingestion**; asthma medication; dogs chewing the inhaler; acute death with large ingestion possible; cardiac arrhythmias, hypokalemia **Amphetamines**; recreational or human prescription; hyperthermia, hyperactivity, circling, hypertension, tachyarrhythmias; acute death with large ingestion possible	**Cardiac disease** **Acute hepatic diseases** **Acute renal disease** **Parasitism** (heavy) internal and external **Congenital problems** **Metabolic disorders** (acidosis, alkalosis) **Neoplasia/cancer** (primary secondary) **Gastric dilatation/volvulus** **Trauma** **Severe hypoglycemia or hyperglycemia** (any cause) **Electric shock** **Excessive Bleeding/hemorrhaging** (due to any reason) **Infectious cause** (endotoxemia/shock)

Major Clinical Abnormality	Common Toxicologic Rule Outs	Nontoxicologic Rule Outs
	Anticoagulant poisoning; internal bleeding 3–5 days post ingestion; signs may not be apparent; acute death due to pulmonary hemorrhage possible	Meningitis (rabies, canine distemper
	Antidepressants (other than tricyclic antidepressants such as SSRI); common human prescription medications; fluoxetine, citalopram, sertraline; acute death possible with large ingestion; CNS and cardiac effects	Shock (anaphylactic; hypovolemic)
		Hypocalcemia/ hypercalcemia (due to any etiology)
	Arsenic: used in ant baits, herbicide; toxicosis uncommon; watery diarrhea, abdominal pain, shock, acute death possible	Marked hypo or hyperthermia (due to any reason hypovolemic)
	Baclofen and other centrally acting muscle relaxants, prescription drug; coma, hypothermia, death with large ingestion	Drowning, near-drowning
	Barbiturates overdose: common anticonvulsant, accidental ingestion of large doses; farm dogs eating flesh/carcass of animals euthanized by barbiturates; coma, hypothermia and death	Hypocalcemia/ hypercalcemia (due to any etiology) Marked hypothermia or hyperthermia (due to any reason)
	Blue-green algae; history of drinking from a lake/pond; algae on the muzzle; collapse, shock, seizures, liver failure, death	
	Botulism; acute death rare; ingestion of preformed toxins from eating a carcass; progressive weakness, paralysis, death	
	Brunfelsia spp ingestion; strychnine-like signs (seizures, stiffness); dogs attracted to fruit/ seed pods/flowers; acute death possible with large ingestion	
	Bufo toad ingestion/mouthing; common in Florida and other southern states; acute collapse, salivation, cardiac arrhythmias, seizures, death	
	Caffeine/theobromin; ingestion of chocolate or caffeine pills; acute death with large ingestion possible; vomiting, CNS signs, cardiac arrhythmias	
	Carbon monoxide poisoning; uncommon, dog confined in garage with car's engine running; bright-red mucous membranes, disorientation, death	
	Cardiac glycoside–containing plants; acute death uncommon; evidence of plant ingestion; lily of the valley, foxglove, oleander, azaleas, kalanchoes	
	Castor beans: acute death unlikely; only possible if several seeds have been ingested, GI signs, liver, kidney damage	

Major Clinical Abnormality	Common Toxicologic Rule Outs	Nontoxicologic Rule Outs
	Cocaine: recreational drug; acute death with large ingestion possible	
	Ethylene glycol: acute death with large ingestions possible; coma, acidosis, ARF; cats more sensitive	
	Garbage poisoning: history of eating garbage; acute death possible with some *Salmonella*, *E coli* toxins; vomiting, progressive shock, dehydration, watery diarrhea, and death	
	Hepatotoxic mushroom (amanita type): vomiting, diarrhea, abdominal pain, shock, liver failure, death	
	Hops (used for beer flavoring): malignant hyperthermia–like syndrome in dogs; acute death possible	
	Ionophores (monencin, lasalocid): dogs eating cattle feed; acute death with large ingestion (premix) possible	
	Iron: prenatal multivitamins; large ingestions, acute death uncommon, vomiting, shock, liver damage	
	Isoniazid ingestion: antituberculosis drug; seizures, acute death due to large ingestions possible	
	Lidocaine and other local anesthetics: uncommon toxicosis; CNS, and cardiovascular effects, overdose likely with injection or sprays	
	Metaldehyde: used as slug bait; seizures, hyperthermia, stiffness, tremors, acute death with large ingestion possible	
	Moldy food ingestion (tremorgenic mycotoxins penitrem A, roquefortine): history of ingestion of moldy food; seizures, hyperthermia, vomiting, acute death possible	
	Nicotine: acute death with large ingestion possible; tobacco products, toxicosis uncommon; GI, CNS, and cardiac effects	
	Organochlorine-type pesticides: lindane, eldrin, dieldrin; use not common anymore; cats more sensitive; seizures, tremors, and acute death	
	OPs/carbamate pesticides: some highly toxic OPs/carbamates like methomyl, aldicarb (tres pasitos), disulfoton; usually SLUD signs present; acute rapid death with large ingestion possible	

Major Clinical Abnormality	Common Toxicologic Rule Outs	Nontoxicologic Rule Outs
	Paint ball ingestion (diethylene and other glycols): ingestion of large amounts; acute death uncommon, seizures due to hypernatremia and other electrolyte changes possible	
	Pseudoephedrine: over-the-counter decongestant; amphetamine-like signs; acute death with large overdose possible	
	Pyrethrins/pyrethroids (permethrin in cats): cats more sensitive; use of concentrated products; tremors, ataxia, seizures, death	
	Sago palm/cycas: acute death unlikely; possible if several seeds have been ingested; GI signs, seizures, liver failure	
	Salt (sodium chloride) poisoning: homemade Play-Doh ingestion; inappropriate use as an emetic; seizures, hypernatremia, death possible	
	Smoke inhalation: history of pet trapped in the house during fire	
	Snake bite: Mohave rattlesnake, Eastern rattlesnake; acute death possible	
	Strychnine: used as a rodenticide bait; rapid onset, seizures, hyperthermia, stiffness, death, quick rigor mortis	
	Tetrodotoxins: acute death rare; ingestion of dried puffer fish, pet salamander; paresis, coma, respiratory failure, death	
	Tricyclic antidepressants: prescription medications; amitriptyline, nortriptyline; acute death with large ingestion possible; CNS and CV effects	
	Water intoxication: history of being on the beach/swimming, hyponateremia, hypochloremia, polydipsia	
	Xylitol ingestion: acute death due to severe hypoglycemia possible; acute liver failure seen 1–3 days after ingestion	
	Zinc phosphide: available as gopher bait; vomiting, CNS effects; acute death with large ingestion possible	

FURTHER READINGS

Beasley VR, editor. Toxicology of selected pesticides, drugs, and chemicals. Vet Clin North Am Small Anim Pract 1990;20(2).

Cote E. Clinical veterinary advisor: dogs and cats. 2nd edition. St Louis (MO): Elsevier Mosby; 2001.

Cote E. Clinical veterinary advisor: dogs and cats. Ist edition. St Louis (MO): Elsevier Mosby; 2007.

Cote E, Khan SA. Intoxication versus acute, nontoxicologic illness: differentiating the two. In: Ettinger SJ, Feldman EC, editors. Ettinger and Feldman's textbook of veterinary internal medicine. 6th edition. St Louis (MO): Elsevier Saunders; 2005. Chapter. 66, p. 242–5.

Fenner WR. Quick reference to veterinary medicine. 3rd edition. Baltimore (MD): Lippincott Williams and Wilkins; 2000.

Khan SA. Intoxication versus acute, nontoxicologic illness: differentiating the two. In: Ettinger SJ, Feldman EC, editors. Ettinger and Feldman's textbook of veterinary internal medicine. 7th edition. St Louis (MO): Saunders Elsevier; 2010. Chapter 144, p. 549–54.

Khan SA. Investigating fatal suspected poisonings. In: Poppenga RH, Gwlatney-Brant SM, editors. Small animal toxicology essentials. Sussex (UK): John Wiley and Sons; 2010. p. 71–6.

Volmer PA, Meerdink GA. Diagnostic toxicology for the small animal practitioner. Vet Clin Small Anim 2002;32:357–65.

Common Reversal Agents/ Antidotes in Small Animal Poisoning

Safdar A. Khan, DVM, MS, PhD

KEYWORDS

- Reversal agents • Antidotes • Poisoning treatment
- Small animal poisoning

Reversal Agent/Antidote	Toxicant/Main Indications	Comment(s)
N-acetylcysteine (Mucomyst)	Acetaminophen (paracetamol) overdose; can be tried for amanita mushroom toxicosis; sago palm toxicosis; xylitol toxicosis	Can be used orally (PO); Injectable (Acetadote) available; in addition, can also use SAMe
Flumazenil (Romazicon)	Benzodiazepines (diazepam, alprazolam, lorazepam, clonazepam) overdose	Can help reverse severe central nervous system (CNS) depression/coma; short half-life; repeat in 1 to 3 hours if needed
Pamidronate (Aredia)	Cholecalciferol; calcipotriene; calcitriol	Treats hypercalcemia and hyperphosphatemia; can cause transient azotemia, may require multiple doses
Cyproheptadine (Periactin)	Serotonin syndrome caused by serotonergic substances (5-hydroxytryptophan; selective serotonin reuptake inhibitors, tricyclic antidepressants)	Can be tried per rectum in animals that cannot take it PO; can repeat once in 8–12 hours

The author has nothing to disclose.
This article was adapted and modified from with permission Khan SA. Clinical veterinary advisor: dogs and cats. 2nd edition. St Louis (MO): Elsevier Mosby; 2010.
ASPCA Animal Poison Control Center, 1717 South Philo Road, Suite 36, Urbana, IL 61802, USA
E-mail address: safdar.khan@aspca.org

Vet Clin Small Anim 42 (2012) 403–406
doi:10.1016/j.cvsm.2012.01.002
0195-5616/12/$ – see front matter © 2012 Elsevier Inc. All rights reserved.

vetsmall.theclinics.com

Reversal Agent/Antidote	Toxicant/Main Indications	Comment(s)
Methocarbamol (Robaxin)	For tremor control in permethrin toxicosis in cats; can also be tried in cats/dogs for tremors resulting from other pyrethrins/pyrethroids	Not an anticonvulsant; works well in permethrin, metaldehyde, tremorgens, and strychnine toxicosis; injectable preferred; PO may be helpful for mild cases
Atipamezole (Antisedan)	To treat alpha-2-adrenergic agonist effects of amitraz, xylazine, clonidine, and brimonidine overdose	Atipamezole and yohimbine have alpha-2-adnergic antagonist properties; atipamezole more specific/preferred
Fomepizole (4-methyl pyrazole; Antizol-Vet)	Ethylene glycol (antifreeze) toxicosis in dogs; some benefit if used within 3 hours of exposure in cats	Good safety margin; does not contribute to acidosis and CNS depression as ethanol does; can use ethanol as an alternative if fomepizole is not available
Calcium disodium EDTA (Calcium Disodium Versenate)	Lead, zinc, cadmium	Injectable; can cause gastrointestinal (GI) signs and nephrotoxicity; do not use if metal still present in GI tract
BAL (British antilewisite; Dimercaprol)	Lead, arsenic, mercury	Injection can be irritating and painful; difficult to obtain; helps remove lead from CNS
Atropine sulfate	For treating muscurinic signs in organophosphates and carbamate toxicosis; certain muscurinic mushrooms	Avoid atropinization (hyperthermia, tachycardia, mydriasis), not for treating nicotinic signs
2-PAM (Paralidoxime)	For treating nicotinic signs in organophosphate toxicosis in dogs, cats	Not useful for most carbamate toxicoses; most beneficial within 24 hours of exposure but may be useful beyond this time; discontinue after 3 doses if no benefit
D-penicillamine (Cuprimine)	Zinc, cadmium, lead, copper, mercury	Used PO; can cause GI signs; do not use when metal is still present in the GI tract
Digoxin immune Fab (Digibind)	Digitalis; cardiac glycosides	Expensive but rapid acting and efficacious; can be used in Bufo toad toxicosis
Deferoxamine (Desferol)	Iron chelator; useful in iron toxicosis	Urine color may turn wine color after chelation with iron
Succimer (2-3-dimercaptosuccinic acid; Chemet)	Lead poisoning in dogs, cats, birds	Used PO; anecdotal reports of renal failure in cats—monitor renal values when using in cats; can be used when object still present in the GI tract

Reversal Agent/Antidote	Toxicant/Main Indications	Comment(s)
Yohimbine (Yobine)	To treat alpha-2-adrenergic agonist effects of amitraz, xylazine, clonidine, and brimonidine overdose	Shorter half-life and less specific than atipamezole; use yohimbine as a second choice if atipamezole is not available
S-adenosyl-L-methionine (SAMe; Denosyl)	General hepatoprotective agent; has been suggested as a supplement	Used as an aid in hepatic damage from various causes (mushroom, xylitol, cycad, acetaminophen, etc)
Naloxone (Narcan)	Opioids/opiates	Can help reverse respiratory/CNS depression; short half-life; repeat in 1 to 3 hours if needed
Vitamin K1 (phytonadione)	Anticoagulants (warfarin, brodifacoum, bromodiolone)	Parenteral use can cause allergic reaction; use PO for 2 to 4 weeks or more as needed; works better with fatty food and in divided doses
Pyridoxine (vitamin B6)	Isoniazid toxicosis in dogs	Difficult to obtain; can be used 1:1 ratio (dose of isoniazid:dose of pyridoxine); 5% to 10% IV infusion over 30 to 60 minutes; use in conjunction with diazepam to control CNS effects
Prussian blue	Thallium toxicosis	Used PO; difficult to obtain; thallium toxicosis no longer common
Leucovorin	Methotrexate overdose	Leucovorin is active form of folic acid; 25 to 250 mg/m^2 every 6 hours IV, IM for up to 72 hours
Intravenous lipid emulsion (Intralipid 10% or 20% solution)	For certain lipophilic drug toxicosis; potential for ivermectin, moxidectin and other avemectins; cholecalciferol and other vitamin D$_3$ analogue; amlodipine; baclofen,; diltiazem; lidocaine; nifedipine; verapamil; severe marijuana toxcoisis; permethrin toxicosis; bupropion; trazodone; phenobarbital and other barbiturates overdose; tricyclic antideprassants; propranolol	Case-control studies demonstrating efficacy and safety not available; 1.5 mL/kg (20% solution) as initial bolus followed by 0.25 mL/kg over 30 to 60 minutes, may have to repeat 2 or 3 times every 4–6 hours provided no hyperlipemia present; lack of efficacy; hyperlipidemia, hemolysis, embolism, infection potential adverse effects

Reversal Agent/Antidote	Toxicant/Main Indications	Comment(s)
Glucagon (GlucaGen)	Used for treating hypoglycemia due to insulin overdose and hypoglycemia agents; beta-adrenergic agents, calcium channel blockers and tricyclic antidepressant overdose for atrioventricular block, bradycardia, and hypotension	Used IV bolus followed by constant rate infusion (CRI); 50 ng/kg IV bolus in 0.9% saline then 5 to 15 ng/kg/min as CRI
Methylene blue	To treat methemoglobinemia from aniline, nitrite, hydroxyurea, naphthalene, and local anesthetic agents	1% Solution injectable solution at 1.5 mg/kg IV, repeat once in 30 minutes if needed; do not give in cats as it can induce methemoblobinemia in cats
Hydroxycobalamin (Cyanokit)	Vitamin B_{12} precursor; used to treat cyanide toxicosis	Hydroxycobalamin combines with cyanide to form cyanocobalamin, which is excreted in urine; used for treating pernicious anemia in humans
Hyperbaric oxygen	Delivers 100% oxygen at pressure >1 atmosphere; used in carbon monoxide, hydrogen sulfide toxicosis; can be helpful for cyanide toxicosis	Hyperbaric chambers may be available in veterinary schools and in some advanced veterinary clinics
Silymarin (milk thistle)	Used as a hepatoprotective agent in acetaminophen and amanita mushroom toxicosis	Used within 48 hours of exposure; may have to be used for several weeks; 20 to 50 mg/kg/d PO
Acepromazine (PromAce)	To control hyperexcitation from amphetamine toxicosis and other similar stimulants; used for seroteneric drug overdose	Can cause hypotension; 0.02 to 0.1 mg/kg IV, IM, or SC; repeat as needed

FURTHER READINGS

Gwaltney-Brant S, Rumbeiha W. New antidotal therapies. Vet Clin North Am Small Anim Pract 2002;32(2):323–39.

Wismer T. Antidotes. In: Poppenga RH, Gwaltney-Brant S, editors. Small animal toxicology essentials. Sussex (UK): Wiley-Blackwell; 2011. p. 57–70.

Index

Note: Page numbers of article titles are in **boldface** type.

Vet Clin Small Anim 42 (2012) 407–422
doi:10.1016/S0195-5616(12)00025-3
0195-5616/12/$ – see front matter © 2012 Elsevier Inc. All rights reserved.

vetsmall.theclinics.com

Moving?

Make sure your subscription moves with you!

To notify us of your new address, find your **Clinics Account Number** (located on your mailing label above your name), and contact customer service at:

Email: journalscustomerservice-usa@elsevier.com

800-654-2452 (subscribers in the U.S. & Canada)
314-447-8871 (subscribers outside of the U.S. & Canada)

Fax number: 314-447-8029

Elsevier Health Sciences Division
Subscription Customer Service
3251 Riverport Lane
Maryland Heights, MO 63043

*To ensure uninterrupted delivery of your subscription, please notify us at least 4 weeks in advance of move.

Printed and bound by CPI Group (UK) Ltd, Croydon, CR0 4YY

03/10/2024

01040457-0002